W9-BZG-232

Understanding Sleep
and Dreaming

Understanding Sleep and Dreaming

William H. Moorcroft

Luther College of Sleep and Dreaming Laboratory and Psychology Department
Decorah, Iowa
and
Colorado State University
Fort Collins, Colorado

with assistance from
Paula Belcher

Department of Psychology
Northwest Christian College
Eugene, Oregon

Kluwer Academic / Plenum Publishers
New York, Boston, Dordrecht, London, Moscow

For my loving wife and friend, Christina, who for over 30 years now has supported and encouraged me in my endeavors. She has also been a wonderful traveling companion in so many ways.

Acknowledgments

There are so many people and institutions to which I owe a big debt of gratitude. Over the years, so many have helped me know and understand sleep and dreams in so many ways. For opening their labs for visits: Alex Borbély and associates Irene Tobler and Peter Acherman in Switzerland; Jim Horne in England; Eva Svanborg in Sweden; Helmuth Rauscher in Austria; Tom Roth and associates in my hometown, Detroit; Ida Karmanova in Russia; Harvey Moldolsky in Toronto; Mark Mahowold and associates, especially Andrea Patterson in Minneapolis; Peter Hauri at the Mayo Clinic; and Mark Solms in London. For so readily corresponding with me by mail or e-mail: Mary Carskadon, Kathy Lee, Mike Bonnett, Monika Woolsey, Bob Stickgold, Eve Van Cauter, Bob Sack, Ernie Hartmann, Lee Kavanau, and Bob Ogilvie. For visiting and speaking at Luther College: Bill Dement, Gayle Delaney, and Peter Hauri. For sharing rooms while at sleep meetings: I. N. Pigarev, Barry Karkow, and Larry Scrima. For extended conversations at meetings: Bill Domhoff, Kelley Bulkeley, John Shepard, Alan Siegel, Jerry Rosen, Carlyle Smith, Henry Lahmeyer, Carol Landis, Bob McCarley, Merrill Mitler, Misha Radulovacki, Tim Roehrs, and Barry Sterman. For hosting me on sabbatical: Roz Cartwright at Rush Medical College in Chicago and Phil Westbrook at the Mayo Clinic in Minnesota. And finally, for the many students over the years who have worked with me on research and asked insightful questions in class.

I also would like to heartily thank Luther College for granting me a sabbatical leave and the Psychology Department at Colorado State University for providing me with an office and wonderful colleagues while I wrote this book. Additionally, I found the technical assistance from CSU psychology staff members Donna Merwarth and Ginger Lacy most helpful.

My thanks also go out to editors Mariclaire Cloutier and Sharon Panulla at Kluwer Academic/Plenum Publishers, for their assistance and guidance. Also to Paula Belcher for carefully editing my writing and giving advice on its content.

If there are others that I have forgotten to acknowledge, my apologies and my thanks.

Wm. H. Moorcroft, Ph.D. (you can call me Bill)
Fort Collins, Colorado
July 4, 2002

PS. I like to hear from instructors and students who have used this book in a course. For that matter, I also like to hear from any others who may have read it, or parts of it. I will endeavor to keep updating the book as new information comes to my awareness and will try to pass it along to those who may be interested. Try contacting me at moorbill@colostate.edu. Meanwhile, I wish you the best of sleep and the most pleasant of dreams.

Preface

As I am writing this, I am anticipating the 50th anniversary of the discovery of REMS. For it was in 1953 that Aserinsky and Kleitman, who, while electronically recording a person's sleep in a University of Chicago lab, were surprised to notice that eye movements occurred periodically even when their subject was, by all indicators, completely asleep. Four years later, Bill Dement—then a student of Kleitman—discovered the connection between these eye movements during sleep and dreaming (Dement & Kleitman, 1957). These startling observations began a whole new era of interest in the laboratory study of sleep, dreaming, and subsequently, sleep disorders. From these pioneering investigations came an explosion of discoveries and surprises, frequently leading to revision, including some outright rejection, of established notions about sleep, sleeping, dreams, and dreaming.

This explosion of new information continues today. The number of articles in scientific journals about sleep, dreaming, and sleep disorders in the last few decades easily outnumbers all those that preceded them. New journals devoted to sleep and dreams have recently been born and a number of very fine technical books have been published. However, nothing written within the last decade is suitable for use by undergraduate students as a textbook or course supplement that adequately covers sleep, dreaming, and sleep disorders. This book is intended to fill that void.

I have written this book from several perspectives. First, from the vantage point of a researcher in each of the three areas of sleep, dreaming, and sleep disorders. I have included the results of some of my research in order to show how knowledge about these many facets of sleep has been discovered.

Second, I have written this book out of my experiences with sleep disorders in sleep disorders centers. I have included many actual experiences with sleep disorder patients so that students can better understand the problems that sleep disorders present to their sufferers.

Finally, I have written this book from my experience as a college professor who has frequently taught courses on sleep, dreaming, and sleep disorders over more than 25 years. This book is written for college students with no prior knowledge of sleep and related phenomena. At the same time, it is not boring for those students that already have some knowledge in these areas. Most people have a natural fascination with sleep and dreams. From this starting place I build to an even greater fascination with, as well as increased understanding of, all aspects of sleep and dreams. I have avoided using technical jargon as much as possible, but some terms, which are included, are critical to know. At the same time I have tried to avoid overgeneralization and oversimplification. In addition, I have endeavored to involve readers as much as possible by talking about all aspects of their sleep and dreaming, as well as taking them to a sleep laboratory during an all-night recording session and having them present while sleep disorder cases are being reviewed in a sleep disorders clinic.

The organization of the book is designed as a journey. Together we will travel first to a modern sleep laboratory to see the cardinal way that sleep and dreaming is studied. It is also intended to both inform readers and heighten their interest in the topic of sleep. From there I will guide you on a climb through the mountains of information that have accumulated about sleep and dreaming. I will take you on an efficient route through these mountains, pointing out the important and scenic highlights along the way. First, we go to the twin peaks of what is known about sleep and what causes us to sleep. Next, we visit the dreams-and-dreaming mountain, after which we travel over to the mountain of sleep disorders. We conclude our journey by climbing to a high vantage point overlooking these mountains of information from which we can explore what might be the functions of sleep and dreaming.

More specifically, the first section of this book starts with a chapter on the basics of sleep (Chapter 1) which describes the specific criteria for sleep and its sub-stages as measured in the lab, what a typical night of sleep is like, and how it changes with age. It includes information on sleep in animals. This is followed by a chapter (Chapter 2) that presents sleep as a recuperative need and as a rhythmic process. Chapter 3 looks at variations of these basics including the effects of sleep loss.

The second section focuses on the brain in sleep and the body in sleep. Chapter 4 presents a brief overview of the structure, basic chemistry, and functioning of the brain, with an emphasis on those aspects most important for sleeping and dreaming. Chapter 5 discusses how sleep affects the body and how the body affects sleep.

The third section turns to dreams and dreaming. Chapter 6 looks at what is known about the nature and content of dreams. Chapter 7 then turns our attention to the process of dreaming. In Chapter 8, the key aspects of the major theories about dreaming, as well as methods of dream interpretation, are summarized.

Section four brings us to sleep disorders. In Chapters 10 and 11 the major types of disorders treated at sleep disorder centers are presented, usually introduced by illustrative case examples that bring the problems to life for the reader. Before that, in Chapter 9, is a look at other difficulties people may have with sleeping and dreaming.

Finally, section five is a summary of what sleep and dreams are all about. On the basis of what has been learned about sleep, dreaming, and sleep disorders, the probable functions of sleep and dreaming are reviewed and discussed. Chapter 12 includes functions of all of sleep and non-REM sleep. Chapter 13 continues with functions of REM sleep and dreaming.

In the end, I hope that readers will gain increasing fascination and knowledge about sleep and dreaming from reading this book. I know I have, while writing it.

About the Author

I am often asked about how I got interested in sleep and dreams. I reply with a little story.

"Everyone in the lab is going to the international sleep meeting in Europe. Why don't you come along? The round trip charter flight is only $180.00. The meeting lasts for 5 days but the flight does not return for another 25 days after that."

I heard this when I was doing postdoctoral research on the maturation of brain waves in baby rats at the University of Nebraska Medical School shortly after receiving a Ph.D. in psychology, actually psychobiology, from Princeton University. I went. I admit that the main reason was to spend a month in Europe. However, what I learned at the meeting, held in the summer of 1971, fascinated me. It was the beginning of a continuing interest in sleep and all of its ramifications.

Shortly after my return from Europe, I began to teach at Luther College and found myself reading and lecturing frequently about sleep. Within a few years, my research interests shifted away from baby rat brains to sleep. Soon I started a sleep research laboratory at Luther College in which I have studied various aspects of sleep and dreaming. I also kept on attending the meetings (some in Europe, others in places like Cap Cod and San Antonio) of what was to become the Sleep Research Society. Later I attended the inagural meeting of the Association for the Study of Dreams (in San Francisco). In 1980, I learned about sleep disorders and did some research in that area while on sabbatical at the Sleep Disorders Center, headed by Rozalind Cartwright, of Rush Medical School in Chicago. My interest in dreaming was piqued during this time, since Dr. Cartwright had already done landmark research in this area. Later, I was on another sabbatical at the Mayo Medical Center's Sleep Disorders Center in Rochester Minnesota. While at Mayo, I again did some sleep disorders research.

I love sleep and dreams, pun intended. I have continued to study, research, lecture, and write about sleep, dreaming, and sleep disorders. And of course, I have to continued to attend those wonderful meetings. My intention is to keep on keeping on with these things until I am no longer able to do so.

Contents

Prologue
A Visit to a Sleep and Dreams Lab

If you were asked to determine if someone is asleep, what would you look for? You probably would check the person's eyes to see if they were closed, see if the person were relaxed and still, be sure they are not very responsive to stimuli, were breathing regularly, and so on. But you, like just about everyone, have at one time or another done all of these things to fool other people into believing you were asleep. Then, too, someone in a coma shows all of these signs, appearing to be asleep. It is apparent that you cannot tell very accurately if a person is asleep simply by observation. Alternatively, you could wake the person up and ask if they were asleep, but you then depend on that person's ability to willingly and accurately tell you and, of course, the person is then no longer asleep. It is rather like the joke my father used to tell: "Says one Englishman to another, 'Were you in the boat when the boat tipped over?' 'No, you blithering idiot, I was in the water!' "

There are two important implications of this inability to observe whether or not another person is asleep. First, until the middle of the twentieth century, there was little scientific study of sleep. Thus, much of what is known about sleep is new knowledge, and some of it is surprising, since it is contrary to popular beliefs. Second, most study of sleep has taken place in a sleep lab where the sleeper is attached to sensitive instruments allowing objective determination of sleep without disturbing it. (Although the development of miniaturized portable equipment has allowed increasingly more sleep research to be conducted outside the lab.) Sleep labs have only been in existence since 1953 when Aserinsky and Kleitman first reported that sleeping people have two different kinds of sleep. Today, there are many sleep labs all over the world

Adapted from Moorcroft, 1993, with permission of the publisher.

engaged in exploring the mysteries of sleep every night. Let me first take you on a visit to a sleep lab before we discuss what is known about basic sleep processes.

A VISIT TO A SLEEP LAB

We arrive at the sleep lab a little before 10 p.m. and walk down a pleasant, carpeted hallway that has several doors on either side. We are directed to an open door leading to a brightly lit room.

The "subject" for tonight's study is a paid volunteer who has changed into her pajamas and is sitting next to a small table partially covered by a clean white towel. On this table are some rolls of medical tape, a few bottles, scissors, a toothpaste-like tube, some gauze, a comb and hair clips, a tape measure, an electrical meter, and other similar things. On the nearby wall hang a dozen or so long wires with disc-like enlargements on one end and metal pins about the size of match sticks on the other end. The 23-year-old subject has short, black hair done in one of the latest styles. She has bright, attentive eyes.

Also in the room is a man in his mid 30s in a white lab coat. He is on the tall side and slender, with a neatly trimmed dark mustache. He pleasantly turns to us and says, "Hi. I'm Sam, the sleep lab technician. This is Joan. She will be our sleeper tonight. Joan has been here before, so she knows what we are about to do. As I get her ready, I will describe what I am doing and why I am doing it."

"First we have to apply several wires to Joan's head. They are called electrodes, but think of them more as antennae." As he is talking, he has us inspect one of the wires. Up close, the disc end looks about the size and shape of half a pea and is hollow." This disc is a gold plated electrode. Other types of wires have plastic ends or thick adhesive tape with just a little silver foil embedded inside. They all work the same, but the metal ones are easier to put on the hairy scalp, while the others work well on bare skin."

Meanwhile, he has started to make precise measurements of Joan's scalp with the miniature tape measure and marks it with a special, soft, red pencil. "The electrodes have to be placed on specific locations on the head several inches above each ear called C3 on the left side and C4 on the right side and another at the back of the head at O1 or O2. The same measurement technique is used worldwide to apply electrodes. That way results from any lab can be directly compared." He carefully marks a spot on each side of the head about one-third of the way down from the center of the top of the head toward each ear. He picks up the comb and several hair clips and parts the hair over the marked area on the right side. Then he picks up a cotton-tipped stick and a bottle of liquid.

"Our bodies are covered with a layer of dead skin plus oil." Turning aside to us with a wry smile on his face, he says in a confidential tone, "That kind of takes the glamour out of looking at a good-looking movie star—all you see is dead skin." Turning back to Joan, he proceeds to moisten the cotton-tip with a gooey solution from one of the bottles and to rub the exposed marked area. "This process removes the dead skin and oils to enable better electrical reception by the electrode." With another wry smile, he turns to Joan and says, "The green color in your hair will grow out in about nine months."

Laughing, Joan replies, "You can't fool me. I've been through this before."

Turning to us, Sam explains, "Actually, all of this stuff is very harmless and easily washes out." He then picks up the toothpaste-like tube. "This substance is electrode gel. It also helps make better electrical contact." As he is talking, he takes the electrode from us and squeezes enough gel into its hollowness just to fill it. Then he carefully places it on the prepared spot on Joan's scalp and has her hold it in place with her left forefinger. Working quickly, he takes the top off a glass petri dish and picks up a moistened piece of square gauze about the size of two big postage stamps. "It's soaked with a biological glue." Sam places the gauze on top of the electrode, being careful not to disturb it. Again, holding all of this in place with his left hand, he uses his right hand to pick up a metal pencil-sized object attached to a small rubber lab hose. While using the dull tip of the object to hold the electrode and gauze in place, he presses a foot switch and a stream of air hisses through the hose and out of the object toward the glue-soaked gauze. Deftly, he pats his fingers on the gauze around the electrode as the glue dries. Fifteen seconds later, he turns off the air stream and sets the apparatus down. "The electrode will stay in place all night now. If I were to give a gentle but firm tug on the attached wire, Joan's head would tilt toward me."

"He thinks I'm a puppet on a string," she playfully complains.

"Not to worry. I will easily remove it in the morning by dissolving the glue."

"What does the electrode do?" you ask.

While repeating the application procedure on the other two marked spots on Joan's head, he tells us, "It allows us to record her brain waves (on what is technically called the EEG or electroencephalogram). As you will see, there are brain waves specific to sleep."

Having finished applying the three scalp electrodes, Sam cleans the skin near the outer corner of the left eye with another cotton-tipped applicator moistened with the gooey solution. He then presses one of the adhesive electrodes onto the prepared spot. Next, he places a piece of hypoallergenic surgical tape over the electrode and surrounding skin. Giving a little jerk on the wire, he says, "That one will also stay in place all night."

As he similarly applies another adhesive electrode at the outer corner of the other eye, he explains, "These electrodes will enable us to measure her eye movements. The eyes are like little batteries with the positive end in front. When the eyes move, the positive front moves closer or farther from the nearby electrode, thus changing the electrical influence on the electrode. In this way, we get what you might call 'eye movement waves' (actually the EOG or electrooculogram). Like brain waves, eye movements help us to determine when Joan is asleep and what kind of sleep she is in."

He then attaches two additional electrodes on Joan's chin as he explains, "These electrodes let us record neck muscle tension. Electrical changes occur when muscles contract. The more contracted or tense a muscle, the more electrical activity. This procedure enables us to assess how relaxed the muscles of the neck are. You see, as long as we are awake, our neck muscles maintain tension in order to hold our head up, even when we are resting our heads on a pillow. This neck muscle tension or EMG (for electromyogram) gives us another indicator of the presence of sleep and the stage of sleep." Turning to me, he asks, "How can you tell when students fall asleep during your lectures, Dr. Moorcroft?"

I reply, "Well, of course they never do." After a few seconds of silence accompanied by stares of disbelief, I continue. "O.K., so once in a while a student may doze off. How do I know? Well, let me see. Ah, they don't answer my questions or take notes and their heads are dropped."

"That's it! Their heads drop because during sleep the neck muscles relax. Also, as we shall see, in one kind of sleep the muscles are almost totally relaxed."

"You mean there is more than one kind of sleep?"

"Yes. We all cycle in and out of different kinds of sleep each night!"

"Is she ready now?" you ask.

"Not quite." Sam replies, as he reaches for three more electrodes. "These pieces of equipment are called ground and reference electrodes." As he prepares and attaches one to the middle of the forehead, he continues, "This one prevents other electrical 'noise' from interfering with our recordings. Have you ever had a portable radio get louder and clearer as you reach out to adjust the knobs?"

"Yes," you reply.

"That happens because you are acting as an antenna for the radio. You see, your body is constantly receiving all sorts of electrical signals – from radio, TV, and all sorts of electrical appliances and motors. Many of these signals are stronger than brain waves and the rest of what we measure. By applying this electrode, we can get rid of this electrical garbage."

He then proceeds to put the final two electrodes on the bony knob behind the bottom of each ear.

"What do those electrodes do?" you ask.

"They are called reference electrodes. Anything we record needs input from two electrodes. Activity on one is actually compared to activity on the other. Sometimes both electrodes are from active areas such as two parts of the brain, and the resulting record is the difference in activity between the two. A lot of other times, it is better if the comparison electrode has no electrical input of its own so that the record shows all of the activity from the active electrode. There is not much electrical activity behind the lower ears, so they work well as comparisons. One of these reference electrodes that I'm applying now is used as a comparison to both eye electrodes and scalp electrodes and sometimes to one chin electrode."

"Wait a minute. What about the other scalp electrode and reference electrode?"

"They're back-ups. We usually don't use all of the scalp electrodes at one time either. The one at the back of the head is useful for determining sleep onset but not of much use otherwise, so sometimes we only use it in the beginning of the night or don't even bother to use it at all. We also only use one of the two electrodes over the ears. If something prevents us from recording from one of these, we can easily switch to the other one without disturbing Joan. Otherwise, we might have to wake her up to attach another electrode."

"Can I go to sleep now?" asks Joan, barely stifling a yawn.

"Soon. Just a few more things to do." He tapes some of the loose wires to her face, directing them all to the back of her head, shaping them into a ponytail with some more tape.

"All set."

"Great. (Yawn) I'm tired."

After Joan uses the bathroom, Sam leads her to another room, with us following. The room resembles a small but cozy motel room with a bed, a nightstand and lamp, a chair, florescent overhead lighting, and carpeting. The bed has a green blanket neatly tucked in at the sides of the mattress and two pillows above the folded end of the top sheet. On the nightstand facing the bed is a speaker with an attached microphone. In the corner of the room opposite the bed is a very small infrared TV camera and infrared light mounted near the ceiling.

After Joan lies down in bed, Sam plugs the color-coded wires into a cable coming through the wall. The wires are long enough to allow Joan to move around easily in bed.

"Are you comfortable?" he asks.

"Very much," she replies.

Sam leads us out of the room and closes the door.

"How can she sleep with all those wires on her?"

"Most people have little trouble, especially after the first night. Think how hard it is to stay awake all night, especially in a quiet room and in a comfortable bed."

We walk across the hall to another room labeled Control Room. As Sam opens the door, we see a room about the size of the bedroom except lined with several computers, TV monitors, and other electrical equipment. There are trails of various colored horizontal lines on the computer screens, some of which are straight and others showing various constantly changing waveforms. "The wires from each bedroom feed into one of these computers. This one here is showing the recordings, called a polysomnogram, from Joan. I previously made careful adjustments and calibrations for the five channels we will be using. The top line is from her left eye, the second line from her right. The third line is the muscular activity from the chin electrodes. The fourth and fifth lines are for the brain waves—one from above one ear and the other from the back of the head."

Sam flips a switch on an intercom next to the computer. "Joan, can you hear me?"

"Just barely." He adjusts the volume.

"How about now?"

"Fine. Real fine."

"O.K. Remember to stay awake while I make adjustments to the machine."

O.K., but don't take too long or I might be gone."

Sam types on the keyboard, the lines on the computer get larger or smaller. The eye movement lines look like mirror images of hills and mountains. The EEGs are small, rapidly, but irregularly, oscillating lines, such as a very nervous person might make if trying to draw a straight line. The EMG does not look like a line at all, but rather a thick band made up of many vertical lines of random heights, somewhat like a magnified side view of a shag carpet. Suddenly, all the lines become wide, irregular, thick tracings. This pattern stops after a second or two as abruptly as it started, and the lines return to their previous patterns of movements.

"What was that?" you blurt out.

"She moved. She probably was trying to get more comfortable. We'll occasionally see that all through the night. It actually is useful, because it tells us how restless the sleep is."

Sam continues to look at the record while making some adjustments using the keyboard. Finally, satisfied, he turns to us and says, "Now, we will see if everything is working as it should." Pulling on the intercom switch he says into the microphone, "Joan, I'd like you to do a few things for me now."

"O.K."

"First, look up." Pause. "Look down." Pause. "Look up." Pause. "Look down." Pause. "Look right." Pause. "Look left." Pause. "Look right." Pause. "Look left." Each time he gives a command, he types a notation of it on the screen. The eye movement lines seemingly respond to his commands, moving toward each other, almost touching when Joan moves her eyes up or to the right and away from each other when the eyes move down or to the left.

"Now blink five times." Again the top two lines move but this time producing what looks like a row of five dunce hats. Again, Sam his instruction to Joan on the screen.

"Now grit your teeth." This time, the thickness of the muscle line triples. "That's fine." Now addressing us he says, "The muscles of the neck contract when a person grits their teeth and the polysomnograph shows it. Next, we'll check the EEG and at the same time get a sample of another kind of brain wave."

"Joan, close your eyes and blank your mind, but don't fall asleep."

"(Yawn) I'll try," came the sleepy voice in return. As Sam makes a notation on the screen, the EEG lines begin to change from their low, fast, random pattern (called beta waves) to higher, slightly slower, but very rhythmic and regular patterns, looking somewhat like a folded ribbon candy viewed from the side.

"These patterns are alpha waves. They occur when a person's mind is awake but relaxed and not particularly concentrating on anything." When he flips the intercom switch and tells Joan to open her eyes, the alpha waves change back to the beta waves.

"Alpha waves also occur when a person is drifting into sleep. What you saw before the alpha waves, and are seeing now, are the beta waves of an awake, alert mind."

"Well, Joan, its time. Call me if you want to get up or need anything, O.K.?"

"O.K."

"Goodnight." he types a notation into the computer as he switches off Joan's sleep room lights with a remote switch near the intercom.

We all watch the screen closely. Not much happens at first other than an occasional body movement. In several minutes, the EMG becomes less thick to about half its original size, more alpha waves appear, and fewer eye movements can be noted. Then the eye channels trace out lines that look like mirror images of rolling hills, and the EEG becomes much more jagged, but the waves are not as rapid as beta nor as rhythmic as alpha. "These waves are the signs of the start of sleep—so called slow rolling eye movements and the replacement of alpha waves with slower, less regular theta waves in the EEG. It's a light sleep called stage 1. She will probably spend very little sleep time in this stage. It's more of a transition between stages."

Soon Joan's eyes stop moving, and the EEG line gradually oscillates less rapidly than before, but it is still rather jagged. Then it more rapidly and regularly oscillates for about a second, producing a wave that looks like compact alpha. "That's a sleep spindle, a sure sign of stage 2 of sleep." Soon there is a sudden, large, upward movement, then down past midline, then back to its previous activity level, resulting in a pattern resembling an upside-down pointed ice cream cone next to a smaller but right-side up cone. "A K-complex, another characteristic of stage 2."

This pattern continues for another 10 minutes—occasional spindles and K-complexes on a background of irregular but slower and slower activity. Then the EEG begins to show occasional large sonorous movements and fewer and fewer spindles and K-complexes. When about 20% of the record is of this pattern, Sam explains, "These are slow waves, also called delta waves. They indicate the presence of slow wave sleep, abbreviated SWS. In many ways, this sleep is the deepest sleep." Soon much of the record contains delta waves and continues this way with little change for about half an hour.

Suddenly, all of the lines become large and blurred indicating a body movement. We confirm this recording when we look up at the TV monitoring Joan and see that she is rolling over. When things settle down, the record again resembles stage 2 with moderate, jagged background and spindles and Ks.

Exactly 93 minutes after sleep onset, the EMG becomes almost a thin, straight line. Suddenly, the eye movement channels burst into activity, showing large, jagged, mirror-image mountains for a few seconds, then falling silent. "That recording is a burst of rapid eye movements. Joan is now in another kind of sleep called REMS (for rapid eye movement sleep). Look closely at the EEG. Notice no spindles or Ks are present and many of the brain waves look like the teeth of a saw blade." Just then there is another burst of eye movement lasting longer than the first. "As you can see, sleep is not a single entity, but is made up of several different states."

The REMS period does not last long. After a few minutes, another body movement occurs and stage 2 returns for 10 to 15 minutes followed by more SWS.

And so it goes throughout the night. Joan cycles between the stages, except there is less and less time spent in SWS (in fact, almost none at all in the second half of the night) and more and more time in REMS. Most time however is spent in stage 2—about half of the night. Around every hour and a half, she starts a REMS period.

It is interesting to observe what is happening to us as we stay up all night to watch Joan sleep. It is especially hard for us to keep awake when nothing exciting is happening, like long periods of stage 2. We have to stand up and keep moving or keep talking. Otherwise, a brief sleep overtakes us. Several times we catch each other drifting off and, in a fun way, scold one another. It seems to get cold in the room between 3 and 5 a.m. We check the thermostat and find that the temperature remained unchanged. We later realized that this time was also the time when it was hardest to stay awake.

At 6:15 a.m., through blurry eyes, we can see that the pattern on the computer screen is changing. Several body movements occur, and the EMG gets thicker again. The EEG becomes low and fast and random, and the eyes start moving, not as rapidly as during REMS and more continuously. "She's awake now," Sam informs us. "Good morning," he intercoms to Joan and turns on the light.

"Ugh—oh, mornin' " (Yawn).

"I'll come in and unplug you now."

"Yeah. O.K."

We follow him in. "How do you feel? Sleep well?"

"Hey, I slept like a log. How about you?"

"Oh, be quiet," he blurts out with a smile.

Now unplugged, Joan is led back to the room with the equipment table. We follow. She sits in the chair next to the table as Sam soaks some gauze in solvent, and then puts a moistened cotton puff over each of the glue-stiffened gauze patches on Joan's head. In about 30 seconds, he lifts both pieces of gauze and the underlying electrode from the left side of her head, and then repeats the procedure on the right side and the back. With another solvent-wet gauze square, he carefully wipes at the area where each electrode rested, then combs the hair back into place. Next, he peels off the tape holding the wires close to her face, and then removes each of the rest of the electrodes in turn. Using a tissue, he wipes off the electrode cream that remains on the skin.

We say good-bye to one another before Joan heads for the shower and Sam returns to the control room to do some post-sleep polysomnograph checks. "See you again tomorrow night," he says as he disappears into the control room. We start to float out of the sleep lab in our sleepless, dazed state, toward our own beds in search of our own quota of that sweet commodity that we have been scientifically observing all night.

A SECOND NIGHT IN THE SLEEP LAB

"I hope you slept well during the day today," I say, "after being up all night."

"Well, I slept but not as well as usual," you reply. "I was kind of restless and woke up a lot, but I'm O.K."

"Sounds typical for daytime sleep. Tonight Sam will awaken Joan at various times during the night to collect dream reports."

"I can't wait. I hope she has some wild ones."

"You may be surprised," I comment, "at just how dull they are!"

"Hi, Sam. Here we are for another night."

"Oh, hi. I just about have Joan ready, so it won't be long now." At that moment she came walking out of the preparation room carrying the ponytail of wires leading from the electrodes on her head and face.

"Not a bad way to earn 75 bucks—sleeping," she says to us.

"It's not all sleep tonight," Sam reminds her. "I will be waking you at various times throughout the night and asking you to report whatever is going through your mind at the time. You may be dreaming or thinking or may have nothing at all going on at that time. That's all right. I just want to know what is going on in your mind when I wake you. All reports are equally valuable."

"Oh well, it's still an easy 75. See ya in the morning."

By now she is in bed and the electrodes are connected to the cable coming from the wall. Soon Sam has turned the machine on, made adjustments, and assured himself that everything is working fine and that Joan is asleep.

"Dreams," Sam says, "can be explored much better in the sleep lab, because we can catch their recall when they are fresh. Tonight, we will wake her three times—first during SWS, then during stage 2, and finally during REMS. Watch for differences in what she reports in each stage. The questions I ask are a bit formal, but they have to be the same every time to be sure we don't miss something.

Soon we see the signs on the moving chart that she is asleep and moving down through the stages. Then at 12:07, ten minutes into the first SWS period, Sam turns on a tape recorder and begins. "Joan ... Joan ... JOAN!"

"Ugh ..., oh-ah ..."

"Joan?"

"Yea." Yawn.

"What was taking place just at the moment you were called?"

"Nothin'. Nothin' was happenin'."

"At that moment would you say that you were awake, drowsy, in light sleep, or in a deep sleep?"

"Deep. It was good sleep."

"Was there any visual imagery? If yes, describe it."

"Well, yeah, kinda. A woods, some trees, you know."

"Were there any distortions in the way familiar people or objects were represented?"

"No, not really. It was kinda vague."

"Were you an active participant in what you experienced or just passively observing it?"

"I just saw it."

"Were there any other persons in this experience?"

"No, none; just trees."

"During this experience were you aware that you were here in the laboratory?"

"No."

"During this experience were you aware that you were observing the contents of your own mind, or did you feel that you were observing or participating in events out in the real world?"

"Sort of real world, but fuzzy."

"How vivid an experience was this: very vivid, moderately vivid, or quite vague?"

"Kinda vague."

"How realistic was this experience: very realistic, a mixture of real and unreal, or very unrealistic?"

"A mixture, I'd say."

"How emotional was this experience: very emotional, only mildly emotional, or very unemotional?"

"Not at all emotional. No emotion."

"How pleasant was this experience: very pleasant, neutral, or unpleasant?"

"Neutral."

"Were you dreaming or thinking?"

"I don't know. Kinda thinking, I guess. But not thinking hard or rationally."

"O.K., you can go back to sleep now."

After Sam turns off the tape recorder, you state, "That wasn't really much of a dream, was it?"

"No." he replies, "That's typical, though, of what you get in SWS sleep—something like a fuzzy photograph. Many times you get nothing."

At 3:10 a.m., ten minutes into stage 2, Sam says, "It's time again," as he turns on the tape recorder.

"Joan."

"Ah, yeah," followed by a strain in her voice indicating that she is stretching.

"What was taking place just at the moment you were called?"

"I (yawn) could not find the classroom where I had to take the final exam. It was like I kept trying one door after another but never finding the room."

"Was there anything else?"

"No, that's pretty much it. It was not real clear."

"What about the visual imagery? Can you describe it?"

"Not very well. I just knew I was opening non-descript doors, looking for the classroom."

"At that moment would you say that you were awake, drowsy, in light sleep, or in deep sleep?"

"I was asleep alright, but it did not seem like it was deep sleep."

"Were there any distortions in the way familiar people or objects were represented?"

"It was not real clear. I just kinda knew what everything was."

"During this experience, were you aware that you were here in the laboratory?"

"No. I thought I was really there, yet it did not seem entirely real."

"During this experience, were you aware that you were observing the contents of your own mind, or did you feel that you were observing or participating in events out in the real world?"

"Neither. It was kinda dreamy. Oh, sorry about the pun."

"That's ok. I understand. How vivid was this experience: very vivid, moderately vivid, or quite vague?"

"It was moderately vivid to a bit vague."

"How realistic was this experience: very realistic, a mixture of real and unreal, or very unrealistic?"

"I did not think about it while I was experiencing it, but reflecting on it now, it seems almost unrealistic. Incomplete."

"How emotional was this experience: very emotional, only mildly emotional, or not emotional?"

"Surprisingly, not very emotional. I was concerned about missing the exam, but I did not feel emotional about it."

"How pleasant was this experience: very pleasant, neutral, or unpleasant?"

"It was O.K. Kinda neutral, I guess."

"Were you dreaming or thinking?"

"More dreaming than thinking."

"You can go back to sleep now."

Sam turns the tape off as he says to us, "That was pretty typical of stage 2. Not much going on but often repeated over and over again. Also, the experience was not real clear. Sometimes, though, we get a real story. That kind of experience is more likely toward the end of the night."

"What happens in REMS?" you ask.

"Just wait."

Five twenty-three a.m., ten minutes into REMS.

"Joan, ..., Joan."

"Ugh ... yea!"

"What was taking place just at the moment you were called?"

"Well, I was in a shed—you know a tin type shed—with many people, some of whom I knew. I was standing on one side of the building around some cars with a couple of middle-aged men and a couple of girls around 20 years of age. Something had happened to one of the cars, an older model, and the girl was upset. At that point my attention was distracted to the other half of the shed where a guy about 20 years of age was showing films of—I guess it was her vacation or something—while others of the same age watched. Right then, the scene shifted to some body of water like a lake or something. I was driving a speedboat, while the male who was showing the film was swimming in a scuba suit. It's crazy, but he was going the same speed as the boat. Then you woke me up."

"At that moment, would you say that you were awake, drowsy, in light sleep, or in deep sleep?"

"Oh, I was asleep alright; it was sound. I guess I would have to say somewhat deep."

"Were there any distortions in the way familiar people or objects were represented?"

"People? No. But, the cars were all funny pastel colors and kinda wavy, shimmering. That's all I can remember."

"During this experience, were you aware that you were here in the laboratory?"

"Oh no. It seemed real, like I was there."

"During this experience, were you aware that you were observing the contents of your own mind, or did you feel that you were observing or participating in events out in the real world?"

"It seemed real at the time, but now that I think about it, things were kind of flat or quiet. You know, not very emotional or something. Like spacey."

"How vivid an experience was this: very vivid, moderately vivid, or quite vague?"

"It was vivid, quite clear."

"How realistic was this experience: very realistic, a mixture of real and unreal, or very unrealistic?"

"It seemed realistic while it was happening, but now not all of it seems like it was real. A mixture I guess."

"How emotional was this experience: very emotional, only mildly emotional, or not emotional?"

"There was some emotion. Kinda like something was not right."

"How pleasant was this experience: very unpleasant, neutral, or unpleasant?"

"It was O.K. Toward unpleasant, I guess."

"Were you dreaming or thinking?"

"Dreaming. No doubt about it, I was dreaming."

"Goodnight. You can go back to sleep again."

"Night."

Turning to us, Sam says, "That experience was a fairly typical dream—like a TV program with action and a sequence of events, but scenes can jump forward, backward, or parallel. I did not have to ask all of the standard questions either, since she had already indicated what the answers would be."

We decide to leave early, since there are to be no more dream reports collected and we are tired from the night before.

"Thanks Sam and say good-bye to Joan for me," you say on your way out of the door.

"I will" he replies. "Good-bye."

Turning to me as we walk down the hall, you ask, "Where was all the sex and violence in the dreams?"

"That's just it. There usually isn't any. Most dreams are pretty dull when you get right down to it."

"Do we always dream during REMS?" you ask.

"People will give a dream report like this one over 80% of the time when awakened during REMS, even if they state before-hand that they never dream."

"Well, thanks again," you call out as you turn to head to your car, "I really appreciate your arranging for me to visit the sleep lab."

"Glad to do it," I respond, "and, oh by the way, ..."

"Yes?"

"Pleasant dreams!"

Part I

Sleep and Sleeping

Anthropologists tell us that sleep and its dreams have been a central focus of many ancient cultures. In some cultures, sleep was seen as a time for the soul to occupy another world (see Chapter 6). Perhaps more common in the history of the Western world was the notion that sleep is a slowing down of the body and brain, even to the point of approaching death. Akin to this idea have been the notions that the brain is forced into sleep by blood filling its vessels (Ancient Greeks), food decomposing in the stomach giving off vapors that ascended to the brain (other Ancient Greeks), the effect of "animal humors" (Middle Ages), blood putting pressure on the brain (18th century), or lack of sensory stimulation (19th century). Around the beginning of the 20th century, a popular notion was that sleep resulted from the buildup of one or another "hypnotoxins" (there were many that were proposed) that supposedly poisoned the brain into sleep when a critical amount had accumulated. During sleep, the hypnotoxin was thought to be eliminated gradually, and eventually wakefulness returned.

A common thread in almost all of these notions is that sleep is viewed as the result of lowered activity of the brain. Waking up is simply the result of the brain being allowed to become fully active again or stimulated into such activity. Only in the middle of the 20th century was there a dramatic shift in thinking; sleep was shown to be the result of active processes within the brain itself (see Chapter 4). This shift occurred 25 years after the first use of the EEG by the German Psychiatrist Hans Berger to establish the presence of sleep without having to awaken the sleeper. By 1960, the stages of sleep had been discovered and named and, with some reluctance, the fact that sleep was an active process was accepted. This acceptance changed the scientific attitude toward sleep and sleeping. Scientists then began asking questions they never thought to ask before such as: What exactly is the nature of sleep? Does it change with age? How much do we need to sleep? How does sleep vary between individuals. This section begins the review of what answers we currently have for these questions. Chapter 1 describes how sleep is measured and what it is like. Chapter 2 explores two major influences on sleep—homeostatic and rhythmic. Chapter 3 looks at some of the common variations of sleep.

Chapter 1

What is Sleep and How is it Scientifically Measured?[1]

If we want to scientifically study sleep, we need to know when a person is asleep and when awake. How do we know if a person is asleep? You might be able with great certainty to determine that the person is awake using criteria such as eyes open, interactive with their surroundings, physically active, appears alert, and so forth. So the absence of these things (little movement, steady breathing, eyes closed, not interacting with surroundings, typical posture) might indicate that the person is asleep. But a person displaying all of these could be awake; you can't be sure. Another way is to ask if they were asleep after they were awakened or were awakened by you. Two problems arise here. First, we cannot be certain that the answer is reliable and, second, the person is no longer in the state of sleep that we wish to study. It was not until the middle of the twentieth century that scientists devised more objective ways of determining if a person was in a state of sleep using technological advances enabling brain waves and other bodily functions to be recorded. To their surprise, they also discovered that sleep is of several types, called stages.

It was not long before these methods, called polysomnography, became refined and universally accepted such that today the determination of states of sleep and wakefulness is reliable and valid. Polysomnography involves the recording of three things—brain waves, eye movements, and neck muscle tension. Polysomnography works because many organs of the body generate small amounts of electrical energy as they perform their functions. Sensors placed near these organs can pick up some of this energy and transmit it via wires to powerful amplifiers whose output is permanently recorded as ink lines on paper or, more recently, as lines on a computer screen and stored in computer memory. Brain waves (or EEG, short for electroencephalogram) are recordings of the waveform and intensity in microvolts of electrical activities of large groups of brain cells. For sleep recording, standard procedure calls for the EEG sensor to be placed on the scalp about 8 centimeters above the right or left ear. EEGs are the most important of all things

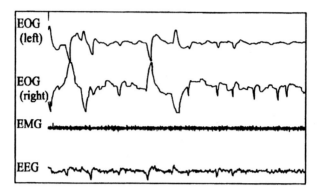

Figure 1. A typical polysomnogram page of 30 seconds duration showing wake. Note the sharp eye movements that resemble mirror images of each other, the high thickness of the EMG tracing, and the not very intense but fast frequency beta waves in the EEG.

recorded for the determination of stages of sleep. The shape of the EEG waves, their frequency, and their intensity are the key components.

Eye movement recordings (or EOG, short for electrooculogram) are possible because the front of the eye is electrically positive. As the eyeballs move, the distance of their positive poles changes relative to sensors placed near the outer corner of each eye. Typically, the movements of each eye are recorded on a separate line on the polysomnogram. It is important to note the presence or absence of any eye movements as well as their shape and frequency when they are present.

For neck muscle tension (or EMG, short for electromyogram), pairs of sensors are placed below the chin or jaw. When muscles contract, they generate some electrical activity whose strength is in proportion to the degree of the contraction or tension that these sensors can pick up. The thickness of the EMG line is what is accessed.

At a minimum, a polysomnogram contains two rows of EOG, one of EMG, and one of EEG (see Figure 1). Additional recordings from brain and other body organs may also be made, and although not essential to determine sleep, may be useful for determination of what else is going on during sleep.

Polysomnographic stages are designated as alert wakefulness, drowsy wakefulness, stages 1, 2, 3, 4 sleep, and rapid eye movement sleep (abbreviated REM sleep or REMS). Stages 1, 2, 3, and 4 are often collectively referred to as non-REMS (abbreviated NREM sleep or NREMS) since, with few exceptions, the physiology of the four stages are very similar. Stages 3 and 4 are also known as slow wave sleep (abbreviated SWS) since the distinction between them is somewhat arbitrary.

THE STAGES OF SLEEP

Figure 2 shows the criteria for the stages of sleep. The components most critical for determining each stage are in bold. Beta waves are irregular, low intensity, and

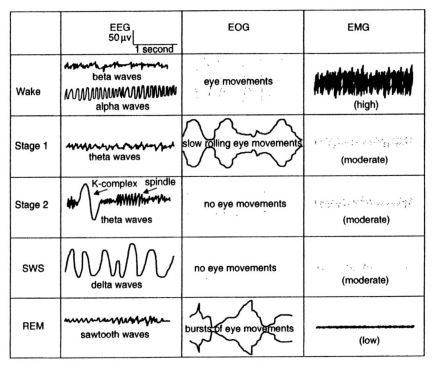

	EEG 50 µv ⌐ 1 second	EOG	EMG
Wake	beta waves / alpha waves	eye movements	(high)
Stage 1	theta waves	slow rolling eye movements	(moderate)
Stage 2	K-complex spindle / theta waves	no eye movements	(moderate)
SWS	delta waves	no eye movements	(moderate)
REM	sawtooth waves	bursts of eye movements	(low)

Figure 2. EEG, EOG, and EMG characteristics of waking and each stage of sleep.

fast frequency (16–25 Hz) that typically occur in an awake, active brain. Alpha waves are regular, moderate intensity, and intermediate frequency (8–12 Hz) that typically occur in an awake but relaxed or drowsy brain. Theta waves are moderate to low intensity and intermediate frequency (3–7 Hz). Delta waves are intense and low frequency ($\frac{1}{2}$ to 2–3 Hz). A K-complex lasts at least $\frac{1}{2}$ second and is a large, slow peak followed by a smaller valley. A spindle is an obvious moderately intense and moderately fast (12–14 Hz) rhythmic oscillation for $\frac{1}{2}$ to $1\frac{1}{2}$ seconds. Sawtooth waves are relatively low intensity and mixed frequency that often have a notched appearance. Left eye movement recordings look like approximate mirror images of the right eye movement recordings. Waking eye movements tend to be relatively constant and have mainly sharp peaks and valleys with some smaller peaks and rounded peaks mixed in. Slow rolling eye movements are mostly large with rounded peaks. The eye movements of REMS usually have sharp peaks and come in bursts of a few seconds each with intervening quiet periods of a few to 10 seconds. The thickness of the EMG line is the key indicator for it.

Figures 1 and 3–6 show typical 30-second polysomnogram pages for each stage.

Although not important for the distinguishing of the stages of sleep and waking, during the 1990s the importance of 20 to 50 Hz gamma waves became apparent.

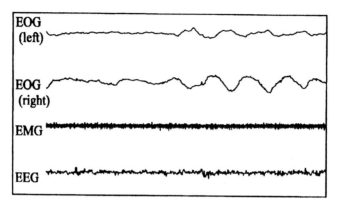

Figure 3. A typical 30 second polysomnogram page showing stage 1. Note the slow eye movements, moderate thickness of the EMG, and theta waves in the EEG.

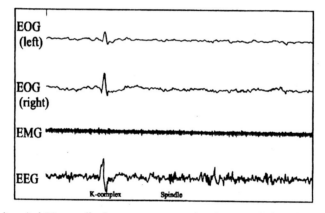

Figure 4. A typical 30 second polysomnogram page showing stage 2 sleep. Note the absence of eye movements (the upward spikes early in the record are from some unknown electrical activity but not eye movements since the one on the first line is not a mirror image of that on the second line), moderate EMG intensity, and theta waves in the EMG with occasional K-complexes and spindles.

These waves are present during waking and REMS. They are thought to be important in synthesizing various aspects of sensory-motor inputs (e.g., size of an object with its color and shape) and/or cognitive processes.

Accurately determining the time of first falling asleep and final awakening is also of great importance. The time between these transitions is called the sleep period. Awakening is easier to determine; it is the sudden shift from a sleep stage to active wake, usually accompanied by a many seconds of movement artifact composed of intense, very high frequency registrations in the EEG, EOG, and EMG recordings

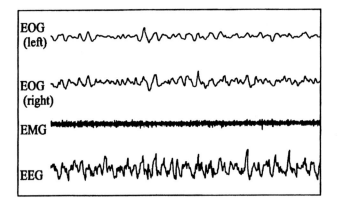

Figure 5. A typical 30 second polysomnogram page showing SWS. Note the absence of eye movements (the peaks and valleys that appear in the EOG records during SWS are not from eye movements since they are not mirror images; rather they are produced by the strong slow wave electrical activity of the brain near the eyeballs), the moderately intense EMG, and the intense but slow EEG activity.

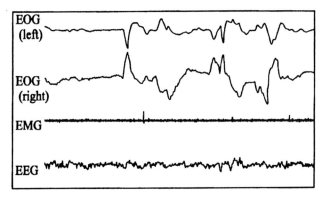

Figure 6. A typical 30 second polysomnogram page showing REMS. Note the bursts of eye movements, the low EMG (but with occasional brief muscle twitches), and the fast frequency, low intensity "sawtooth" pattern of the EEG.

(see Figure 7). Sleep onset is more difficult, because we do not simply drop off to sleep. Instead, the transition from wake to sleep is gradual, with complex successions of changes beginning with relaxed drowsiness, going through stage 1, and ending in the first couple of minutes of stage 2. Furthermore, a person typically briefly dips in and out of sleep several times before maintaining it. Different sets of criteria are used to pinpoint the time of sleep onset, but most involve the replacement of drowsy waking EEG (typically alpha waves) with sustained theta waves plus the other indicators of stage 1 or stage 2. In practice, the time of sleep onset can usually be determined within a range of several seconds.

As can be seen in Figures 2 and 6, REMS is a very unique state. The EEG very closely resembles that of wakefulness, yet it is clear from behavioral criteria (see below) and subsequent subjective reports from the person that they are asleep. Furthermore, during REMS, the muscles controlling body movements are paralyzed into a very relaxed state as shown by the very low EMG level. During REMS, the EOG shows bursts of rapid eye movements with seconds of quiescence between bursts. (You might want to see this phenomenon for yourself even without the aid of a polysomnograph by looking at the bulge of the eyeballs moving under the eyelids in a sleeping person early in the morning. Just be sure the person knows that you will do this in case they awaken only to be startled with your face a few inches away! Actually, this exercise is easier to do with a baby.)

It is useful to distinguish between the components of REMS that are tonic and those that are phasic. The tonic components are those that are constant, such as the EEG and the muscle paralysis. The phasic components are the relatively short-lived clusters of events, such as the rems[2] and a number of changes in the body to be discussed in Chapter 5.

NREMS is what most people think sleep is and ought to be. The brain waves, especially in SWS, are those of a brain that is idling. At the same time, the body is relaxed but capable of movement.

Let's put all this together now by following a typical young adult, Rita, as she sleeps through the night. Shortly after she turns out the lights, intent on going to sleep, her EOG is flat and her EEG begins to show less aroused beta waves and more drowsy alpha waves, while her EMG shows her muscles relaxing. A few minutes later, she begins to show signs of stage 1—slow eye movements appear on her EOG, while her EEG alpha waves are replaced by theta waves mixed with other low voltage, fast waves. However, the alpha waves reemerge a few times before disappearing completely. If we were to ask, she would quickly say that she was not quite asleep but less conscious, maybe experiencing something like floating. On other occasions, she might say she had had a simple, short dream.

A short time later, usually less than 10 minutes, we see the first sign of stage 2, a K-complex or perhaps a spindle in her EEG. If we now were to ask if she were asleep yet, it would take longer to get a response, and she would seem a bit groggy at that, but her reply would be affirmative. The slow eye movements shortly thereafter disappear. After another 20 or so minutes go by, we begin to see large, slow delta waves that quickly begin to dominate the EEG. We now know she is in SWS. Awakening her now would be more difficult and result in obvious grogginess. A good half-hour later, the delta waves diminish and signs of stage 2 reemerge for about another 10 minutes.

It is now about 80 minutes since the onset of Rita's sleep and we notice that the EMG has become almost a thin, flat line. Shortly thereafter, there are sawtooth waves

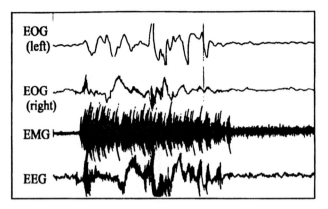

Figure 7. A typical 30 second polysomnogram page showing movement artifact. Note the very thick EMG and obliterated EEG and partially obliterated EOG.

in the EEG, and suddenly the EOG dances with a burst of rems signaling the appearance of REMS. We could have awakened her at this point more easily than when she was in SWS but less easily then stage 1. If asked, after being awakened from REMS, she probably would have said she was dreaming.

After only a couple of minutes of REMS, the lines on the polysomnograph computer get very intense and scrambled. Rita has moved. Around thirty seconds later, she settles down again but is no longer in REMS. A brief interval of stage 1 is followed by solid stage 2 followed by a bit more SWS before again entering REMS.

This sequence continues throughout the night with the interval between REMS periods gradually increasing to closer to 100 minutes, the indictors of REMS on the polysomnogram getting more obvious, and the duration of each successive REMS period increasing until the last one is a half hour or more. As changes are taking place, the amount of SWS quickly diminishes such that it is hardly visible in the later half of the night. From this point on, most of the rest of her NREMS is stage 2 with some brief arousals, counted as awakenings only if lasting more than 30 seconds, and periods of stage 1 mixed in. Movements, often at the point of stage change, occur about 50 times during the 8-hour sleep period.

DEFINITION OF SLEEP

In spite of all of this description, we have not yet defined sleep. Polysomnograms are a convenient way to measure sleep accurately but say little about what sleep is. For centuries, most people seemed to accept the intuitive notion of sleep—the body, including the brain, are slowed down or even stopped. Science has shown that this belief is wrong. For example, the discovery that there are different stages of sleep that alternate in a lawful way showed that something very active must be going on to produce sleep. Today the accepted definition of *sleep is simply a reversible behavioral state of low attention to the environment typically accompanied by a relaxed posture and minimal movement.* The sleeping person does not sense their surroundings nor respond to them anywhere near the degree they do when awake. This finding has been verified in experiments like the following.

Sleepy subjects in a quiet environment were asked to continue doing a simple behavioral task, such as alternating tapping or attending to words, visual patterns, or sound patterns. They began to falter greatly at the time the polysomnogram showed clear stage 1 patterns. For example, Ogilvie (c.f. Ogilvie, Wilkinson, & Allison, 1989) had people press a button each time they heard a sound. When awake, they performed at or near 100% accuracy but only at about 5% when in stage 2 and at 0% in SWS and REMS. Importantly, as soon as they showed signs of stage 1, they averaged about 60% (ranging from 0 to 75%). In contrast to these behavioral observations, a person's self-perception of being asleep does not regularly agree with polysomnographic indicators of stage 1 or even sometimes stage 2 sleep.

Although the sleeping persons do not sense their surroundings nor respond to them anywhere near the degree they do when awake, there is not a total lack of sensing and perceiving external stimuli. Intense, discomforting, or especially meaningful stimuli can cause a sudden awakening.

Not only are there several states of sleep rather than a unitary state, as our intuitive experience would have us believe, they also alternate in a lawful pattern. NREMS is replaced about every 90 to 110 minutes (10 minutes shorter the first time) with REMS of increasing duration as the night progresses. The first REMS period of the night lasts only a few minutes. This time gradually increases with each successive REMS period such that the last one is 30 or so minutes in duration. Additionally there are changes in NREMS as the night progresses. Early in the night, there is considerable (in the neighborhood of 60 minutes) SWS that rapidly diminishes in time and intensity in an exponential fashion such that there is little to be seen in the second half of the night. Stage 1 sleep occupies only about 5% of the sleep period and, other than at sleep onset, mostly follows the two to three one-minute awakenings scattered during the sleep period. Overall stage 2 sleep occupies 50% of the sleep period, but there is less of it early in the sleep period and more as SWS diminishes. Figure 8 and Table 1 summarize these facts and others. The sleep period is the time from when a person first falls asleep through last awakening. Sleep efficiency is the proportion of sleep period spent asleep rather than awake. Sleep latency is the time it takes to get to sleep.

We sometimes talk about deep sleep. In one sense, this term usually means our sleep was relatively uninterrupted, and we awakened very refreshed. Yet, in another sense, it is not very meaningful. It is a holdover from the notion of deep sleep as being furthest away from wakefulness. In fact, neither REMS nor NREMS are quantitatively deeper sleep. Rather, they are qualitatively different kinds of sleep. Instead of thinking

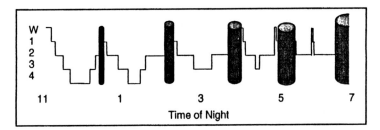

Figure 8. Idealized sequence of sleep stages through the sleep period in an average young adult. W = waking, 1 = NREMS stage 1, 2 = NREMS stage 2, 3 = NREMS stage 3, 4 = stage 4, and the cylinders = REMS. Note that the first REMS period comes after about 80 minutes of NREMS and then NREM and REMS alternate about every 90 minutes thereafter. Also note that SWS occurs mainly early in the night and REMS gets longer as sleep progresses.

Table 1. Average (and Range of) Percents of Sleep/Wake Stages in the Average Young Adult

Stage	Percent	Range
W	1	0–3
1	5	1–10
2	50	40–60
SWS	20	10–35
REM	25	15–35

Stage shifts	35 (about)
Efficiency	.96
Sleep latency	10 min.
Time in bed	7 hrs & 20 min.
Total sleep time	7 hrs
Number of awakenings	2
NREM–REM cycle	90 min.
Number of REM periods	4–5

of sleep as being toward the lower end of a ramp leading from waking, we should think of it as being like different rooms in a house. Just as a kitchen differs from a family room that differs from a bedroom, so too does wake differ from NREMS, and both differ from REMS. Yet, we can accurately talk about the depth or quality of sleep in general. It is measured by such things as greater intensity of delta waves, less stage one, fewer arousals, and so forth. Research has shown that sleep punctuated by arousals lasting 3 to 15 seconds that occur more frequently than every 20 minutes fragment sleep enough to reduce its quality resulting in sleepiness the next waking period. Arousals are indicated by bursts of faster frequency EEG or alpha waves sometimes accompanied by increases in EMG. Typically, these arousals do not result in awakening. The overall quality of sleep is often represented as the sleep efficiency index (SEI)—a number ranging from 0.0 to 1.0 that is the proportion of the sleep period spent asleep.

Box 1

Sleep in Animals

As far as we know, all mammals and many other animals have some form of sleep. Sleep in over 90 species of mammals has been studied, extensively in a few species like the cat, rat, mouse, and, of course, human, but otherwise only slightly studied in only a very small proportion of all the animals alive today. As a result, there are large gaps in our knowledge of animal sleep, and often what we can conclude is based on broad inferences from scant data. However, at least a few representatives from each of the 17 mammalian orders have been studied. There are enough data available to make some observations about sleep in animals.

There are great variations in the sleep of animals. Those animals closer to us on the evolutionary tree have sleep that more closely resembles ours, but the amount of sleep per nychthemeron[3] varies greatly. For example, the length of sleep per nychthemeron ranges from 1.9 hours in the giraffe to 19.9 hours in the little brown bat. Other examples include Asiatic elephants at 3.1 hours, baboons at 9.4 hours, lions at 13.5 hours, and eastern chipmunks at 19.9 hours. The amount of sleep per nychthemeron bares no affinity to the degree of relatedness between species. Cows, sheep, deer and other grazing animals sleep only up to 2 hours per nychthemeron and even that is divided into multiple occasions. Dogs may sleep for 8 hours. Cats and mice spend about 13 hours asleep divided into several periods. Possums, baboons, and bats may sleep close to 20 hours per nychthemeron. It appears that several factors interact to influence sleep length in mammals with some factors being more important than others for individual species. These factors are thought to be:

- the degree to which the species is predator or prey; the more likely an animal is to be preyed upon, the less it can afford to sleep. However this factor is controversial because it is hard to measure.
- the quality, quantity, and availability of the food supply that the species typically eats; animals who do not have an abundant supply of highly nutritious food need to spend more time awake finding and consuming it.
- the type of sleeping habitat the species has; an animal with a safe sleeping place can safely sleep more than one that does not.
- if the species is warm or cold blooded; cold blooded animals may use sleep as a time to avoid becoming too warm or too cold.
- the degree to which the brain is developed at birth in the species; REMS seems to facilitate brain development (see Chapter 12). Thus animals relatively immature at birth need to spend more time in this state.
- the body size of the species; large animals are at less risk for loosing or gaining too much body heat during sleep, thus can sleep for longer periods at a time.
- events and activities; sleep increases around the time of brooding, hibernation, injury, copulation, and other activities.

The distribution of sleep in the nychthemeron varies greatly between species, too. Diurnal animals, such as humans, sleep mainly at night, while nocturnal animals do the opposite. Other animals sleep during both the day and night. Even within these patterns there are variations. Some animals, like humans, pretty much have a single, consolidated period or two of sleep. Others have many small periods of sleep per nychthemeron. Then there is the crepuscular pattern of sleep like that of the bat—asleep except at dawn and dusk.

The habits, places, and postures of animal sleep likewise vary greatly. Some animals, such as rabbits, sleep in burrows; some animals, such as gorillas, make nests to sleep in; while others, such as zebras, sleep in the open. Horses sometimes sleep standing up; some birds can apparently sleep while flying; foxes sleep curled up. Some humans have even been observed to sleep sitting at a desk in a classroom! You can probably add to the list other varieties of animal (and student) sleep habits.

All of the mammals so far tested, except the sea-dwelling dolphins and birds, cycle between some form of REMS and NREMS. Only a small percent of the sleep of most birds is REMS, but avian predators (e.g., eagles, hawks) have a much larger percent of sleep. For a while it appeared that the Australian Spiny Anteater, echidna, did not manifest REMS. This observation was of considerable theoretical interest, because this animal is an egg-laying mammal of very ancient origin. It was thought to give a clue of how sleep developed over the ages; specifically that REMS is a newer type of sleep than NREMS. However, careful study in the 1990s by neurophysiologist Jerry Siegel (of UCLA and the VA Center in Sepulveda Medical Center in California) and colleagues (see Siegel, 1997) using newer kinds of techniques revealed that the echidna shows signs of rudimentary REMS mixed in with its NREMS. They also found that another ancient egg-laying mammal, the platypus, has copious amounts of obvious REMS (Siegel, 1997).

Smaller animals generally sleep longer than larger ones and have a shorter NREM–REM sleep cycle. Birds have much less REMS in their sleep than do mammals. Most primates have the same four NREM stages of sleep that we have. Non-primate mammals seem to have two or just one stage of NREMS. Not all animals show all of the signs of REMS that are seen in humans. Some animals, such as rabbits, dogs, and most birds, do not show complete muscle paralysis. Rems are absent in or minimal in animals, such as moles, opossums, and owls, that do not move their eyes when awake. Yet, in all of these animals, there is some kind of regular cycling between NREM and REMS. All mammals and birds that have REMS have more of it early in life.

Some mammals and birds show patterns of sleep not seen in humans. Some carnivores, ungulates, and insectivores spend part of their nychthemeron somewhere between sleep and wake in what is called dozing (also called drowsiness, but not to be confused with human drowsiness as discussed in Chapter 3). This state is characterized by relaxed body position, partially closed eyes, slightly less responsiveness to stimuli, and a mixture of activated EEG waves and slow waves. You may have noticed cats spending a lot of time in this state, but, contrary to appearances in class, college students have not been documented to exhibit this kind of drowsiness.

Mammals that live in the sea and birds that migrate over oceans have a problem. They cannot settle down to rest while sleeping. The sea mammals need to surface periodically to breathe, and the migrating birds have no place to stop. One way some of these animals have solved the problem is to sleep half of their brain at a time. Bottlenose dolphins and porpoises have been most studied by the Russian scientist L. M. Mukhametov of the Severtsov Institute of Evolution, Morphology and Ecology of Animals in Moscow. He and his colleagues have found that both sides of the brain in these animals may simultaneously show a small amount of stage 2-like sleep, with the animal surfacing to breathe without awakening, but such complex, continuously coordinated activity is not seen during SWS. Rather, EEGs show that while one half of the brain sleeps, the other half is awake. When in this state, the wake half enables the animal to surfacing periodically, then take a breath. This pattern can persist for over an hour at a time followed by awakening, before the other half takes its turn to sleep. However, the total amount of sleep that each side of the brain gets is seldom equal. Additionally, studies have shown that each side has its own quota of sleep each nychthemeron and that one half cannot sleep for the other half. (Other sea mammals compensate differently; they hold their breath while sleeping for up to $\frac{1}{2}$ hour at a time, then awaken to surface and breathe before returning to sleep.)

Many species of birds have also been found to sleep half a brain at a time. Additionally, several other variants of sleep are found in birds. Vigilant sleep found in birds is intermediate combination of NREM and REMS. Gaze wake in birds is sleep with low voltage, fast EEG, and reduced muscle tone but with open eyes manifesting slow, unique eye movements. Pigeons and other birds sometimes peep, something like a reverse blink, while sleeping. The frequency of blinks in individual pigeons is increased by predators being nearby but decreased by the presence of other pigeons or by sleep deprivation.

Even less is known about the sleep of lower animals, but of those that have been studied, the signs of sleep are even more different from those found in humans and other mammals due to their more primitive brains. In most cases, behavioral criteria are relied upon to study sleep in these animals. These criteria include (1) periods of quiescence in a typical posture that are easily reversed by intense or sensory stimuli indicating a potential threat, and (2) a compensatory increase in this state following a period of its deprivation. These indicators of sleep have been shown in at least some representatives from all orders, including lower vertebrates (reptiles, amphibians, and fish) and invertebrates (for example, scorpions, cockroaches, and fruit flies). However, no signs of sleep have been found in other representatives of these orders.

Sleep has been clearly seen in many but not all reptiles that have been studied. Some amphibians appear to have some form of sleep, but others apparently do not. Some fish and some invertebrates have clearly been shown to have states resembling sleep. Interesting animal sleep research has been done by Biological Sciences Dr. Ida Karmanova, Professor and retired Director of the Laboratory of Wake-Sleep Evolution at the I.M. Sechenov Institute of Evolutionary Physiology and Biochemistry in St. Petersburg, Russia (Karmanova, 1982; Karmanova & Oganesyan, 1999). This research has not been widely attended to in the West. She and her associates have data that strongly suggest that reptiles have two kinds of sleep that are forerunners of NREM and REMS in more advanced animals. Even lower vertebrates demonstrate wakefulness plus three other states of immobility or "protosleeps" according to these Russian researchers. These states are not sleep per se, but sleep as seen in higher vertebrates develops out of one of these (c.f. Karmanova & Oganesyan, 1999).

Hibernation and torpor seem in some ways to be related to sleep and other ways to differ from it. Hibernation is an extended period of quiescence, while the body temperature and metabolic rate are greatly lowered with periodic bouts every several days to every several weeks of increases in muscle tension, more than a few deep breaths, and other activity. Torpor is a similar state but not as intense and only lasting part of a day. EEG, body temperature, and arousability all line up in a continuum from quiet wake to sleep to torpor to hibernation. Torpor consists mainly of low amplitude SWS, but there are no recordable brain waves during hibernation. However, hibernation is usually achieved by going through SWS and then through torpor. During sleep there is typically a slight drop in body temperature, a moderate one during torpor, and a great drop during hibernation. Arousal is slower from torpor than from sleep and even slower yet from hibernation. On the other hand, when animals come out of hibernation, they sleep for a long time as if they are sleep deprived. The longer the duration of the hibernation, the longer the subsequent sleep.

SLEEP CHANGES WITH AGE

What we have been describing pertains to the "average young adult" (who is approximately between 20 and 50 years of age). This pattern of sleep forms the basis from which comparisons can be made to different ages and unusual sleep. It is convenient to contrast sleep in average young adults with that of newborns and infants, children, teenagers, and the elderly.

Sleep in Newborns, Infants, and Children

Sleep in newborns and infants is markedly different from that of the average young adult. Newborn sleep does not fit the polysomnographic criteria used at other ages, because the newborn brain is too immature to produce the kinds of brain waves we have just reviewed. They are so different that the stages have their own names, quiet sleep (QS) characterized by EEG similar to that of SWS in adults plus the absence of body movements, active sleep (AS) characterized by low voltage, irregular brain waves and body movements and occasional vocalizations, and indeterminate sleep (IS) which is something between quiet and active sleep. Newborns sleep 16–18 hours of every nychthemeron[3] of which 50% is AS. AS constitutes as much as 75%

of the sleep of late term fetuses and premature newborns. QS and AS alternate in a 60-minute cycle, and newborns frequently go directly into AS.

Another difference at this age is the distribution of sleep and wake across the nychthemeron. Rather than the typical adult pattern of a long period of sleep, typically at night, altering with a long period of wake, every nychthemeron plus maybe an afternoon nap, newborns alternate between sleep and wake many times during a nychthemeron. In a relatively short period of time during infancy, AS comes to resemble REMS more and more (it can be called REMS at 12 weeks of age), and QS morphs into NREMS. This process is similar to the maturation of the coos and babbling of infants into adult language; the coos and babbling are not adult speech but are the important, immature precursors of it.

Furthermore, the amount of REMS per nychthemeron drops to adult level by about 2 years of age. Eventually—the sooner the better in the view of the parents—the infant begins to "sleep through the night" supplemented by a couple of daytime naps. The total sleep time drops to 14–15 hours per nychthemeron by 16 weeks of age and gradually continues to drop to 10–12 hours between ages 3–5. Napping diminishes until there is typically one per nychthemeron and then none.

When toddlers and pre-school-aged children fall asleep, they quickly (within 10 minutes) go into deep stage 4 sleep from which it is difficult to awaken them. They often stay in this stage for about an hour at which point the child's brain waves shift into a mixture of sleep and arousal. Children may change positions and show other movements such as stroking their face, vocalizing, blinking. They may even awaken briefly. Attempts to enter REMS at this point are often unsuccessful, and we say they have "skipped" the first REMS period. Usually within a minute or two, they are back in NREMS, mainly SWS. Now they go into 10–20 minutes of REMS. The rest of the sleep period is filled with alternations of NREM and REMS every 60 minutes with the duration of REMS increasing to around 35 minutes in the middle of the sleep period thereafter gradually decreasing to 20–25 minutes. There may be some return of NREMS toward the end of the sleep period.

During the rest of childhood, the changes in sleep continue but more slowly. By grade school, the NREM-REM sleep cycle is at adult levels, and by age 10, the sleep stage amounts begin to assume adult proportions, but the total sleep time remains higher at about 10 hours. It appears that the sleep of older children is the most intense of any other age. It is easy for children of this age to fall asleep, and they have fewer awakenings. Also, it is very difficult to awaken a preteen child from NREMS.

Sleep in Teens

The sleep of teenagers also differs from that of the average young adult. Although the need for sleep per nychthemeron remains higher than that of the adult, at 8.5–9.25 hours, teens in the Western world typically get much less than this amount, especially males. Let's look at the source and implications of these statements more closely.

Bill Dement (physician and one of the long time, most active, and most influential sleep researchers, now retired from the Stanford University sleep research labs) and Mary Carskadon (PhD, former student and then colleague of Dement at Stanford and now Director of Sleep and Chronobiology Research at E.P. Bradley Hospital and Professor of Psychiatry and Human Behavior at the Brown University School of Medicine) did a series of experiments with teens at what they called summer "sleep camp." The campers were monitored with the polysomnograph while required to spend 10 hours in bed every night. They were then tested for alertness and behavioral functioning in various ways during the day. It was found that, separately from the amount of sleep obtained, daytime sleepiness gradually increased from the onset to the middle of puberty then stayed level through the rest of the teen years. When given the opportunity, teens consistently slept more than the average young adult. In subsequent studies at this camp, the amount of time in bed was shortened by varying degrees. When sleep was restricted to less than the amount needed, increased signs of fatigue and drops in behavioral abilities were found during the day, especially in the morning (see Chapters 2 and 9 for more on the effects of sleep deprivation). Subsequently the amount of sleep teens were getting in their home situations was found to be considerably less than the campers demonstrated was actually needed.

So we know that Western teens need much more sleep than they think they need and actually get. There appears to be a noticeable drop in sleep obtained in the early teenage years. There are $2\frac{1}{2}$ hours less sleep than needed on school nights and over 1 hour less on non-school nights. Another drop of an additional half hour occurs in college freshmen. (It is not known for certain what happens to the sleep of like-aged teens who do not go on to college, but it is thought they too undersleep to some degree.) Further complicating matters is the irregularity of sleeping in teens who often go to bed later but "sleep in" on non-school mornings. The net results of sleeping less than really needed are signs of sleep deprivation including daytime sleepiness resulting in automobile accidents, decline in grades, moodiness, and impulsivity (see Chapter 9 for more on this). Napping returns for many adolescent and college students as schedules permit. For example, during a 10-year study of a group of German adolescents, at any given time, between 50% and 75% expressed the desire for more sleep. And it wasn't always the same students who expressed this desire every time. To round matters out, during the rest of the college years there is a gradual drift toward the average young adult patterns.

Sleep in the Elderly

Sleep in the elderly is best characterized as fraying (Webb, 1975). The end of a tightly wound rope might fray over time. Some ropes fray a lot, but others fray very little. In a similar way, the tightly defined sleep of the average young adult may come apart with age. For some, it frays a lot, and for others, it frays hardly at all. A consequence of the varying degrees of fraying results in great individual differences in the sleep of the elderly. These changes actually begin during mid to late middle age but become more intense and noticeable in the elderly.

Sleep onset is often reported to be more difficult and nighttime awakenings more prevalent in the elderly. Sleep at night decreases to an average of 6–7 hours, but total sleep in the nychthemeron may not decrease from average adult levels when napping is included. Even so, the sleep obtained by the elderly tends to be lighter. It is fragmented by more and sometimes longer awakenings and is more easily interrupted by noises and other stimuli. As a result, sleep efficiency has gradually declined starting at about age 30 from a SEI of 0.96 to the low 0.80s in the elderly.

SWS sleep is greatly diminished to only 5–10%, especially in males, because the intensity of the delta waves has diminished (the culmination of a gradual decline that begins in early adolescence). But even if the intensity requirement of delta waves for scoring SWS is lowered, the amount of SWS is still somewhat lower than that of the average young adult.

The total amount of REMS does not change much, but there is a noticeable decrease in the number of rems during REMS. However, there is more REMS earlier in the night and the duration of the REMS periods may not change much as the night progresses. Accompanying these changes is a proportional increase in stage 1 sleep. As a result of all of these changes, the elderly frequently report that their sleep is less satisfying than when they were younger.

Another issue is the amount of sleep that the elderly need. It turns out the answer is not obvious, and there is not consensus among sleep experts. As mentioned above, both self-reports and polysomnographic studies agree that older people tend to sleep less at night than when younger. However, if naps are included in the count, then it appears that there is much less difference per nychthemeron. Also, an objective test for daytime sleepiness, the MSLT (see Chapter 2), and other data suggest that the elderly are sleepier during the day than when they were younger. This finding can be interpreted to mean they are not getting enough sleep at night. Another way of combining these data is that the elderly need just as much sleep as they did when younger but more evenly distributed over the nychthemeron. Supporting this conclusion are studies with elderly animals that also show a more even distribution of sleep per nychthemeron. On the other hand, elderly people are less affected by the loss of sleep than younger people, suggesting less of a need for sleep. Certainly the elderly's sleep/wake pattern changes, and the intensity of both sleep and wakefulness lessens, but the meaning of these facts is not obvious.

Other changes are common in addition to these changes. Circadian rhythms advance (see Chapter 3) causing early evening sleepiness and early morning awakenings. Perhaps you have noticed this fact in grandma and grandpa. Additionally, sleep disorders such as sleep disordered breathing and periodic limb movements in sleep are more common, causing sleep fragmentation. Also, illnesses common in the elderly and medications often used by this population can contribute to complaints of insomnia.

Box 2

Sleep in other Cultures

There has been surprisingly little cross-cultural study of sleep. Most of what we know of sleep is from study of sleep in the Western industrialized world where people typically sleep at somewhat regular times, typically alone or in pairs, in isolated, quiet, climate-controlled indoor bedrooms. In contrast, many people from primitive cultures sleep in shared spaces with constant noise and great variations in heat and cold and humidity. Rather than sleeping in bedclothes between blankets on mattresses, they may be sleeping in what they have been wearing for many days between skins on mats, wooden platforms, or the ground. Bedtimes tend to be determined by the darkness of night, but sleep may not be consolidated. Western Europeans of 200–500 years ago are reported to have slept in two phases at night. "First sleep," lasting several hours was followed by a "watching period" before the "second or morning sleep." Thomas A. Wehr, psychiatrist at the National Institute of Mental Health in Bethesda, Maryland, had subjects spend weeks of 14-hour nights, during which time, they had to be in bed. They soon settled into a pattern of taking a long time to fall asleep, sleeping for 2–5 hours, lying quietly in bed for 1–3 hours, then sleeping for 2–5 hours (c.f. People in Traditional, 1999). Moreover, they awakened after each REMS period. During the watching period, people often stayed in bed to contemplate, pray, converse with one another, have sex, or simply just let their wandering minds enjoy this semiconscious state.

CONCLUSION

One of the things that you should get out of the information presented in this chapter is that sleep is not as simple as it seems. Prior to the scientific study of sleep, people believed that sleep was a passive phenomenon. Our brains and bodies simply seemed to reduce their levels of functioning as we went to sleep. Indeed it seems that way, because things like noises, pains, or thoughts that keep our minds or bodies aroused can keep us from sleeping. Also, in spite of dreaming, it was believed that not much is going on mentally when we sleep. The discovery of REMS changed all that. The existence of more than one kind of sleep and the regular cycling between the stages of sleep showed that there must be active mechanisms controlling sleep as well as wakefulness. Also, REMS is anything but an inactive state. The EEG shows the brain is very activated. The only reason we remain quietly in bed during REMS is because our muscles of movement are paralyzed.

With the change in the notion of what sleep is came a whole new scientific attitude toward it. New questions were asked that no one ever thought to ask before. More interest, especially in REMS, was generated. More scientists turned their research attention to sleep. More research money became available. More sleep research was done. With this increase in research came even more surprise discoveries about sleep—and even more understanding of how much more there is to learn. Much of the rest of this book is filled with the knowledge and understanding, much of it surprising and some counterintuitive, gained as a result of the new attitude and understanding about sleep. Read on.

Chapter 2

The Need to Sleep[4]

The need to sleep is compelling. You feel sleepy at regular times and even sleepier if you go without it. Bernie Webb, a psychologist who had a long and distinguished career in sleep research at the University of Florida prior to his retirement, called sleep a "gentle tyrant." By this statement, he meant that we are regularly compelled to sleep, yet we are not absolutely compelled to sleep at a given time. As we shall see, both time awake and time of nychthemeron play interacting roles in the urge to sleep (which we call sleepiness). But first, we shall explore each of these factors separately.

SLEEP AS HOMEOSTATIC[5]

Measuring Sleepiness

The longer we are awake, the greater our need to sleep. The first several hours awake we do not notice the urge, but as the amount of continuous time we are awake approaches 16 hours (sooner if we are sleep deprived), we become aware of some sleepiness. If our time awake goes well beyond 16 hours, we feel the urge to sleep getting stronger and stronger until about 30 to 50 hours without sleep have elapsed, when we seem to be as sleepy as we can be.

Subjective scales of sleepiness may not always be accurate because a person may not be aware of their true sleepiness or not wish to divulge the feelings. The study of sleep requires more exact ways of measuring sleepiness than casually asking people how they feel. A better way is to have people indicate on a standardized scale how sleepy they feel. The **Stanford Sleepiness Scale** or SSS (shown in Figure 9), on which a person selects one of seven items to describe the current state of alertness, is well validated on average people for just this purpose. While it has been shown that sleep deprivation does increase SSS scores, there are no norms available to which to compare responses. The **Epworth Sleepiness Scale** (shown in Figure 10) asks questions about falling asleep in situations that typically promote sleep. It has been validated on populations

Chose one of the following to describe your current state:

1. Feeling active and vital, alert, wide awake
2. Functioning at a high level, but not at peak, able to concentrate
3. Awake, but relaxed; responsive but not fully alert
4. A little foggy, not at peak, let down
5. Fogginess, beginning to lose interest in remaining awake, slowed down
6. Sleepiness, prefer to be lying down, fighting sleep, woozy
7. Almost in reverie, sleep onset soon, lost struggle to remain awake

Figure 9. The Stanford Sleepiness Scale.

How likely are you to doze off or fall asleep in the following situations, in contrast to feeling just tired? This refers to your usual way of life in recent times. Even if you have not done some of these things recently try to work out how they would have affected you. Use the following scale to choose the most appropriate number for each situation:

0 = no chance of dozing
1 = slight chance of dozing
2 = moderate chance of dozing
3 = high chance of dozing

1. Sitting and resting
2. Watching television
3. Sitting, inactive in a public place (e.g., a theater or a meeting)
4. As a passenger in a car for 1 h without a break
5. Lying down to rest in the afternoon when circumstances permit
6. Sitting and talking to someone
7. Sitting quietly after a lunch without alcohol
8. In a car while stopped for a few minutes in traffic

Figure 10. The Epworth Sleepiness Scale.

of people complaining of a sleep problem. Various analog scales have also been developed on which a person indicates how they feel by placing a mark on a line between most alert at one end and most sleepy at the other (see example in Figure 11).

More objective measures of sleepiness include various performance measures—usually repetitive tasks such as number substitution or pressing one of several buttons in response to the nature of a light or sound pattern—that are scored for speed and accuracy. A different kind of objective sleepiness measure with very good validity and reliability is the **Multiple Sleep Latency Test (MSLT)**. A person is given a 20-minute opportunity to fall asleep in a quiet, comfortable sleep lab room every

> Place an X on the line that best describes how you feel right now.
>
> Almost asleep _____ Extremely alert

Figure 11. An analog sleepiness scale.

2 hours during the day. They are instructed to allow sleep to occur by not resisting. An average of more than 10 minutes to get to sleep is considered acceptable sleepiness while less than 5 minutes is considered pathological. It should be mentioned that they are awakened once they fall asleep so that their sleepiness is not diminished because of the test.

The MSLT is thought to measure physiological sleep need. Sleepiness may not always manifest itself on performance tests or in real life, because a stimulating environment or competing motivation can mask it. Sleepy people often might fall asleep watching a movie but seldom do when watching an exciting basketball game. Arousing environmental circumstances can compensate for or "mask" physiological sleepiness. Put another way, a quiet, warm, boring environment will not cause you to fall asleep, unless you have physiological sleepiness but such environments can "unmask" such a need. It is felt that the MSLT more directly measures the pure physiological need to sleep, because it eliminates conditions and motives that might otherwise prevent sleep. On the other hand, the MSLT may not show the degree to which sleepiness in an individual may be manifested in real life situations.

The Effects of Continuous Sleep Deprivation

The list of the effects of continuous sleep deprivation that have been reported is long and includes changes in emotions, behaviors, and mental processes as well as biological effects (see Table 2). Sleep deprivation also reduces the amount of alpha waves when awake, increases both slow waves and theta waves during sleep, but leaves waking beta waves unchanged. Additionally, sleep deprivation reduces the time it takes to fall asleep and increases sleep efficiency. The effects of sleep deprivation wax and wane, resulting in periods of good alertness alternating with periods of decreased alertness, slowed reactions, and errors. This pattern is similar to your flashlight periodically getting dim. However, while the number and intensity of the effects increases as the degree of sleep deprivation increases, the manifestation of the effects can be influenced by the situation. For example, the psychomotor behaviors (thinking and decision making which lead to movements to execute these decisions) most affected are long, monotonous, externally paced, newly learned tasks requiring use of memory but without providing any performance feedback.

There is another effect of sleep deprivation on behavior. Microsleeps[6] may cause brief absences of attention called lapses. These phenomena are equivalent to your flashlight suddenly going dark for several seconds. The frequency of microsleeps increases

Table 2. Effects of Sleep Deprivation

SUBJECTIVE	perceptual distortions &
lethargy	hallucinations
less ability to experience pleasure	greater indecisiveness
sense of partial loss of control	slowing of mental processes such
disorientation	as reaction time
irritability and negative moods	decrease in short-term memory
even paranoia in some	decline in logical reasoning ability
BEHAVIORS	for complex problems
less spontaneous	decrease in creativity and mental
over responsiveness	flexibility
decrease in vigilance	decrease in integrative ability
decreased sense of humor	lapses of consciousness
less desire to socialize	*BIOLOGICAL*
microsleeps	heart palpitations
less able to deal effectively with	fall in body temperature (by about
unfamiliar situations	$\frac{1}{2}$ °C or 0.8 °F)
decreased psychomotor	droopy eyelids
performance	itchy eyes
clumsiness	tremor
MENTAL PROCESSES	weight gain
difficulty concentrating	

with the degree of sleep deprivation and after about 40 continuous hours without sleep they are unavoidable without sustained mental effort and strong external stimulation. Serious delusions and depersonalization may occur after four continuous nychthemerons without sleep, especially in persons of weak psychological stability.

Some things do not appear to be affected by mild sleep deprivation. Objective measurements show that shear physical exertion and exercise not requiring much mental effort (such as weight lifting, running, or swimming) do not seem to be diminished by mild sleep deprivation. However, sleep deprived people *feel* that they are doing worse or exercising harder than they would if they had had adequate sleep, and the exercise takes more effort as reflected in increase heart and respiration rates. In contrast, sports that require more attention, thinking, and rapid changes in coordination (such as basketball, tennis, or soccer) are more likely to be negatively affected by sleep deprivation.

You may not entirely agree with what you have just read, because many people do not notice any performance decrements when doing certain tasks during sleep deprivation. In fact, until the late 1950s, scientists were not able to demonstrate any performance deficits resulting from sleep deprivation. This lack of evidence was because they were not looking at the right kinds of tasks. Only when they used tasks whose timing was not determined by the subject that went on for longer than 10 minutes and were rather boring and repetitive, did the effects of sleep deprivation become noticeable. A typical experiment would use the five-choice reaction time task. For this task, subjects were seated before five buttons for 20-minutes and required to press the button that corresponded to the lighting of one of five lights, with a new light turning on as soon as the button for the previous light was pressed. Compared to non-deprived subjects, the sleep deprived ones gradually became slower and slower in their response times. Furthermore, while their best responses were as fast as those of the controls, they had more slow responses and later outright lapses during the last 15 minutes.

The effects of sleep deprivation can, however, be overcome (or, more technically, masked) by things like activity, bright light, noise, temperature, posture, stress, and motivation. Experiments something like the following have been done. During the first 36 hours of sleep debt, while doing a vigilance task rewarded with money for being correct but fines for false alarms, performance was maintained at a higher level than in sleep deprived subjects doing the same task for no rewards. During the next 24 hours the performance decreased in the incentive group but was still above that of the no incentive group. As sleep deprivation continued beyond this point, no difference occurred between the incentive and no incentive groups.

Notice what all these findings say: not all performance is detrimentally affected by sleep deprivation, and when the effects are present, persons do not experience only a general slowing down. Furthermore, sleep deprived subjects can compensate for short periods of time even on tasks that are affected if they apply extra effort, especially when motivated by being given an incentive or immediate feedback of how they are doing. However, the ability of people to compensate by applying extra effort diminishes with greater sleep deprivation. Interestingly, external stimulation, such as loud noise when doing the five-choice reaction time task, impairs the performance of non-sleep deprived subjects but improves the performance of sleep-deprived subjects. The noise is distracting to the non-deprived subjects but arousing to the deprived ones.

Paradoxically, sleep deprived people are both more easily distracted and more easily irritated by irrelevant stimuli, yet often fail to attend to important stimuli outside of their immediate focus. For example, when in a simulated bridge of a commercial cargo ship with various radios and computer screens for radar, weather, and visual views, sleep deprived subjects, like those with adequate sleep, performed well when everything was routine. However, unlike those with adequate sleep, the sleep deprived subjects had trouble determining and focusing on the most important source of data during a crisis. Additionally, they often ignored a new source of information about impending danger.

Chapter 9 further explores the effects of sleep deprivation, especially how it can disrupt people's lives.

The Effects of Partial Sleep Deprivation

More common than missing an entire night of sleep is getting some sleep but not enough. In self-report surveys, most adults describe averaging $7\frac{1}{2}$ hours of sleep per nychthemeron and one-third admit to $6\frac{1}{2}$ hours on weeknights, with attempts at make-up sleep on weekends. If these reports are true, the average person is not sleeping enough, because in experiments where adults are allowed to sleep as long as they want, they eventually settled into an average of $8\frac{1}{2}$ hours per nychthemeron.

The effects of multiple nights of partial sleep deprivation accumulate. Most people can function well the next day after a couple of nights of missing an hour or two of sleep, but the effects are increasingly noticeable for most people when the amount of sleep per night drops below 6 hours or as the missed sleep night after night accumulates.

In many ways, the effects of partial sleep deprivation are similar to those of total sleep deprivation. Sleep onset generally becomes quicker, and sleep is more efficient. The most noticed effect is a decline in mood, but there is also a noticeable decline in mental skills similar to those found with total sleep deprivation.

In other ways, partial sleep deprivation is somewhat akin to selective REMS deprivation, because it is the end of the night that is cut off (see below). Yet, with successive nights of partial sleep, REM pressure accumulates, and there tends to be more REMS occurring early in the night. Nevertheless, the total amount of REMS is still diminished.

Figure 12, from Dement and Carskadon, 1981, shows the effect on sleepiness of obtaining partial sleep. They had subjects sleep in the lab for two successive nights.

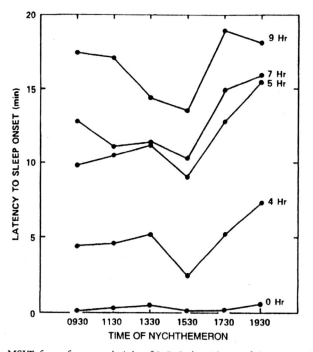

Figure 12. MSLTs from after second night of 9, 7, 5, 4 or 0 hours of sleep per night. (Reprinted from Kryger, Roth, & Dement, *Principles and practice of sleep medicine*, pg. 18, 1989, with permission from Elsevier Science.)

Some were allowed to sleep for 9 hours, others 7, 5, 4, or 0 hours. The data shown are from MSLTs done after the second night. It can be seen that sleepiness increases as the length of sleep decreases. However, this trend is not linear; for example, there is little difference between the 7- and 5-hour groups but a big jump in sleepiness in the 4-hour group. Also apparent is the mid afternoon dip in all but the 0 hour group who were bottomed out across all time trials—something called a basement effect. They may have been even more tired than the test is capable of showing. Finally the 5- and 4-hour groups were sleepier in the morning than they were at almost all other times except during the mid-afternoon dip, whereas this result was not seen in the 9- and 7-hour groups.

To illustrate the cumulative effects of partial sleep deprivation, Dement and Carskadon (1981) had young adults sleep for 5 hours each nychthemeron for 7 consecutive nychthemerons. Each day they underwent a MSLT. Figure 13 shows the results—the subjects became sleepier as the sleep deprivation accumulated. This observation was especially true during the morning and the mid-afternoon except following day 7. Analysis of their nighttime polysomnograms showed that they had little reduction in total NREMS, but REMS was greatly curtailed. Also as they got sleepier, their sleep efficiency greatly improved.

In another experiment, subjects spent 20 days in the lab, getting either 4, 6, or 8 hours sleep per nychthemeron. During the day, they were tested on a battery of vigilance, cognitive, and performance tests. The greater the sleep deficit over time, the worse the subjects did on the tests. For example, on a digit substitution task and a psychomotor vigilance task, the 8-hour sleep group learned, the 6-hour sleep group did not improve much, and the 4-hour sleep group after some initial improvement plateaued and then did progressively worse over time. In spite of their performance,

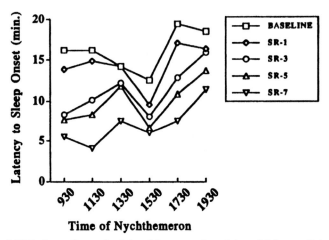

Figure 13. MSLTs from after each night of 7 consecutive nights of 5 hours of sleep. (Figure kindly provided by Mary Carskadon from data from Dement and Carskadon, 1981.)

the deprived subjects reported that the sleep deprivation affected them at first, but they successfully adapted to it.

A very different type of experiment involved studying cumulative, partial sleep deprivation in military personnel. Least affected were tasks requiring manual effort. Greater problems, up to 50% following four days of sleep deprivation, were experienced with tasks requiring mental effort. A specific example comes from the study of U.S. Army Rangers in training who averaged 3.2 hours of sleep per nychthemeron for 8 weeks. After a few weeks, their instructors said it was not unusual to observe what they called "droning"—unresponsiveness and the inability to process information while performing a task. Similar behavior is more commonly called "automatic behavior" when it has been observed in night shift workers, such as nurses.

Until recently, only relatively minor effects of sleep deprivation on the body have been reported. For a long time research showed that mild sleep deprivation has a small but measurable negative effect on the immune system (see Chapter 5). It was also shown that going without sleep for over a week results in things like mild vibration of the eyeballs from side to side, hand trembling, some slurring of speech, drooping eyelids, greater gagging, and increased sensitivity to pain, all of which quickly reverse with sleep. More recently, careful studies by Eve Van Cauter and colleagues of the Department of Medicine at the University of Chicago have shown more serious and potentially permanent effects of chronic sleep deprivation on hormones levels (see Chapter 5).

Many people desire to learn how to sleep less. Some claim they have been successful by shortening their nights of sleep. (You probably have tried it; were you successful?) Careful psychometric and psychomotor testing following multiple nights of partial sleep restriction strongly counters what these people believe. In one experiment, subjects were asked to decrease their sleep by $\frac{1}{2}$ or 1 hour every few weeks. After a few weeks, they were asked to maintain their sleep at this new level before returning to whatever amount of sleep they desired. Each time the subjects made a reduction, they reported feeling sleepy but said this passed after a few days. By the time they had reduced their sleep by $1\frac{1}{2}$ to 2 hours (to about 3 NREM/REMS cycles), they voiced complaints about having trouble waking up in the morning, but their sleep onset times decreased, and their sleep efficiency increased. Tests of performance revealed no deficits. Several weeks after the experiment ended, some of the subjects were again studied, revealing they were getting about 1 hour less sleep than before they started the experiment. (See Box 3 for more on this experiment and learning to sleep less.)

The Effects of Deprivation of Selected Stages

REMS Deprivation

Following the discovery of REMS, there was considerable interest in determining the effects of depriving people of it. The theoretical basis for this interest was the

Box 3

Are We Chronically Sleep Deprived?

Most sleep experts would answer this question in the affirmative. In fact, most say sleep deprivation is a chronic and serious problem in the U.S. They cite data that say the average young adult needs 8.2 hours of sleep per night (some individuals need more, others less; Van Dongen & Dinges, 2001) to be thoroughly rested, but far too many get less. The data cited include needing alarm clocks to awaken (see Chapter 3), not feeling well rested upon awakening, short sleep onset times, and high sleep efficiency. Additionally, people average less sleep than they did at the turn of the 20th century. Given the opportunity, people will and do sleep more, mood is elevated by more sleep, and MSLT scores rise with more sleep. These experts point out that not sleeping enough results in chronic symptoms of sleep deprivation with potentially serious consequences.

Psychologist and prominent sleep researcher, Jim Horne of Loughborough University in England, has argued against this notion (c.f. Harrison & Horne, 1995). He questions the data presented above, saying it is either flawed or can be explained in other ways. For example, the evidence that we sleep less than at the turn of the century prior to the widespread use of electric lights when people reported sleeping for 9 hours compared to $7\frac{1}{2}$ hours today is based on one survey report from 1910–1911, but ignores a number of other surveys from that era that does not show such a high average amount of sleep. In addition, it is not clear that similar groups of people are being compared. Along another line, he points out that although people, given the opportunity to sleep more, can and will do so does not necessarily mean that they need this extra sleep. People given the opportunity to eat more food will often do so but not necessarily because they are staving. He calls such extra sleep "optional sleep" that is beyond physiological need which he calls "core sleep" (see Chapter 11 for more on this theory). While core sleep is necessary and highly beneficial, the benefits of optional sleep beyond this amount are minimal—such as a slight improvement in MSLT and performance scores—given the costs of less wake time, longer time to sleep onset, and increase in waking during sleep. Further, a short 20-minute or so mid-day nap will give the same benefits as extended nighttime sleep (see Chapter 3). Likewise, although he does concede that the afternoon dip could be attenuated with more sleep, the same effect could also be achieved by a nap.

Horne (1988) also cites several experiments showing that people can learn to sleep less, such as the one reported earlier in this chapter. Horne interprets these results as being able to successfully reduce sleep. However, others look at these same data and question this conclusion. It took several weeks of following rigid schedules of sleep without napping (although some subjects admitted that they did nap at times) or sleeping in on weekends. They had to endure bouts of discomfort from sleepiness and difficulty getting out of bed in the morning. Also, there was a lot of encouragement and attention from the experimenters for the subjects to continue. It is doubtful that persons not involved in a formal experiment could achieve the same results, especially if they could not discipline themselves to rigidly adhere to the schedule. These studies also point to the effects of sleepiness on the body (see Chapter 5) and the increase likelihood of having a serious accident (see Chapter 9) when sleep deprived. Finally, in one experiment of this type, the subjects reported that their extra time awake was wasted on nothing important; in the end, they actually felt they had gained little.

Psychologist Michael Bonnet (of Wright State University School of Medicine and the Department of Veterans Affairs Medical Center in Dayton, Ohio), like most other sleep researchers, has countered Horne in other ways. He contends that the data dismissed by Horne does indeed support the need of an average of more than $8\frac{1}{2}$ hours of sleep. For example, people who regularly get that much sleep, report feeling more energetic, happier, and less fatigued. However, his real focus seems to be on the about one-third of adults in the United States who are averaging less than $7\frac{1}{2}$ hours and thus are chronically, seriously sleep deprived. Research shows that six to seven nychthemerons of 6 hours sleep each is equivalent to one full night without any sleep and reduced to just three nychthemerons with only 4 hours sleep, with severe microsleeps occurring in subjects in the 4 hour per nychthemeron condition.

Bonnet also points to the statistics supported by lab research on the negative consequences of such cumulative sleep deprivation. For example, a study suggests sleepiness is a leading cause of automobile and other accidents. In the lab, most people averaging less than $7\frac{1}{2}$ hours of sleep per nychthemeron have an average MSLT of less than 5 minutes, are considered pathologically sleepy (see Chapter 11), and perform poorly on driving simulation tasks. More recently, researchers such as Eve VanCauter, PhD, research associate and professor at the Department of Medicine of the University of Chicago, have shown the negative physiological effects of chronic sleep deprivation on the physiology of the body (see Chapter 5).

Given the difficulty and the risks of sleep deprivation, I don't advise you to try shortening your sleep.

---

association of REMS with dreaming and the prevailing notion (from psychoanalytic theory) that dreaming was a safety valve necessary to keep us from going crazy (see Chapter 8). Researchers saw REMS deprivation as a chance to test this theory. As sometimes happens in science, the theory was wrong, but the data the research on it generated were useful in other ways.

Interestingly, some of the earliest research on sleep deprivation (considered dream deprivation at the time) seemed to support the psychoanalytic theory. A commonly cited example is the experience of Randy Tripp (see Box 4). Subsequently, the research went into the sleep lab where subjects could be selectively deprived of REMS by awakening them every time the polysomnogram showed them entering this stage. This task is difficult, because the frequency of attempts to initiate REMS increases seemingly exponentially as the deprivation procedure proceeds. For example, one

Box 4

Classic Sleep Deprivation Reports

Sometimes research gets poorly reported and then repeated so often that it becomes a kind of legend. The sleep deprivation "experiments" done by Peter Tripp and Randy Gardner are examples of these kinds of studies, the first of which is used as evidence of the grave psychological problems that result from sleep deprivation and the second as evidence exactly the opposite.

Peter was a New York disk jockey in the late 1950s who went without sleep for 200 hours as a fund raising effort as psychologists and physicians monitored him. The reports emphasized the mental deterioration he experienced, including irrationality, hallucinations, and outright paranoia, yet ignoring the fact that he did his radio show every night so well that listeners could not tell any difference. And, following 13 hours of sleep that terminated the marathon, he awoke without any of these symptoms. Reports of Peter's experience with sleep deprivation tend to conclude that people will "go crazy" without sleep.

Randy was a high school student in the early 1960s who decided, as a science fair project, to set the Guinness world record for going without sleep. After he was underway, the local press did a story that caused a team of local physicians and sleep researchers to get involved observing and testing Randy. Most reports of his efforts to stay awake successfully for 264 continuous hours (that's 11 days) offer glowing accounts of how easy and relatively uneventful it was for Randy to accomplish this task. Based on the casual observations of one of the researchers who spent much of day 10 with Randy doing normal things, it was concluded that Randy did not hallucinate, have other sensory problems, or experience any negative mood changes. Among other things, near the end of his sleep deprivation, Randy beat one of the researchers at a game of pinball. In contrast, the actual scientific reports of the experiment lead to quite different conclusions. Careful psychological and neurological testing showed that Randy was greatly affected while sleep deprived. A partial list includes trouble focusing, uncoordination, moodiness, problems concentrating, hallucinations, muscular weakness, difficulty speaking, and occasional paranoia. He recovered completely following one night of extended sleep.

You can see that the truth is somewhere between the contradictory way these two famous attempts at sleep deprivation are usually reported. Continuous long duration sleep deprivation is not easy, comfortable, or without temporary psychological and neurological effects. Yet, the problems all go away quickly, leaving no apparent permanent damage as soon as ample sleep is obtained.

study required 17 awakenings from REMS on the first night, 42 on the fourth, and 68 on the seventh. This happening has come to be called REM pressure. Another indicator of REM pressure occurs during recovery sleep following REMS deprivation when there is a dramatic increase of REMS over baseline with a higher density of rems.

Apparently, we need REMS but not for the psychoanalytic reasons. Although some bizarre things happened in REMS deprived people, their symptoms resolved quickly with the resumption of REMS. Today, it is agreed that REMS deprivation may result in any one of a number of temporary symptoms, including changes in emotions, increased liveliness, greater appetite, more interest in sex, and memory impairment. One curious finding is that REMS deprivation can temporarily lessen the degree of depression in some depressed individuals. More information of the effects of REMS deprivation, especially on learning and memory, can be found in Chapter 12.

SWS Deprivation

Although there has been greater initial interest and research activity directed toward the deprivation of REMS, subsequently, there has also been some research done on the effects of SWS sleep deprivation. It is a bit harder to do, because if you awaken the subjects every time they initiate SWS, the amounts of other sleep, especially REMS, are also greatly disrupted since NREMS normally is the doorway to REMS. (Before reading on, what do you think is the solution to experimentally depriving subjects of SWS while minimizing REMS disruption?)

Instead of awakening a sleeping person, a tone is sounded just loud enough to drive them out of SWS but not loud enough to awaken them. With this procedure, considerable REMS is obtained, as are stages 1 and 2 sleep. It takes about 6 times as many sleep interruptions to eliminate SWS sleep as it does to eliminate REMS. The result is an increase in SWS pressure—increasing attempts to begin it, a temporary increase in the density of delta waves, and some increase in SWS time on the first night when unimpeded sleep is again allowed to occur. (Interestingly, there typically is also an increase in REMS on recovery nights 2 and 3.) SWS deprived people do not report experiencing any behavioral deficits but complain about being lethargic and having muscle aches. Yet, they do tend to be more subdued and withdrawn.

Deprivation of Stages 1 and 2

It would be nice to do studies of deprivation of stages 1 and 2, but so far nobody has determined just how to do it without awakening the sleeper and disrupting other stages of sleep. There might be a bit of fame for you if you can figure out a way to do either of these studies and then determine the effects. Meanwhile, we will keep watching the research literature in the hopes that someday, someone can get the job done.

Recovery from Sleep Deprivation

Only sleep can reverse the effects of lost sleep. Caffeine, exercise, stimulation and the like can ameliorate the effects a bit but not reverse the loss. However, the make up sleep does not have to equal hour for hour the time lost, since recovery sleep is of greater intensity and efficiency. Recovery sleep is more intense sleep in the sense that it is harder to awaken the sleeper. Additionally, SWS intensity is shown by the percent and amplitude of the delta waves. The increased frequency of rems is thought to indicate greater REMS intensity. Total sleep time is somewhat longer if there are no external limits on time in bed.

Recovery from sleep deprivation is relatively quick and complete. It typically takes 1 to possibly 3 nights—shorter if the recovery nights are extended, longer in proportion to the degree of sleep deprivation. The early recovery sleep emphasizes SWS, so much so that REMS may be less than normal. Rate of recovery of SWS follows a saturating exponential curve (Jewett et al., 1999); that is, there is proportionally more recovery in the first few hours of SWS than the last few hours. Later in the night or even during the next night or two, REMS recovers. Its recovery seems to depend on increasing the amount of time in this stage more than increasing its intensity.

In spite of the fact that recovery of NREMS takes priority over recovery of REMS, studies that have experimentally curtailed the amount of SWS during recovery fail to show that it is what is most important for sleep debt recovery. Likewise, with REMS, so why NREMS takes precedence during recovery remains a mystery.

Extended sleep can contribute to recovery from sleep deprivation, but sometimes people extend their sleep even when not deprived. What are the effects of extending sleep? First, the extra sleep itself has a low efficiency and contains little, if any, SWS unless sleep is extended beyond 12 hours, at which point some SWS begins to reoccur. Instead of making people super-alert and able to function at above normal levels, the opposite appears to be true. Too much sleep on one night has been described as making people "under responsive, lethargic, and 'thick-headed.'" (Do these effects sound familiar to you?) Additionally, such extended sleep results in emotional letdown and irritability plus deficits of performance. People who had extended their sleep made non-preservation errors when doing tasks like the Wisconsin Sort Test. In contrast, they make preservation errors when sleep deprived.

These effects may be an exaggeration of what is called sleep inertia (see Chapter 3). Sleep inertia gradually diminishes over several minutes (although there is now some evidence that some effects are present for hours) after awakening. It is more severe following awakening from SWS and includes feelings of disorientation and lack of alertness accompanied by impairments in performance and thinking. In severe cases, there may be no memory later for what was said and done during the state of inertia that follows awakening from deep sleep.

So, overall, there appears to be an optimal level of sleep. Indeed, people who regularly obtain $8\frac{1}{2}$ hours of sleep per night, not less or more, report feeling happier, more energetic, and less fatigued (National Sleep Foundation, 2001) as well as performing better.

SLEEP AS RHYTHMIC

Most animals seem to have fairly regular sleeping schedules during the nychthe-meron. We humans, tend to be most tired at night and, more often than not, sleep then. This pattern is an important example of the circadian rhythms of the body, near 24-hour cycles of behavior and physiology. Not only is our sleep influenced by circadian rhythms, but so also is our sensory processing, short term memory, cognitive perform-ance, alertness, and many other behaviors. Likewise, our body temperature (which, as we shall see, is important for sleep), hormones, urine production, and other biological processes are also on a circadian schedule. Our internal biological clock(s) enable us to be in synchrony with the 24-hour external world just as the clocks on our walls and wrists enable us to synchronize our schedules with those of many individuals for collective work and social activities. In fact, our circadian rhythms enable us to have an internal biological (subjective) day and night that usually enables us to mirror and prepare for the forthcoming change between external (objective) day and night.

Before we go any further, become familiar with the terms shown in Figure 14. They are useful for describing circadian rhythms. Next, let us look at how the circa-dian rhythms for sleep and wake are studied.

For many experiments, there needs to be a situation in which the subject can be isolated from environmental time cues. The original experiments were done in caves, but, more recently, special sleep labs with no windows, clocks, radios, phones, or any other direct links with the outside world that could give an indication, however sub-tle, of the time have been used. Inside these labs, one of three types of experiments can be undertaken: free-run, forced desynchrony, or constant routine.

Free-run experiments were the earliest to be done. The subjects are free to sleep whenever they feel like it. They have control over the lighting and when they eat meals. Studies typically go on for weeks, and, without any time clues, the subjects rely on their own internal circadian clocks. Free-running subjects eventually have an average circadian period of about 25 hours.

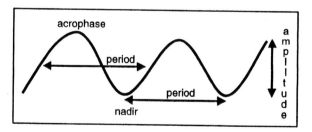

Figure 14. Important terms for describing circadian rhythms. Also: phase = relative position of the curve—often determined by its peaks—relative to some other curve or to time.

In contrast, **forced desynchrony** requires subjects to be on a sleep/wake (plus dark/light and meal) cycle that is outside the bounds of what most people are capable of achieving (often 28 hours) for a number of days or weeks. This sequence causes the sleep/wake cycle to become desynchronized from the circadian temperature cycle (which remains closer to 24 hours) meaning that subjects will be sleeping and awake at different phases of their temperature cycle over the weeks of the experiment.

In the **constant routine**, the subject remains in quiet, lying in bed or in a semi-recumbent position, but awake, with the illumination low and constant. Small meals are eaten every hour. Constant routine studies are typically done for more than 24 hours but less than 48.

Another research method for studying circadian rhythm of sleep in an ordinary laboratory is to have people maintain a schedule of **very short sleep/wake cycles**. The most common are 90- or 20-minute nychthemerons both with a $\frac{1}{3}$, $\frac{2}{3}$ ratio of sleep to wake. Thus, on the 20-minute cycle, the subject has to be in bed trying to sleep for seven minutes. Then they must get out of bed and be awake for 13 minutes before returning to bed. Most subjects cannot tolerate this routine for very long. Thus, the duration of sessions is between 24 and 48 hours. The amount of sleep obtained during each in-bed portion is measured. The advantage of these protocols is that they produce enough data points to quickly see the circadian cycle of sleepiness without the masking of the build-up of long wake time. However, there appears to be some sleep deprivation in subjects on the 20-minute nychthemeron. The ultradian cycle (see below) can also be discerned in the 20-minute nychthemeron.

There are a number of major findings about our circadian sleep rhythm. The sleep/wake cycle is dependent on the circadian clock, not vice versa. Left to its own devices, our internal sleep/wake cycle would be something greater than 24 hours. Freed of external influences in constant routine studies, it runs precisely 24.18 hours (Czeisler et al., 1999). There is greater variation with a mean closer to 24.5 hours in many blind people and closer to 25 hours in individuals in free-run conditions who have control over the lights in the room.

Most of us live successfully in a 24-hour world because our internal rhythms are regularly reset (technical term, **entrained**) primarily by stimuli from outside the body acting as **zeitgebers** (German for time giver). Entrainment is like if you, the zeitgeber, were to daily reset your watch that runs fast or slow. The major zeitgeber for our sleep and wake cycle is the nychthemeral alternation of light and dark that occurs on the planet we inhabit. Things like activity, social stimulation, mealtimes, and bedtimes can also help but play a relatively minor role compared to light. The right amount of properly timed light can either **phase advance** (move the phase to an earlier time) or **phase delay** (move the phase to a later time) our circadian rhythm for sleep and wake to any new phase in usually two to three nychthemerons. The brighter the light, the greater the entrainment effect. Recent research has shown that even room light, which is generally 20 times dimmer than outside light on a somewhat cloudy day, can also have a weak entrainment influence. Our Circadian rhythm for sleep/wake can be easily entrained to shorter (up to 22 hour) or longer (up to 26 hour) periods, and periods even longer or shorter if approached gradually.

Pause for a moment and try to predict what would happen to your sleep in the absence of any strong zeitgebers.

Answer: Your sleep/wake rhythm would become "desynchronized" with the 24-hour world. You would alternate maybe every couple of weeks between wanting to sleep during the day and wanting to sleep during the night. If you were to try always to sleep at night, you would have a week of good sleep followed by a week of fair sleep, then a week of poor sleep, then a week of fair sleep, and so on. This pattern is in fact what happens to many blind people. For the other one-fourth, either other zeitgebers are strong enough to entrain their circadian rhythm, or they have a type of blindness that allows some light information to get through to the brain even though they have no awareness of light sensation (see Chapter 4). About half of totally blind people have a melatonin cycle that influences their sleep (see Chapter 4) that is very precise within individuals, averaging 24.5 hours but ranging from a bit less than 24 hours to 25 hours.

A phase response curve (PRC) shows the times when we are sensitive to a zietgeber being able to entrain the circadian clock as well as the direction and intensity of the change. Figure 15 shows a PRC for light in humans. Exposure to light for a few hours before and after our regular time of falling asleep will delay the clock, but exposure a few hours before and after our regular arising time will advance the clock. PRCs are related to our body time, not the real time, but since most people sleep when it is dark out, it has become common to describe the phases of the PRC in terms of subjective night, subjective dawn, subjective day, and subjective dusk. Some, but not all, researchers also see a "Dead Zone" during much of the subjective day where the light has no effect.

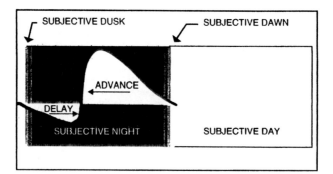

Figure 15. A phase response curve, PRC, for light in humans.

Take a careful look at the PRC for light in Figure 15. Notice that at subjective dawn we are nudged a bit toward phase advance and at subjective dusk we are nudged a bit toward phase delay. Each of these effects is stronger in subjective night after subjective dawn and in subjective night before subjective dusk. In the midst of subjective night, there is a sharp "crossover point" where the effect quickly changes from one to the other. This crossover point is close to the core body temperature nadir. Typically, since our bodies tend to run slow (i.e., longer than 24 hours) we need to be advanced a bit more than we need to be delayed every nychthemeron to keep in phase with our external, objective world. In special circumstances, such as when we take a jet across time zones, we need a much greater delay (when flying West) or advance (when flying east). (See chapter 9 for more on jet lag and related topics.)

The circadian rhythm for sleep actually has two peaks and two nadirs every cycle in most, but not all, people. This pattern is shown in Figure 16, a composite summary of several kinds of research, especially experimental 20-minute nychthemerons, MSLT studies, and some free-running conditions. It also reinforces the subjective reports of many people. Notice that about 12 hours after maximal sleepiness at night, there is a less intense increase in sleepiness that is called the "midafternoon dip" because of a dip in alertness that accompanies the increase in sleepiness. (It is also called the "post-lunch dip," which is a misnomer since it has nothing to do with lunch.) It is much easier to fall asleep and stay asleep during the times when sleepiness is high but more difficult when sleepiness is low. Notice that there is a sharp transition in just a couple of hours between our time of maximal alertness early in the evening and our time of maximal sleepiness during the night.

The effects of our circadian rhythm for sleep may not always be obvious—both in everyday life and in the research lab—because of masking. Masking occurs when extraneous influences intervene between the clock and behavioral effectors to reduce

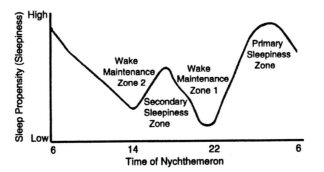

Figure 16. Typical sleepiness during a nychthemeron. (From Moorcroft, 1993 with permission of the publisher.)

Box 5

Other Rhythms

Circadian rhythms are not the only kind of rhythm involved with sleep and wake. The rhythmic cycling that occurs between NREMS and REMS about every 90 minutes is called an ultradian, meaning less than a day, rhythm. It is thought to be a more obvious part of the basic rest activity cycle (BRAC)—a 90-minute rhythm that occurs throughout the nychthemeron regardless of waking or sleeping. This 90-minute cycle has also been dubbed the biological hour. Although not always obvious, careful testing has revealed that we cycle between highs and lows about every 90 minutes on such diverse things as our level of fantasies, stomach activity, resting heart rate, eye movements, EEG frequencies, sexual arousal, eating, as well as sleepiness.

---

greatly the effect of the clock. Things like activity, meals, and posture can mask the circadian rhythm for sleep.

Our circadian rhythm influences some aspects of sleep more than others. Generally speaking, REMS is strongly influenced, but NREMS is not. REMS latency, duration, and propensity are all strongly influenced by the circadian rhythm, but rem density is not. Affected REMS components are at their peak in the early morning hours when circadian sleepiness is at its peak. Additionally, there is a weak effect of sleep length on REMS propensity that has a non-additive interaction with the circadian influence. Things are much the opposite for SWS, however. SWS propensity and strength is strongly affected by the amount of preceding wakefulness but only weakly influenced by circadian phase.

INTERACTION OF HOMEOSTATIC AND CIRCADIAN EFFECTS

By now you may be asking yourself how do the homeostatic drive to sleep and the circadian control of wakefulness both influence our sleep at the same time? One answer comes in the form of a model. Models are used in science to summarize and integrate a great deal of data in an attempt to show the way things are and how they work. The best models are based on more facts than assumptions. Good models are then used to formulate new research to attempt to verify some of the predictions of the model. Subsequently, models tend to be modified to encompass new data or abandoned if the new data simply do not fit.

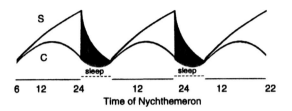

S

C

sleep   sleep

6   12   24   12   24   12   22

Time of Nychthemeron

Figure 17. Borbély's "two process model" of sleep/wake propensity. (From Borbely, A. (1982). A two process model of sleep regulation. *Human Neurobiology, 1,* 195–204, with permission of the author and the publisher, Springer–Verlag).

Alex Borbély of Switzerland formulated what is currently the most widely accepted model of sleep called the "**two process model**" of sleep/wake propensity (see Figure 17). One process in this model is homeostatic, labeled **process S**, and the other is circadian, called **process C.** You can think of the level of process S as the intensity of sleepiness accumulated during wakefulness and strength of sleep when asleep. Process S builds up in a saturating exponential function (note shape of S in Figure 17) while awake but declines in a similar, but more rapid, manner during SWS. Empirically, the characteristics of process S in this model are derived from the effect of accumulated waking and accumulated sleeping on the amplitude of slow waves.

Process C is a circadian process that is in phase related to the core body temperature rhythm (see chapter 5), but its exact shape and phase were derived empirically from sleep propensities at different circadian phases. You can think of process C as represented in Borbély's model as intensity of alertness. However, there is some disagreement if process C is simply a wake drive all the time or a wake drive during the day and a sleep drive at night; either way the outcome is the same for our purposes.

Think of each process in this model as a different kind of timer. Process S is like an hourglass indicating degree of sleepiness with a 30- to 50-hour capacity. When awake, sand flows from one end to the other, but, unlike most hourglasses, the rate at which the sand flows is fast at first but diminishes as the top chamber empties; sleep is like inverting the hourglass so that sand flows the other way but twice as fast. Process C is like a 24-hour wall clock that displays the current level of circadian strength of alertness instead of what time it is. The degree of sleepiness, the likelihood of sleep, and sleep duration at any time result from the interaction of both timers.

A revised version of the model (Figure 18) shows several changes that were made to accommodate new data. The shape of both process S and process C more accurately reflect their true nature. The staircase shape of process S during sleep reflects the fact that we go into and out of several bouts of SWS during a night of sleep. Parallel process Cs were added—one as an awakening threshold and the other as a sleep threshold. The tendency to fall asleep is strong when process S rises above the sleep threshold of process C. We tend to awaken when process S touches the wake threshold of process C. We tend to stay in whatever state we are in when S is between

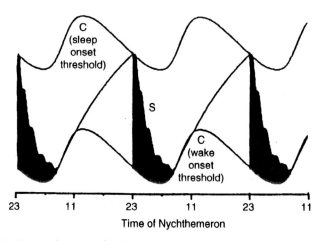

Figure 18. A revised version of Borbély's "two process model" of sleep/wake propensity. From Achermann P & Borbely AA (1990). (Permission to use this figure granted by the Copyright Clearance Center, Inc. on behalf of the American Journal of Physiology.)

the two C thresholds. Work across the model now to see how it describes sleepiness and sleep duration at different times. People who go without sleep for more than a nychthemeron usually report a "second wind" in the morning. Can you see from the model why it happens? Hint: although process S continues to increase, what happens to its distance from the wake threshold in the morning?

The two-process model has gained considerable empirical support. It is consistent with recovery from sleep deprivation, how sleep duration changes with the phase of the circadian rhythm, characteristics of rebound following sleep deprivation, and more. For example, it is consistent with the analysis of data from a forced desynchrony experiment of Derk-Jan Dijk (a Dutch psychologist who has been a part of the research endeavors in several laboratories in Europe and the US including Borbély's lab in Zurich and Czeisler's lab at Harvard) and Czeisler (a MD/PhD sleep researcher at Harvard Medical School) in 1994. Eight young males were individually required to maintain a 28-hour forced desynchrony protocol and encouraged to sleep during the one-third of the cycle (9.33 hours) that was dark. The subject's circadian sleep/wake cycle soon became desynchronized (at 24.18 hours) from this dark/light schedule. As a result, they were initiating sleep at different phases (3+ hours later each cycle) of their circadian cycle, yet prior wakefulness length had minimal variation, since they spent most the night portion asleep. This finding allowed Djik and Czeisler to unmask the circadian influence from the homeostatic influence and vice versa so that the contribution of each to sleeping and waking could be assessed. Sleep propensity was maximal when circadian alertness was at its minimum and gradually decreased as circadian alertness increased. Sleep propensity was also directly proportional to the

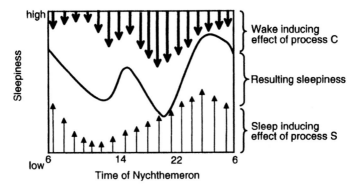

Figure 19. How the opposing influences of process S and process C cause our nychthemeral pattern of sleepiness.

length of the preceding period of wakefulness and diminished in proportion to the length of subsequent sleep, both non-linearly.

If you look only at the circadian drive, it seems paradoxical that its arousal influence is greatest just prior to the normal sleep period and lowest prior to awakening. Likewise, if you look only at the homeostatic component, it seems paradoxical that we continue to sleep near the end of the sleep period when homeostatic sleepiness is very low. But when considered together, it can be seen that the circadian and homeostatic factors oppose each other for long periods of time, thus allowing one long period of sleep to be followed by one long period of wake during each circadian cycle (see Figure 17). Several hours of sleep happen when you fall asleep at the normal time, because the homeostatic sleep drive is great but, as the sleep drive diminishes, the circadian wake drive gets weaker, also. The net result is that you stay asleep until both homeostatic sleepiness is weak and circadian alertness begins to increase. Likewise, when you are awake, the homeostatic sleep drive builds up, but the circadian wake drive also gets stronger, opposing it until it starts to weaken again about the time sleep onset starts. Without the circadian influence, the total sleep amount would not change during the nychthemeron, but it would be taken in multiple naps rather than all together at night.

Djik and Czeisler (1994) also showed that SWS propensity is almost independent of circadian phase but that the REMS propensity is strongly influenced by it (with peak close to habitual waking time) but also mildly inhibited by homeostatic sleep need. Can you see that unlike sleep propensity, during normal sleep/wake cycles SWS propensity and REMS propensity tend to supplement one another? The occurrence of sleep spindles are governed by weak circadian influence (high when circadian arousal drive is lowest) and strongly inhibited by sleep need. Since they function to help prevent sounds and lights from awakening us, they, too, contribute to our sleeping in one long, consolidated period.

Chapter 3

Normal Variations of Sleep[7]

Now that we have reviewed many basic aspects of sleep in Chapters 1 and 2, we can explore its normal variations and related factors. Sleep problems and pathologies will be discussed in Chapters 9 and 10. In this chapter, we will explore the nature of sleepiness, what constitutes good sleep, long and short sleepers, morning larks and night owls, problems teens experience with sleep, how the sleep of women differs, naps, and sleep inertia.

SLEEPINESS AND TIREDNESS

We all have used the terms sleepy and tired and alert and awake and have a notion of what these terms mean. But in science we need to be precise in the terms we use. Otherwise, we may find that we are really dealing with somewhat different things. Bill Dement, MD/PhD, longtime, notable sleep researcher and retired Director of the Stanford University Sleep Disorders Center, suggests the following continuum:

Awake ⇔ Sleepiness ⇔ Drowsiness ⇔ Sleep

He uses this continuum to distinguish ordinary sleepiness from what precedes sleep. **Drowsiness** is the period of awake with heavy eyelids that occurs just prior to sleep and is accompanied by a strong urge to sleep. Conscious effort is needed during drowsiness to stay awake and keep eyes open. Additionally, he points out that alertness is an antonym to sleepiness, and tiredness is a broader category than sleepiness. Tiredness includes sleepiness but also fatigue from muscular or mental exertion. Fatigue may also result from tedium, boredom, apathy, and general lack of interest.

Dave Dinges, research psychologist specializing in sleep at the University of Pennsylvania School of Medicine, has described the factors that can lead to a subjective sense of sleepiness:

1. Prior Sleep. Both too little and too much recent sleep can cause a person to feel sleepy.

2. Amount of Wakefulness. The greater the time awake since prior sleep, the greater the likeliness of feeling sleepy.

3. Circadian Phase. The current time of the nychthemeron influences sleepiness.

4. Health Status. Illness usually causes sleepiness.

5. Age. Beginning with middle age, people generally sleep less well and, thus, often feel sleepier.

6. Drugs. Some drugs influence sleepiness.

7. Surroundings. Stimulating, novel, exciting situations can reduce the sense of sleepiness. In contrast, situations that are warm, boring, quiet, and so forth may heighten the sense of sleepiness. Such situations do not cause sleepiness as commonly believed. Rather, as the bodily need for sleep increases, the influence of environmental factors increases. An exciting situation, such as a football game, may keep a sleep deprived person from feeling sleepy, while a boring lecture won't put a fully rested person to sleep but can unmask sleepiness in a sleep deprived individual.

Box 6

Sleep Needs and Accumulating Sleep Deprivation

Given the data on the average amount of sleep needed and sleep obtained and the effects of the accumulation of partial sleep deprivation, what is the bottom line for us? In my opinion, the evidence is strong that too many of us—especially most college students—who are averaging less than $7\frac{1}{2}$ hours of sleep a night are not getting enough sleep and this deprivation is having serious negative consequences. For most of us, getting $8\frac{1}{2}$ hours would be even better. Think right now how much better off you would be with more sleep and how you can get it.

Note: it is an open question if *everyone* needs $8\frac{1}{2}$ hours of sleep per night or this amount is just an average, with individual amounts distributed along a bell-shaped curve as are most psychobiological things. Older research, conducted with less sensitive instruments available prior to the MSLT, suggested such a distribution is true. However, it is possible the short sleepers in these studies would have been shown to be sleepy on the MSLT; but then again, perhaps not. Only research will provide the answer.

Meanwhile, forget the numbers. How are you functioning during the day? Is it hard to get up in the morning? Do you struggle to stay awake? Do you fall asleep in class, when reading, or in quiet situations? (Remember, it is not dull, monotonous lectures or warm, dim classrooms, or boring books that put you to sleep. It is only your own individual sleep need that does so.) If your answers are affirmative and you do not have a sleep disorder (see Chapter 10), you need to get more sleep and possibly more regular sleep. For a week, try increasing your nightly sleep by 15 minutes and getting up at about the same time every day, including weekends. Do this again and again until you are no longer sleepy during the day. This task accomplished, notice how much better you feel and how much more productive and successful you are. Congratulations!

GOOD SLEEP

Some mornings we may awaken eager and ready to get going. On such mornings, we may think, "That was a good night of sleep. I feel great." But on other mornings, our experience may be quite different. We find it hard to awaken, may hit the snooze button a few times, and finally have to drag ourselves out of bed. Such experiences may cause us to wonder just what makes for good sleep and how we can get more.

Unfortunately, only some of the factors that contribute to a good night of sleep are known at this time. Quality of sleep is primarily a subjective thing. While we can distinguish some poor sleepers by the polysomnogram, others who say they slept poorly show nothing unique in their record. One factor is amount of sleep—both most recently and for the last several days. If we have not allowed our bodies and brains to get the sleep they need on a given night, then we will awaken feeling unrefreshed. Also, as mentioned in the last chapter, partial sleep deprivation tends to accumulate, and, even after a single night of what would ordinarily be an adequate amount of sleep, we may still feel less than totally refreshed. Van Dongen and Dinges (2001) report that people who are alike on amount of sleep need per night during the identical circadian phase can differ by as much as an order of magnitude when sleep deprived. That is, there is a kind of individual trait vulnerability to sleep loss. So one aspect of good sleep and how to get it is simply to be sure you as an individual get enough.

But total sleep time alone is not enough. **Sleep continuity** has also been found to be important. When our sleep is fragmented by multiple **arousals**—awakenings but also changes in our EEGs toward lighter stages of sleep—then our sleep is less satisfying and effective. Michael Bonnet, has done excellent research on this topic (c.f. Bonnet, 1986; Downey & Bonnet, 1987). He noted a common factor in people with several different types of sleep disorders (to be more fully discussed in Chapter 10). Their sleep was punctuated with brief arousals. He tested his hypothesis by stimulating sleepers in his lab just enough to change their EEG briefly at various intervals throughout the night. He then tested their levels of sleepiness and performance the next day. He found that arousal intervals of greater than 20 minutes had little effect on subsequent sleepiness and performance, but people aroused every minute tested the same as people who were totally sleep deprived. Partial effects were seen with intervals between 1 and 20 minutes, with greater intensity of effects the closer the interval was to 1 minute. The conclusion: an important component of good sleep is sleep continuity, and anything that fragments sleep such as noise, pain and other discomforts, stress or anticipated stress, too warm or too cold of a room, a snoring or restless sleeping partner, stormy weather, and so forth can lead to poor sleep.

As we also learned in Chapter 2, there are times of the nychthemeron that we are able to sleep more easily and other times when sleep is more difficult to obtain and sustain. Sleep obtained during our subjective night and our mid-afternoon dip is much more likely to be good sleep than sleep obtained at other times. As we shall see in Chapter 9, the experiences of shift workers demonstrate the problem of getting good sleep during the day.

Regular wake-up times (and to a lesser extent, bedtimes) have also been shown to be important for obtaining good sleep. When we go to sleep and get up at greatly different times, such as staying up late on weekends and sleeping in the next morning, we tend to disrupt the phase of our circadian rhythms. Not only do we try to sleep when our circadian rhythm urges us to be awake, when we try to return to our weekday schedule, we have delayed the phase of our circadian rhythm for sleep, such that we are now trying to sleep when our body expects us to be awake. This experience has even been given a special name—Sunday night insomnia. The end result is several days of poor sleep resulting in daytime sleepiness and impaired performance.

Note that we have said nothing about the different stages of sleep. While we know from Chapter 1 that typical sleep contains specific proportions of each stage and that a pressure occurs when sufficient amounts of either REMS or SWS are not obtained, it has not been demonstrated that the typical proportions and cycling of NREMS and REMS are related to good sleep. There are some suggestions that inadequate REMS may result in poorer mood the next day, yet good sleep seems more related to the quantity of uninterrupted sleep than the amounts or continuity of the specific stages.

Peter Hauri, clinical psychologist and retired director of the Mayo Clinic Sleep Disorders Center, has talked about good sleep in terms of the balance of the sleep and wake systems in the brain (see Chapter 4). Typically, one becomes active while the other becomes inactive, but not always. They are not like ends of a teeter-totter, such that as one goes up, the other necessarily goes down; rather, they are somewhat independent. If the wake system remains active (higher heart rate and other physiological measures sometimes show this) while the sleep system becomes active, then we may not be able to get to sleep easily, and, if we do get to sleep, we do not have quality sleep.

LONG AND SHORT SLEEPERS

Chapter 1 discussed sleep in the average young adult. The average young adult needs about 8 hours of sleep per nychthemeron, and 68% of people report they average between $6\frac{1}{2}$ and $8\frac{1}{2}$ hours of sleep. Therefore, quite a few people are getting considerably more or less than an average amount of sleep. Many of those getting less sleep are sleep depriving themselves, but others may not need any more sleep than they are getting. Likewise, many people getting more than the average amount of sleep may biologically need it. Although definitive evidence is lacking, there are suggestions that degree of sleep need may be inherited, just as while most people are close to average height, some are much shorter and others much taller for inherited biological reasons. Identical twins (raised together or apart) have more similar sleep characteristics, including length, than non-twins. There are a few documented individuals who do perfectly well with 3 or even 1 hour of sleep and are otherwise normal and healthy. Reports of people who never slept have been shown to be untrue or caused by very rare diseases that disrupted more than sleep.

An individual can tell how much sleep they need by how they feel and perform during the day. Outside of undergoing a MSLT, there is really no other way. If you have trouble waking up in the morning and getting out of bed, if you feel sleepy during the day and have to fight off sleep a lot, if you fall asleep in warm, quiet, boring situations or when driving, you may not be getting enough sleep (or you may have a sleep disorder—see Chapter 10 for additional signs and symptoms of sleep disorders). Try getting more sleep by going to bed 15 minutes earlier each night—or more if you are sleeping much less than eight hours per night and have severe daytime sleepiness—for a week at a time and seeing how you feel the next morning. Maintain the sleep level that enables you to feel alert for much of the day.

Some of you may be trying to sleep too much. While this is not as likely in the Western industrialized world as not sleeping enough, it does happen. This problem, too, may be due to a sleep disorder, so see Chapter 10 first. If you take a long time to fall asleep, wake up often, and are not sleepy during the day, you may want to try to reduce your bedtime by 15 minutes per week until you are sleeping better and notice slight signs of sleepiness the next day. At this point, go back to the previous step and stay there.

What is known about people who genuinely need much more or much less sleep than the average person? Ernest Hartmann, psychiatrist at a sleep disorders center in Newton, Massachusetts, published research in 1973 on groups of sleepers who either needed less sleep than average, the short sleepers, and those that needed more than average, the long sleepers. He was careful to include only people who really needed less than $5\frac{1}{2}$ hours or more than 8 hours, with 9 hours spent in bed to feel rested. He excluded insomniacs and people who were sleep depriving themselves or willfully oversleeping. Then, using clinical interviews supplemented by psychological tests, he looked for characteristic profiles of people in the two extremes. While no individuals necessarily displayed all of the characteristics, collectively the short sleepers differed from the long sleepers.

In the sleep lab, the sleep stages and NREM–REM sleep cycle were not unusual, but the long sleepers got more REMS and stage 2 sleep than the average young adult, and the short sleepers got less. The long sleepers had twice as much REMS as the short sleepers, and the sleep efficiency of the long sleepers was poorer than that of the short sleepers. Also, in other experiments, long sleepers have been shown to recover more quickly from sleep deprivation.

The main differences he found were psychological. In many ways, short sleepers seemed to be the opposite of long sleepers. Short sleepers were more likely to report that they were generally self-content, full of energy and proficient, and desire to be productive. Short sleepers were also more socially sophisticated. Long sleepers tended to be more introverted and worry about things, yet some were very creative. They often were active politically in a critical and non-conformist way.

Psychological tests revealed additional differences between long and short sleepers. Long sleepers tended, as a group, to show mild to moderate neurotic traits. Some of them were not very self-confident and others anxious, inhibited, and depressed. They manifested more bodily aches. Short sleepers were more conforming and had a tendency to deny problems. They also tended to have a lot of ambition, be decisive, and were out-going.

Their attitudes toward sleep differed also. Short sleepers tended to view sleep as a waste of time while long sleepers reported they liked sleep and felt it necessary to get a sufficient amount. Aeschbach and colleagues (2001) report that short sleepers tolerated being sleep deprived better than long sleepers.

When awakened near the end of each REMS period (see Chapter 7 for more on this procedure), long sleepers showed a change as the sleep period progressed. Early on, they reported that they felt quiet and passive, but this turned to active and energetic by the end of the night. The short sleepers demonstrated no such change. Hartmann interpreted these results to mean that the long sleepers were experiencing psychological change during the night that the short sleepers were not.

These data are intriguing but are correlational, making it impossible to determine if the personality/lifestyle determined the sleep characteristics or vice versa. In an effort to determine causality, Hartmann (1973) also studied a very rare group of sleepers. These people are like short sleepers in terms of sleep and personality/lifestyle for weeks or months at a time, and then are like long sleepers for weeks or months at a time. When things were going well in their lives, they were short sleepers, but when experiencing stress, job uncertainty, physical demands, or emotional strife, most resembled long sleepers. Importantly, Hartmann found that the personality/ lifestyle changes preceded the changes in sleep, suggesting that longer sleep serves a psychological function. Hartmann believes that what happens to variable length sleepers is an exaggeration of what happens in most people. He points out that during emotional tumult, average sleepers increase their REMS to a modest but significant degree.

Other researchers have not supported Hartmann's findings regarding long and short sleepers. However, some of these researchers (e.g., Webb, 1975) used college students as their subjects, which may have influenced the results, since college students have atypical sleep patterns to begin with. Another set of researchers (Stuss & Broughton, 1978) only weakly supported Hartmann's findings in six adult, very short sleepers. A different criticism of Hartmann's research on long, short, and variable length sleepers is that he did not directly determine if the length of sleep was what the sleepers actually needed or was self-imposed sleep deprivation or oversleeping. Measures like the MSLT were not available at the time to assess these factors. This research needs to be replicated using newer techniques.

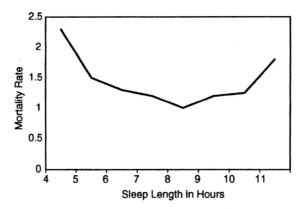

Figure 20. Mortality rates and length of sleep in over one million adults. (After Kripke, Simmons, Garfinkel, & Hammond, 1979.)

Related research is also very interesting. In 1959–60, the American Cancer Society did a survey of 1 million people over the age of 30. One of the questions asked had to do with amount of sleep typically obtained. Six years later, they did a follow up study of these individuals and found that more of the self-reported long and short sleepers had died than those who obtained near an average length of sleep (see Figure 20). The greater the reported sleep deviated from 8 hours, the greater the mortality rate. At this point, hopefully, you are asking if this finding is an artifact caused by other factors. The authors, too, thought of that possibility and statistically factored out age, sex, exercise, diet, and smoking from the data but still got the same results. There was no difference in the causes of death between the long sleepers, the short sleepers, and the average length sleepers. So the reasons why people who slept less than average or more than average were more likely to die remain an intriguing mystery.

MORNING LARKS AND NIGHT OWLS

Some people's sleep is **phase shifted.** By this term, we mean that the shape of the circadian rhythm curve is the same (see Figure 16 in Chapter 2), but the whole thing is shifted to the left for **phase advance** and to the right for **phase delay.** The degree of the shift is usually less than an hour, but this time is enough to make a noticeable difference.

You may have noticed that Grandma and Grandpa tend to go to bed earlier than younger people, but they also get up much earlier. It's not just that they are party poopers; rather, their circadian rhythms are phase advanced. In contrast, the circadian rhythms of teenagers tend to be phase delayed. Many other people, regardless of age, may also be phase shifted. We commonly call those who are phase advanced "morning larks" and those who are phase delayed "night owls," although the technical terms are **morning types (MTs)** and **evening types (ETs)** respectively. Most of us are between them and are sometimes referred to as NTs for **neither type.**

It is important for research, as well as for other uses, to have a simple and fast way to identify people who have certain characteristics such as being MTs and ETs. Fortunately, there is a valid questionnaire developed by Smith, Reily, and Midkiff (1989) that distinguishes between ETs, MTs, and NTs. It consists of a page of 13 questions about the time of day that you typically get up, what time of the day you feel at your best, how you would feel if you had to sleep at different times, and so forth.

Research has shown that in addition to being more alert in the morning and sleepy in the evening, MTs generally fall asleep more easily than ETs and have better moods after awakening but awaken more during sleep than NTs and ETs. The circadian temperature of MTs peaks about 1 hour earlier in the nychthemeron than ETs. ETs feel more alert and believe that they perform better later in the day and on into the evening. The difference between ETs and MTs is typically a two-hour phase shift. However, when this shift interacts with process S (see Chapter 2) the result is a possible difference of 4 hours in time of peak alertness (Van Dongen & Dinges, 2001). Not only do ETs tend to go to bed later and get up later, they tend to be more irregular in their bedtime habits, especially on non-work nights from nychthemeron to nychthemeron but average the same amounts and patterns of sleep as ETs and NTs. ETs also experience less jet lag and tolerate shift work better.

There are some noticeable changes in the circadian rhythm that occur in the elderly that supplement the discussion of sleep changes with age that were discussed in Chapter 1. Most elderly are morning larks tending to arise early and go to bed early. In older elderly persons, this tendency is more noticeable in women than men. This change actually is the culmination of changes that begin in middle-aged persons. Additionally, the amplitude of the circadian rhythm for sleep/wake is lower in the elderly, and there appears to be an attenuation of response to zeitgebers. Some research also suggests that the period of the circadian rhythm for sleep is shorter in the elderly, but other studies have failed to confirm this.

What causes some people to be MTs and others ETs? It is not entirely clear, but some things are known. It is not easy for either group to adopt the sleep habits of the other type, suggesting that it is not merely a matter of choice. Yet, of people the same age, more workers than students are MTs, suggesting that there is some flexibility given demands of work. Still, many of these workers expressed the desire to be able to go to bed later and get up later, so maybe they are going against their internal or other dispositions. Also, as just indicated, age plays an important role in that younger people who tend to be ETs gradually become NTs and then MTs as they get older. Although it is often the elderly who are notorious MTs, recent evidence suggests MT characteristics are also noticeable by middle age.

Box 7

Awakening without an Alarm (Part 1)

What determines when we awaken from sleep? For most of us it is an alarm clock or some other external means such as a radio, another person shaking us or throwing water in our face, or a cat kneading our stomach. But alarm clocks are a relatively recent phenomenon in the history of human existence. Prior to their invention and widespread use, many people, we might imagine, used to wake up on their own after their body had had enough sleep. But circumstances, such as the need to tend to some chore or social obligation, may have necessitated arising at a particular time regardless if enough sleep had been obtained.

Is it possible to awaken oneself at a time determined prior to going to sleep? Anecdotally, there are people who say they can accomplish this task. Occasionally, over the last century, there has even been research directed at determining the extent of this ability with usually positive results. However, the existence of this ability has not been widely recognized, and the extent of the ability is not clear. In the 1990s, several of my students and I undertook to do new research on this question (Moorcroft, Kayser, & Griggs, 1997).

We first did a random telephone survey of 269 adults in the upper Midwest of the United States. To our surprise, we found that approximately one-fourth of those surveyed never used an alarm clock or other external means to awaken. Another one-fourth set their alarm but regularly awakened before it; they just did not trust their ability. Then there was the one-fourth who needed their alarm and often more to awaken on time. The remaining one-fourth expressed no consistent pattern. We asked those who said that they self-awakened without or before their alarm how they did so, but no consistent model emerged. Prior to going to bed, some visualized a clock set to the desired time, others repeated the time to themselves, and so forth. Many said they did nothing special; it just happened.

We next selected 15 people who said they regularly self-awaken, and then objectively tested for this ability in their own beds for three consecutive nights while choosing their own wake-up times. Each subject wore an actigraph—a wrist-watch size devise that is able to store data that can discriminate sleep from wake in normal sleepers on a minute by minute basis—to bed for three consecutive nights. From this method, we were able to compare intended awakening time, which each subject recorded in a journal before going to bed, to actual awakening time. The mean difference between actual and intended awakening time was +4.61 minutes. That is, after hundreds of minutes asleep, they were able to self-awaken within 5 minutes of their target. Five awakened within 10 minutes of their target time (mostly before) on each night, five did so on two of the three nights, and of the remaining five, four did so on one night. Choice of target times varied considerably within subjects but more so for those who were more successful. Taken together, these results show that many people have the ability to regularly awaken themselves from sleep at a desired time and that such an ability is of practicable utility.

How can people awaken themselves at a desired time? Part of the answer was given in subsequent research by Born and colleagues (1999). They found that the level of the hormone adrenocorticotropin increased during the hour before they were told they would be awakened early the next morning but not if told they would be awakened later in the morning. Perhaps this change in this hormone level helps awaken a person. Still unexplained is the cognitive time keeping process during sleep that causes the release of this hormone at the proper time.

PROBLEMS TEENS EXPERIENCE WITH SLEEP

A great deal of focus has been directed toward the sleep of teenagers in the United States and other countries such as Italy and Brazil. As mentioned, they tend to be strongly phase delayed, which can present many of them with real problems when they have to be in school early in the morning. In the United States, many teenagers have to be in class before 8 a.m., meaning many are arising an hour or two earlier than this hour. Yet, their bodies do not want to fall asleep until around 11 p.m. Adding to this problem, are the demands of work and the desire to socialize that may make bedtimes even later. The result is all too often chronic sleep deprivation in teenagers. "It is not unusual to see students sleep in class, especially in the morning," say both high school students and their teachers. Even when awake, they are so "out of it" that paying attention and learning suffer.

Do delaying school start times to 8:30 or 9:00 make a difference? Apparently, yes, according to University of Minnesota's Center for Applied Research and Educational Improvement (School Start Time Study, 2000). For several years, some of the schools in and around Minneapolis, Minnesota, have been using such start times for their high schools. Reports of the effects have begun to become available, showing many benefits and few problems. Generally, better results have been found in suburban Edina High School than the urban Minneapolis schools. The students starting school later are more alert according to teachers, student sleepiness decreased as they average an extra hour of sleep each nychthemeron, school counselors and nurses report fewer students seeking help for emotional and physical complaints, and there is better attendance and less tardiness. Students report earning higher grades, and statistical analyses of records found a slight increase. Student behavior has also shown improvements (e.g., quieter hallways, better lunchroom behavior). Many students report that they are more able to do their homework during school hours, because they are more alert. Parents report their teens are "easier to live with" and that they now have "connection time" with their teens over breakfast. Participation in after-school sports and extra curricular activities has not been negatively affected.

But all of the sleepiness of teens cannot be explained by the phase delay in their circadian rhythms and remedied by delaying school start times. There are also social demands and, with the increasing number of teens with part-time jobs, the demands of work. It is the opinion of researchers in this area that parents and teens themselves could do more in getting to bed earlier, especially on weekends, and recognizing the importance of adequate amounts of sleep taken at regular times.

COLLEGE STUDENT SLEEP

The sleep of college students is worse than that of high school students, at least for freshmen college students in their late teens. Although not as rigidly bound to school start times, most college freshman get even less sleep than high school seniors, because they choose to go to bed so much later. Delayed bedtimes not only shorten their average night of sleep by about half an hour more than their prior amount but also tend to make them even more phase delayed. And things seem to be getting worse over recent years; there has been a dramatic increase in the number of college students who report less stability in their sleep habits and less satisfaction with their sleep over the last couple of decades (Hicks, Johnson, & Pellegrini, 1992).

The typical college freshman is considerably sleepy during the day, causing significant impairment. To particularly compensate, and because a less rigid schedule allows it, napping becomes common. As students continue their college careers, their sleep deprivation gradually reverses, apparently because of earlier bedtimes and needing less sleep. Seniors typically are much less sleepy than freshmen.

Box 8

Yawning

Beware: Reading this may cause you to yawn.

Yawning, an involuntary, slow, deep breath accompanied by wide gaping of the mouth is found in all mammals, maybe all vertebrates. Even human fetuses yawn. Once started it cannot be stopped, but it can be stifled. However, stifled yawns are not satisfying—only a gaping yawn is. (Try this: When you feel like yawning, force it through your nose or clench your teeth and note how you felt about this yawn compared to the full-blown variety.) The functions of yawning are not conclusively known but seem related to respiration, heightening alertness, and non-verbal communication.

A common notion is that yawning serves to increase the oxygen in the blood. It is true that yawning does include extra expansion of the lungs resulting in more oxygen intake and carbon dioxide being expelled. It also increases return of blood to the heart and more blood going to the cortex of the brain. However, breathing pure oxygen does not decrease yawning, nor does breathing a higher concentration of carbon dioxide increase it. Neither does increasing respiration rate have any effect. Thus, the reason for yawning cannot be to increase oxygen in the blood.

It is also common knowledge that yawning is related to sleepiness and alertness. Yawning is common before going to sleep or after awakening (but not during sleep). It is noticeable when feeling drowsy. Its lowest occurrence is mid-afternoon. Stretching sometimes accompanies yawning. The need to be vigilant in a non-stimulating situation will also increase yawning. Yawning does cause a temporary increase in heart rate, may restore tone to the muscles involved, and may cause reflexive stimulation of the arousal centers in the brain. Yet yawning also occurs before and after eating, after drinking alcohol, and in the midst of a stressful situation.

Yawning also is a form of non-verbal communication. Animals communicate threat and aggression with a teeth-showing, eyes-wide-open yawn. It also can signal dominance or the readiness for sleep, but, in this case, the eyes are shut. In humans, yawning most often signals boredom or the readiness for sleep.

Yawning among humans is also highly contagious. Seeing others yawn greatly increases yawning or the urge to yawn. Even if the face of the yawner is rotated 90° or 180°, it still has this effect. Surprisingly, the gaping mouth is not the most important facial feature to cause this contagion. A gaping mouth alone will have no effect, but viewing the facial features of someone who is covering a yawning mouth is sufficient. But that's not all. Hearing a yawn will produce contagion. Hearing *about* yawning will also cause this effect. (A colleague says she never lectures about yawning until near the end of the class period for just this reason.) Reading about yawning will cause yawning, too. (Are you yawning yet?) It is speculated that yawning is contagious in humans because it helped synchronized bedtimes in our early ancestors.

HOW THE SLEEP OF WOMEN DIFFERS

Until now we have said nothing about the differences in sleep between men and women for two reasons. First, the sleep of men and women is nearly identical, especially the nature of the stages, the homeostatic and rhythmic components, and changes with age. Second, when sleep research was emerging in the mid 20th century, researchers were faced with many questions and wanted to answer the most basic ones first, such as what sleep is like in general in humans. For this reason, they controlled for the menstrual cycle by only looking at the sleep of women during their follicular phase, assuming, we can suspect, that someone would get back to questions about how sleep might differ between men and women and how the reproductive hormones influence women's sleep. Surprisingly, with a few notable exceptions, only in the late 1980s did researchers finally focus on how the sleep of women might differ from that of men.

For example, Reyner and Horne (1995) found some differences between the sleep of men and women previously unrecognized. Women go to bed earlier than men and fall asleep sooner. As a result, the sleep period is much longer for women. However, women do not sleep as well, with more awakenings and time spent awake during the sleep period. These differences become greater with advancing age, plus older women take longer to fall asleep. The National Sleep Foundation poll of 2001 found that adult women are more likely than men to get eight or more hours of sleep per workday but no differences on non-workdays.

Other researchers have noted that the main difference between the sexes is that the fraying of sleep in the elderly tends to occur sooner in males by about 10 years. For example, some elderly females still show classical SWS, but few elderly males do. Additionally, women have twice as many sleep spindles then do men, more SWS, and differences in their delta waves, such as a slower decline with age. Further, things like sleep deprivation, drugs, shift work, and jet lag may magnify the differences in the sleep of women compared to men.

Even greater attention has been paid to conditions distinctive in women, notably changes in their reproductive hormones and related developmental status. Menarche, the menstrual cycle, pregnancy, and menopause all have been found to have effects on sleep quality and quantity. (Much of this research has been done by Kathryn Lee, PhD, a nurse with the Department of Family Health Care Nursing, School of Nursing, University of California, San Francisco, and her associates: Lee, McEnany, & Zaffke, 2000; Lee, Zaffke, & McEnany, 2000; Baratte-Beebe & Lee, 1999.)

The effects of menarche on sleep have not specifically been studied, but the menstrual cycle, whose onset it heralds, has been. First, we must realize the considerable difficulty in investigating this question. For example, there are great differences both within and between women in the length of each menstrual cycle, but the results have to be coordinated by cycle phase (menstrual ⇨ follicular ⇨ ovulation ⇨ luteal ⇨ menstrual and so on). Second, not all women have the same changes in their sleep during the menstrual cycle. Third, ovulation may not occur with each cycle, changing subsequent hormone production. Fourth, the use of oral contraceptives changes hormone levels and thus sleep. Fifth, data from research using retrospective methods are easier to obtain but much less reliable than data obtained using prospective designs. To this point, enough research has been done to make the following points but not always with clear consensus.

Significant sleep disturbance is reported by about 15% of cycling women, but even more report milder disturbance. Up to half of menstruating women report that bloating disturbs their sleep for two or three days resulting in less rest from it. The increase of progesterone after ovulation causes an increase in body temperature and also causes some women to feel sleepier, fall asleep more quickly, awaken less, decrease the latency to REMS, and increase stage 2 sleep. Subsequently, when the level of progesterone is falling just prior to menstruation, some women find it more difficult to fall asleep, experience poorer sleep in the form of more awakenings, have lower sleep efficiency, spend more time in bed, get less SWS, recall more dreams that are more vivid, and are sleepier during the day. Women who experience premenstrual dysphoric disorder, have been reported to experience differences in their sleep throughout their entire menstrual cycle including insomnia, or hypersomnia, daytime sleepiness, more unpleasant dreams, more stage 2 but less stage 3 and REMS, shorter REMS latency, and greater difficulty awakening in the morning.

Sleep and sleepiness also change during the course of pregnancy. Overall, upwards of 75% of women report their sleep was more disturbed during pregnancy than at any other time in their lives. Specifically, 13% of women report experiencing sleep changes during the first trimester, 19% during the second trimester, 68% during the third trimester, and 11% during the entire pregnancy. The most noticeable change during the first trimester is a conspicuous increase in sleepiness and sleeping, both at night and in napping. One of the probable causes is an underlying decrease in both SWS and sleep efficiency with some insomnia. Things seem to get back to normal during the second trimester, although there may be an increase in the number of awakenings. Sleep becomes decidedly more difficult to obtain during the third trimester. The number of awakenings that started to increase both in frequency and duration by mid-pregnancy reaches four or more by the end of pregnancy, contributing to insomnia, less total sleep time, more daytime sleepiness, and often more napping. However, some women report that their sleep seems to return to normal during the last month of pregnancy.

Studies in the sleep lab have also revealed changes within sleep during pregnancy. REMS has been found to either decrease or increase during the middle of pregnancy but almost always decreases later. Changes in REMS latency seem to vary from woman to woman but often diminish toward the end of pregnancy. SWS amount gradually declines during pregnancy, frequently approaching total absence during the third trimester. As SWS decreases, stages 1 and 2 increase. Sleep efficiency begins a decline during the second trimester that continues during the third trimester. For some women, all of these things tend to come close to normal levels during the last month.

The causes for these changes in sleep include hormonal changes, metabolic changes, physical discomfort, including muscle cramps and lower back and joint pain, leg discomfort, nausea and heartburn, sinus congestion, increasing urge to urinate, fetal movements and uterine contractions, and emotional changes—especially anxiety and depression. For example, there is an increased need to urinate during the first trimester as the increase in progesterone causes the smooth muscle of the ureters to relax and dilate. Urinary frequency declines during the second trimester as the uterus moves up from the pelvis to the abdomen. However, the fetus now begins to move, which, along with the emergence of other discomforts, may cause some awakenings. During the third trimester, pressure on the bladder from the increasing size of the fetus causes the return of the need to urinate frequently. Also progesterone, which increases during pregnancy, causes sleepiness.

What happens to sleep in the month following pregnancy is less clear. Most obvious is fatigue and the disruption of sleep caused by the need to attend to the needs of the newborn (which also may affect the sleep of the father and other caregivers). But factors like recovery from the delivery, breast-feeding, postpartum depression complicate the picture. Generally it appears that sleep efficiency declines further (to near 0.80), the latency to REMS is greatly reduced, and SWS increases while stage 2 decreases. There is a decline in mood, especially with more confusion/bewilderment that correlates to the degree of sleep disturbance including deficiencies in REMS amount. By the third month after delivery, there is a recovery of most aspects of sleep, but sleep efficiency is still low and the number of awakenings high.

There are some differences depending upon if it is the first or a subsequent pregnancy. Even if their children are sleeping through the night, women who have already borne a child have more awakenings resulting in lower sleep efficiency during and after pregnancy. Also, it is interesting to note that it has been estimated, that in the first year with a new baby, parents lose 400–750 hours of sleep.

Box 9

Co-Sleeping/Bedsharing

In the modern Western industrialized world, infants sleep in their own bed located in their own separate bedroom. It is assumed that this is both natural and necessary. Also the wealth of the Western industrialized world renders this practice feasible. However, in most other areas of the world and even more widespread in earlier times, co-sleeping is the norm. Co-sleeping is when the infant sleeps in the same room or area with one or more caregivers.

A specific form of co-sleeping is bedsharing where the infant sleeps in the same bed as the caregiver, usually the mother. In places like Japan, India, and Africa, it is usual for families to sleep together in one family bed. However, the Catholic Church outlawed bedsharing in the 13th century because of reports that many infants had been smothered when a sleeping adult rolled over on it. (Actually the incidences most likely were intentional infanticide by mothers.) This fear is expressed by many in the Western world who look aghast at bedsharing. But Anthropologist James J. McKenna, director of the Mother-Baby Behavioral Sleep Laboratory at the University of Notre Dame, maintains that there is no evidence that it is detrimental and may even be beneficial if the infant is laying on its back on a firm mattress, not over wrapped, and its head not covered by blankets. His research shows that the sleep of the infant is longer but lighter with more arousals and movements; also the heart rates, respiration, and sleep stages of infant and mother become synchronized. Furthermore, mothers and babies tend to wake each other up during the night, which may prevent long breathing pauses in babies that contribute to sudden infant death syndrome. There is also some suggestion that bedsharing might be more soothing to infants as well as be stimulatory for their brain development.

Co-sleeping occurs more frequently than is commonly believed (Thiedke, CC 2001). Anywhere from 35 to 55% of preschoolers and up to 23% of school-aged children co-sleep with their parents. Co-sleeping is more common among Hispanics (90%) and African-Americans (70%). It is well accepted among Pacific and Asian cultures, also.

It should be noted that the American Academy of Pediatrics Task Force on Infant Position and SIDS (Does Bed, 1997) states the following: "There is no basis at this time for encouraging bedsharing as a strategy to reduce SIDS" (p. 272). Also, the U.S. Consumer Product Safety Commission has stated, "children younger than 2 years should sleep in cribs" (Nakamura, Wind, & Danello, 1999, p. 1023). Drago and Dannenberg (1999) made a similar recommendation. However, these conclusions have been severely challenged as being based on weak or misinterpreted evidence while ignoring the positive evidence for bedsharing (McAfee, 2000; Rosenberg, 2000; McKenna & Gardner, 2000).

The end of the reproductive years in a woman is marked by menopause when the production of progesterone and estrogen begin to fall and eventually remain low. One of the consequences, hot flashes during sleep, is reported by over a third of women. They contribute to an increase of brief arousals during sleep. In extreme cases, severe hot flashes can result in hundreds of awakenings per night. Even a moderate level can result in an increase in stage shifts and lower sleep efficiency. On the other hand, the number of hot flashes during just the two hours prior to sleep correlate with the amount of subsequent stage 4 observed. During menopause, women complain of fatigue, lethargy, and mood problems (however the mood problems do not correlate with the quality of sleep) but not daytime sleepiness, general problems of falling asleep, or getting less sleep. Following menopause, many women complain of difficulties in getting to sleep and of waking more during sleep.

NAPS

Naps are periods of sleep that are shorter than usually taken by the individual or typical of the species. They also have been called sleep without pajamas taken during the day. Most human naps range from 20 minutes to 2 hours; the average is 70 minutes. Napping is encouraged by many cultures in the world, most typically in the afternoon in warm climates, but tends to be discouraged in adults in Western industrialized nations who view it as slothful. All told, about half of the people in the world take an afternoon nap.

As we saw in Chapter 2, there is a natural, biological tendency to become sleepy in mid-afternoon suggesting that napping is normal. Also, naps can help to relieve the effects of sleep deprivation. Napping, or at lease the urge to nap, increases in proportion to amount of sleep debt. Age has a great influence on napping. As we saw in Chapter 1, the sleep of newborns can be considered to be distributed in a series of naps. Even when infants begin to sleep through the night, they still take naps during the day. Napping in young children continues for several years. Napping reappears in teenagers and young adults, especially those in college, at least half of whom nap at least once a week. This daytime sleep pattern is due to both changes in biological sleep needs and too little sleep at night. Napping reemerges in the elderly, but the reasons for it are not clear. It may be that the elderly now have the time and opportunity to nap, and/or it may be a change in the regulation of sleep that occurs during the later years of life. Morning people gain more benefit from short naps than evening people.

Adults nap for one or a combination of reasons. Many naps are compensatory—making up for sleep debt. Naps increase during illness and seem to have a recuperative function (see Chapter 5). Environmental factors, especially hot weather, may promote napping. The circadian mid-afternoon dip is a biological factor contributing to napping. Some napping may be recreational—simply for pleasure. Finally, prophylactic napping, napping in anticipation of sleep deprivation, long periods of wakefulness, or even being awake during the typical sleeping hours is thought by some to be highly beneficial, even more beneficial than napping after sleep debt has accumulated. Afternoon classroom naps by college students are a good illustration: "frequently compensatory, certainly environmental, influenced by biological rhythms, sometimes [prophylactic], and mainly recreational" (Moorcroft, 1993).

Naps are usually highly beneficial but can also have negative consequences. A short nap of about 20 minutes can be refreshing and increase alertness. Even if not perceived as refreshing, they usually enhance performance such as the ability to pay attention, to respond rapidly, to remember better, to think more clearly, and so forth. This performance enhancement usually lasts about 3 hours but can extend out even to 18 hours. However, naps, especially longer ones, can cause several minutes or more of sleep inertia upon awakening (see below). It has been suggested to limit naps to about 20 minutes, because longer than an hour brings less additional benefit but greatly increases sleep inertia. Twenty minutes of napping generally brings optimal general refreshment and improvement of performance. It is necessary to sleep for longer than 90 minutes for serious sleep debt recovery.

An example of research on naps is that done by Masaya Takahashi, DMSc, and Heihachiro Arito, DMSc, of the National Institute of Industrial Health in Kawasaki, Japan (Takahashi & Arito, 2000). They had 12 young, healthy students limit their sleep to only 4 hours for one night, on two occasions. The following day, using a counterbalanced design, each subject had no opportunity to nap on one occasion or 15 minutes in bed available to nap right after lunch (from 12:30 to 12:45 p.m.) on the other occasion. Both before and after lunch, at intervals of about $1\frac{1}{2}$ hour, subjects completed tests of memory and logical reasoning and rated their own subjective sleepiness. After a nap averaging 10 minutes in duration as confirmed by sleep polysomnography, they felt less sleepy and performed better on logical reasoning than without a nap.

There is no unique kind of sleep that occurs during naps; naps contain the same kinds of sleep as occurs during the night. However, REMS is more likely during morning naps. The amount of REMS obtained during a nap has no effect on the amount of REMS during subsequent night sleep. However NREMS obtained during naps does reduce subsequent NREMS.

Claudio Stampi, M.D., director of the Chronobiology Research Institute in Newton, Massachusetts, has researched management sleep in extreme conditions through the use of napping (Mason, 2000). For example, he has studied and advised solo world sailors who engage in 90 or so days of continuous racing. He found that they can get by on $4\frac{1}{2}$ to $5\frac{1}{2}$ hours of sleep per nychthemeron, but less than this seems to present problems. For the times when even this limited amount of sleep is not possible, the best strategy is to try to get whatever sleep possible in 1-hour naps, especially when experiencing a wave of sleepiness.

In Stampi's lab studies, where subjects were allowed 3 hours of sleep per nychthemeron, three 1-hour naps caused less performance detriment than two $1\frac{1}{2}$-hour naps or one block of 3 hours of sleep. He also found that 50% of stage 2 sleep and 50% of REMS is lost using such a strategy, but only 5% of SWS is lost. Often stages 1 and 2 are virtually skipped. ETs do better on such a schedule than MTs. However, Stampi finds that relentless training can improve either type's ability to utilize such polyphasic sleep.

SLEEP INERTIA

Sometimes people experience bleariness, confusion, and less of an ability to perform immediately after awakening from sleep. This experience, called **sleep inertia**, may be apparent for several or more minutes, but actual performance decrements are now known to last up to several hours. Both the subjective feelings and the objective performance effects dissipate exponentially. Sleep inertia is much more noticeable following awakening from NREMS than REMS and has a greater effect on cognitive tasks, especially those depending on memory, than psychomotor and perceptual tasks. For example, a person might not remember a phone call in the middle of the night or might turn off an alarm clock and return to sleep without awareness of having done so later. It is easier to return to sleep during sleep inertia.

Sleep inertia is less noticeable following gradual morning awakenings following a full night of sleep than if abruptly waking from a short night of sleep, abruptly awakened after 30 or more minutes of SWS, or when waking from a nap, especially a longer nap. The more difficult it is to awaken a person, the greater will be their sleep inertia. Extending night sleep beyond typical amounts will result in sleep inertia if there was no prior sleep debt but not when extending sleep to recover from sleep deprivation. On the other hand, uncompensated sleep deprivation seems to worsen sleep inertia.

SLEEPY VS. ALERT PEOPLE

Peretz Lavie, psychologist at the Sleep Laboratory, Faculty of Medicine, Technion-Israel Institute of Technology, Haifa, Israel, was presented with a problem by the Israeli military a number of years ago: a few soldiers frequently fell asleep when on night guard duty. No amounts or types of sanctions were able to alter the problem. Lavie tested these individuals in several ways and found that they were genuinely sleepier than most people and were just not able to remain awake at night. Further, he found that these people were not only sleepier than most people, but extending the amount of sleep per nychthemeron made no difference in their sleepiness. They fell asleep more quickly at night and when napping, slept more efficiently, but found it hard to stay awake.

Lavie concluded that their sleepiness was a trait—a fixed individual characteristic—rather than a state—a variable characteristic depending on circumstances; they are simply chronically sleepy people. He also found some people with the opposite characteristics—alert by day but with trouble getting to sleep at night; he called them "alert." Most of us are somewhere in between. The difference may be in the relative strength of the wake producing and sleep producing parts of the brain (see Chapter 4).

Part II

What Causes us to Sleep?

If you are like most of my students, after reading the first three chapters, you may be thinking that sleep is more complicated than you had imagined. Then you may begin to think about what causes us to sleep and what effects sleep has on the body.

Look again at the introduction to Part I. Notice that prior to the 20th century, notions of what sleep was like and how it was produced were intertwined. Also, it was assumed that sleep was a passive phenomenon. During the 20th century, it became apparent that sleep was an active phenomenon rather than passive, with considerable complexity. This knowledge of sleep was shown by the discovery of REMS and its regular cycling with NREMS, which could only be accomplished by active control mechanisms. Once this information became apparent, scientists began looking for the mechanisms that control sleep and paying more attention to what effects sleep has on the body. Chapter 4 reveals the basics of what is known about the involvement of the brain in sleep and Chapter 5 does the same for the rest of the body.

Chapter 4

The Brain in Sleep[8]

In order to fully understand sleep, it is necessary to understand how the brain produces it. It used to be thought that the brain simply reduces its overall level of activity and arousal as the way of producing sleep. We now know this is not true (see Box 10). As Pittsburgh psychiatrist and sleep and brain researcher, Eric Nofzinger, (personal communication, June, 2000) said, rather than a general reduction in activity, "the brain is functioning under a different set of rules during sleep." It functionally reorganizes during sleep such that some areas become more active during sleep, and others become less active. It is necessary, therefore, to have a basic understanding of brain anatomy and brain functioning to understand sleep fully.

Box 10

Discovery of Sleep as an Active Brain Process[9]

For centuries, sleep was assumed to be a passive process. It certainly seems that way to many today. To get to sleep, you have to allow your brain and body to relax their activity and arousal. You cannot actively do so; you just have to let it happen. And anything, whether it is noise, light, pain, discomfort, thoughts, and so forth, that interferes can prevent sleep. During the 20th century, several scientific findings changed this notion, at least among scientists, to one of sleep being actively produced. Among these findings was a chain of research involving laboratory experiments on the cat brain.

The story begins with experiments done by a Belgian physiologist, Frederick Bremer (Bremer, 1935, 1936). He made a cut between the brain and the spinal cord (cut C in Figure 28) in cats knowing that this procedure would cut the brain off from arousing stimuli from the body. Without such stimulation, he reasoned the brain would remain continuously asleep. Of course, the body was paralyzed, but Bremer

---

could observe signs of sleep and wakefulness in the head, such as what was happening in the eyeballs and the types of brainwaves produced. He noted more sleep than usual, but there were periods of wakefulness. He reasoned that the brief wakefulness occurred, because there was still sensory input via the cranial nerves in the brainstem that transported sensory information from the head. When he made a similar cut higher in the brain between the midbrain and the forebrain (cut D in Figure 28), input from most cranial nerves was also cut off except for smell and vision. These cats slept almost continuously, but could be awakened briefly by strong lights or smells. His conclusion from these experiments was what everybody knew already: sleep is a passive phenomenon and wakefulness is produced by sensory input arousing the brain.

In 1949, Giuseppi Moruzzi & Horace Magoun of Italy published their famous paper that named the ARAS (ascending reticular activating system). They showed that stimulation of the reticular formation, but not the sensory pathways next to it, resulted in long lasting activation of the EEG typical of wakefulness. The next year, Don Lindsley and colleagues at UCLA found that lesions of the reticular formation, but not the sensory pathways in the brainstem, resulted in permanent signs of sleep such as cortical slow waves and immobility that only strong stimuli could briefly change to waking. But notice that the conclusion from these findings only modifies how the brain passively produces sleep; it is not the sensory information itself that awakens the brain but activity in the ascending reticular formation. Sensory stimulation is still important, though, since sensory input to the brain has an activating effect on the ascending reticular formation. Nevertheless, this process is not the only way the ascending reticular formation becomes activated.

Then, in 1958, Batini and colleagues published a report that showed sleep was the result of an active brain process. They did an experiment similar to the one done by Bremer except that they placed their cut through the middle of the pons (cut E in Figure 28). These cats never showed any signs of sleeping. Since Bremer's animals showed sleep when the cut was a bit lower, Batini and colleagues concluded that something in the lower brainstem was necessary to produce sleep and must do so actively. This finding reinforced the implication of the discovery of REMS in humans at the University of Chicago by Eugene Aserinsky and Nathaniel Kleitmann a few years before (1953).

Once it became apparent to scientists that sleep was active rather than passive, they began to ask what in the brain actively produces sleep. For example, Villablanca in Mexico (1965) replicated part of the Bremer experiment by again cutting the forebrain at its junction with the midbrain (cut D in Figure 28), only this time he wanted to know what was happening below the cut as well as above it. He placed recording electrodes inside the brain at locations in the brainstem as well as in the forebrain. He had newer technology and was able to observe the animals for much longer than Bremer. He found that, after a week, the forebrain showed alternations of waking and sleep, but only NREMS. The brainstem showed evidence of alternations of waking and sleep, but only REMS. Furthermore, the state of the brain in front of the cut was often different from the state behind the cut; for example, the brainstem could be asleep, while the forebrain was awake. These observations showed several things. There are areas in the forebrain that can also produce sleep, but only NREMS. There are parts of the brainstem that can actively produce sleep, but only REMS. Both parts of the brain can produce wakefulness. The normal synchronization of the two parts of the brain is by neural connections, not chemicals in the blood, since both parts of the severed brain still shared the same blood supply.

In subsequent experiments, the cut was made even higher above the thalamus, causing a dramatic reduction in both REMS and NREMS (Villablanca & Marcus, 1972), or the thalamus itself was removed (Villablanca & Salinas-Zeballois, 1972), again diminishing the amount of sleep but also producing some dissociation of EEG and behavior such as slow waves during waking. These observations showed that both the brainstem and forebrain have sleep/wake mechanisms and that the thalamus normally couples these. These observations opened the door for scientists to ask even more specific questions about exactly what areas of the brain help produce each state and how they do it. The results of these experiments and many that followed have given us the understanding of the brain's involvement in sleep that we have today.

The key cells for brain functioning are neurons. Neurons can become electrically activated via chemical processes. When activated, neurons send electrical impulses, called action potentials, down frequently long extensions called axons. When the action potential arrives at the end of an axon, it can increase or decrease the activation level of other neurons situated close to it by the release of chemicals called **neurotransmitters**. Neurons also release neuromodulators that have no direct effect on other neurons but can cause the effect of recently released neurotransmitters to be enhanced or diminished. There are many neurotransmitters and neuromodulators, but we shall focus only on those that are known to be important for sleep and wakefulness. There are other chemicals found in the blood and in the cerebral-spinal fluid that is located in canals and spaces around and within the brain and spinal cord that can influence the sleep/wake systems of the brain.

The cells of the brain are organized in numerous areas and subareas, each with their own names. We will concentrate only on the areas most important for sleep/wake. It is important to realize that these areas do not operate in isolation but influence and are influenced by other areas via the axons from the cells in them. Importantly, even though these connections via axons are physical, their degree of activity at any time may vary greatly, meaning that some interactions between cells and areas may be functionally more important at one time than at another. This source is the functional reorganization of the brain that underlies sleep/wake.

Before looking specifically at how the brain is organized in waking, NREMS, and REMS we shall take an overview of first the chemistry of the brain.

THE CHEMISTRY OF SLEEP/WAKE

Waking

There are several neurotransmitters known to be involved in waking (see Table 3). Norepinephrine, and its chemical relative dopamine, both enhance arousal but may not be necessary for it. The drugs in the amphetamine family cause heightened arousal through their effects on these neurotransmitters. **Acetylcholine** is a key neurotransmitter for the arousal of waking as well as REMS. **Histamine**, too, plays a role in waking as demonstrated by the drowsiness produced when it is blocked by antihistamines. **Glutamate** is a primary neurotransmitter for arousal but also plays a role in producing the brain waves seen in SWS. **Orexin** (aka hypocretin) is a newly discovered substance that is also involved in waking. It has two names, because it was discovered at about the same time in two different labs, each of which gave it a different name (see Box 11).

Table 3. Some of the Neurotransmitters most Important for the Production of Waking and Sleeping

	Acetylcholine	Adenosine	GABA	Glutamate	Histamine	Norepinephrine, Dopamine	Serotonin
Waking	↑	accumulates		↑	↑	↑	↑
NREM sleep	↓	diminishes	↑	↑	↓	↓	↑↑
REM sleep	↑	diminishes?			↓↓	↓↓	
Sleep Deprivation		accumulates				Turnover↑	

Relative increase is represented by the up arrows and relative decrease by down arrows. The number of arrows represents the degree of the change.

Box 11

Discovery of Orexin/Hypocretin[13]

During the late 1990s, two different research teams working on two different research problems discovered a chemical in the brain that is important for waking. Masashi Yanagisawa with the help of his colleagues was working with a newly discovered peptide produced in the lateral hypothalamus that influenced food intake in rats. He named it orexin from the Greek work for appetite. He and his colleagues then created a strain of mice that were unable to produce orexin and were studying them for feeding abnormalities by using an infrared camera to record their night time feeding. They were surprised to see that these mice would suddenly fall down while doing ordinary things like moving about or grooming. Suspecting that the rats were having seizures, they monitored their brainwaves and discovered instead that they were suddenly falling asleep just as humans with narcolepsy (see Chapter 10) do.

At the same time, Emmanuel Mignot and colleagues at Stanford University Medical School had been studying a group of Doberman pinschers that suffered from narcolepsy and were narrowing the search for the genes responsible for the disorder. They focused in on genes responsible for production of receptors for a recently discovered peptide produced in the lateral hypothalamus that was named hypocretin, because it was produced in the hypothalamus and chemically resembled another peptide called incretin. Just two weeks after the Yanagisawa and colleagues mouse narcolepsy discovery was published, Mignot and colleagues published their narcoleptic dog discovery. These publications stimulated more research that strengthened the link between orexin/hypocretin and narcolepsy, this time in humans.

In a short time, orexin/hypocretin was shown to be important for the normal control of waking/sleeping. It was found to be released onto cells in many of the areas of the brain important for the control of sleeping/waking. It was shown to be especially involved in regulating REMS. Then it was found that Mignot's dogs had narcolepsy, not because of a lack of orexin/hypocretin, but because of a lack of receptors to this substance. Now it appears that orexin/hypocretin is a neurotransmitter important for maintaining normal wakefulness.

Many substances found in the cerebral-spinal fluid have also been implicated in waking (and some also with REMS). They include things like corticotropin releasing factor, vasoactive intestinal peptide, and neurotensin. Finally, some substances found in the blood have likewise been implicated in wakefulness, including thyroid stimulating hormone, adrenocortical tropic hormone, and various glucocordoids.

NREM Sleep

Serotonin was previously thought to be very important for NREMS (see Box 12) but now is thought to help only sleep onset by dampening the brain's response to sensory inputs. Tryptophan, the substance used by the brain to manufacture serotonin, can mildly facilitate sleep onset. The inhibitory neurotransmitter GABA is widely used in the brain during NREMS to damp down neural activity and reduce arousal. It also plays a key role in the production of spindles and delta waves. Many prescription sleeping pills act by enhancing the action of GABA. The progressive buildup during waking of adenosine, a byproduct of the use of certain energy releasing molecules, was shown in the late 1990s to be a strong contributor to sleepiness and sleep need. The adenosine is packaged by some neurons and used as a neurotransmitter. The greater the level of adenosine at sleep onset the greater the amount of SWS and delta waves during sleep. The levels of adenosine in the brain progressively diminish with sleep. Adenosine may very well be the cumulative meter of brain activity during waking that influences when and how much sleep is needed. The affects of adenosine on sleep are attenuated by caffeine. As mentioned above, glutamate is used in the process of producing slow waves and spindles. Key neuromodulators for NREMS include several peptides such as somatostatin and substances related to opiates. Substances in the blood that facilitate NREMS include cholecystokinin, prostaglandins, interleukins, growth hormone, and prolactin.

Box 12

Serotonin and Sleep (Jouvet, 1999)

From the late 1950s to the early 1970s, the neurotransmitter serotonin was believed to be the neurotransmitter of sleep, because drugs that interfered with serotonin in the brain caused insomnia, whereas drugs that facilitated serotonin caused stronger and longer SWS. Also, long time sleep researcher, Michel Jouvet, MD of Claude Bernard University in Lyon, France, showed that damage to the raphé, the area of the brain that is the source of serotonin, produced insomnia in proportion to the degree of damage. Subsequently restoring serotonin with drugs could then reverse this insomnia. In humans, sometimes when brain damage caused insomnia, the damage included the raphé.

During the late 1970s and early 1980s, the notion that serotonin is the neurotransmitter of sleep fell into disfavor, because experiments showed that recovery of sleep eventually occurred following either damage to the raphé or destruction by drugs of the capability of the brain to manufacture serotonin. Also, it was found that both the electrical activation in the raphé and its release of serotonin was high during waking compared to during sleep—just the opposite of what would be required for it to be a "sleep center." Additionally, researchers could not find any areas of the brain where direct application of serotonin resulted in sleep. So the hypothesis that serotonin was the neurotransmitter for sleep was abandoned.

Then in the late 1980s, the role of serotonin in sleep was revived. Based on research that showed that stimulation of the raphé by electrodes could quiet behavior and reduce sensory responses, it was hypothesized that rather than being the neurotransmitter of sleep, serotonin is a part of what causes sleep onset. Additionally, Jouvet posited that serotonin is involved with process S (see Borbely's model in Chapter 2). Indeed, following sleep deprivation, if serotonin is interfered with, the normal rebound of SWS is suppressed. Serotonin was found to influence the ascending reticular activating system and the VLPO to produce its effects on sleep onset. Thus, it now appears that when the raphé releases serotonin into the brainstem and the VLPO, NREMS is initiated.

REM *Sleep*

The key neurotransmitter for the production of REMS is acetylcholine. Turning off REMS is accomplished by neurons using norepinephrine and serotonin. Glycine is an inhibitory neurotransmitter that is used to produce the muscle paralysis of REMS.

Circadian Rhythm

Melatonin is a hormone released by the pineal gland located within the approximate center of the brain. It is a mildly sleep promoting substance that also acts as a zeitgeber. It is released during the subjective night of the nychthemeron, but sun or room light blocks its release (see Chapter 5).

BASIC BRAIN ANATOMY AND FUNCTIONING

All brain areas are involved in sleep/wake, but we shall concentrate on those that are in control of or otherwise particularly important for these states. Think of the brain as being like the planet earth. There are large portions, such as the **brainstem** and **forebrain, that are like continents** (see Figure 21). The brainstem is at the very core of the brain and is like a long tube with bulges here and there. On top and covering the upper sides of the brainstem is the very large forebrain. Within each of these continents, there are known areas that are equivalent to countries. Some areas, like some countries, have obvious physical boundaries, but some of the boundaries are not obvious but nonetheless real. Within the areas are subareas and subsubareas just like there are states, cities, regions, and so forth on the earth.

The brainstem can be divided into several regions (see Figure 22). At the very bottom is a long relatively narrow portion, the **medulla**, on top of which is a bulge called the **pons**. Attached to the back of the pons is another bulge known as the cerebellum. On top of the pons is the relatively short and narrow **midbrain**. Running up the interior of almost the entire brainstem is a region called the **reticular formation**.

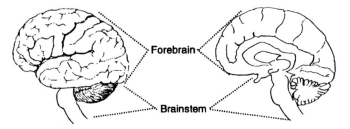

Forebrain

Brainstem

Figure 21. A diagram of the human brain showing the left side (on the left) pulled away from the right side revealing the internal surface of the brain (on the right).

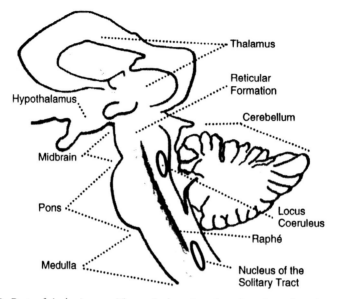

Figure 22. Parts of the brainstem. The geniculates (not shown) are located on the outsides of the thalamus.

Close to the reticular formation is another region that runs up the very middle of the brainstem, the **raphé.** There are areas (equivalent to cities) in the brainstem that are important for sleep/wake, especially the **nucleus of the solitary tract** in the medulla and the **locus coeruleus** in the top of the pons. At the very top of the brain stem is a pair of bulbs, one on the right and one on the left, known as the **thalamus.** Toward each back and side of the top of the thalamus is a **geniculate nucleus.** A small but very important area lies below the thalamus and is known as the **hypothalamus.** A very small part of the bottom of the front part of the hypothalamus is the suprachiasmatic nucleus.

The forebrain is dominated in size by the wrinkled **cerebral cortex** on its surface. The cerebral cortex is divided into four regions (see Figure 23) on each side known as the **frontal cortex** in the front, **parietal cortex** in the middle, **occipital cortex** at the back, and **temporal cortex** at the side. Below the cerebral cortex are several important forebrain areas. A pair of ram's horn-shaped structures, called the **hippocampus,** lay to either side of the thalamus (see Figure 24). Below the center, running front to back of the cerebral cortex is the **cingulate cortex.** There is an **amygdala** beyond the far left and another beyond the far right toward the back of the thalamus (see Figure 23).

Encompassing various aspects of the forebrain is something like a group of islands called the **limbic system.** To the naked eye, some of these islands appear to be physically connected with one another, while others seem to be isolated but are

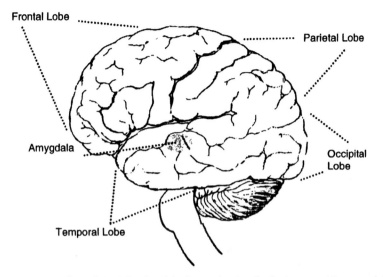

Figure 23. The surface of the left side of the brain showing forebrain areas. The amygdala is more interior and thus is shown as a shadow.

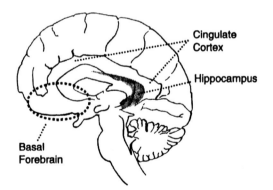

Figure 24. The inside of the left half of the brain showing the locations of two forebrain structures—the cingulate cortex and a shadow of the hippocampus which lies more to the outside.

actually functionally connected by axons. Key components of the limbic system include hippocampus, amygdala, cingulate cortex, parts of the hypothalamus, and portions of the frontal cortex.

Finally, there is a loosely defined region known as the **basal forebrain area**. It is located on the lower front sides of the forebrain but includes parts of the anterior hypothalamus (see Figure 24).

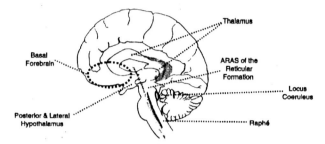

Figure 25. A view of the inside of the right side of the brain showing areas important for producing wakefulness.

Waking

To remain awake, your brain depends on activation from a few key areas in the brainstem (see Figure 25). This activation puts neurons in your cerebral cortex and other parts of your forebrain in a state of readiness to receive information and to respond to it quickly. Without this level of activation, your brain would drift off into a slow, dull state. The anterior portion of the reticular formation has become known as the **ascending reticular activating system (ARAS)** because of this key role. It receives input from most of your sensory systems and much of the forebrain, too. Its output activates the cerebral cortex via two routes using the neurotransmitters glutamate, norephinephrine, and acetylcholine. One route goes to a portion of the thalamus termed non-specific since, unlike the output of much of the rest of the thalamus, its output is not directed at a specific part of the cerebral cortex. During waking, there is a pattern of constant firing in the thalamus. The other route from the ARAS goes to (1) the posterior hypothalamus that in turn uses histamine to activate the cerebral cortex and (2) the basal forebrain area that uses acetylcholine to excite the cerebral cortex and hippocampus.

The locus coeruleus and the raphé also stimulate wakefulness. The locus coeruleus uses norepinephrine to activate the entire forebrain but especially the sensory and integrative areas; this area is also a key for controlling what aspects of sensory input are attended to when awake. The raphé uses serotonin to activate the forebrain. There are additional brainstem areas that use dopamine also to help activate the forebrain.

The newly discovered substance orexin (aka hypocretin) is produced in the neurons of the lateral hypothalamus. These neurons release it from the ends of their axons located in many other areas of the brain to facilitate wakefulness. The neuromodulators involved in wakefulness include substance P, vasoactive intestinal polypeptide, neurotensin, and others.

NREM Sleep

The key area for NREMS is in the basal forebrain, but areas in the brain stem also have a contributory role (see Figure 26). The basal forebrain area uses the inhibitory

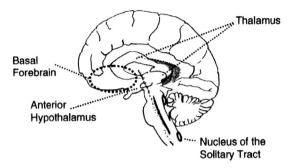

Thalamus

Basal
Forebrain

Anterior
Hypothalamus

Nucleus of the
Solitary Tract

Figure 26. A view of the inside of the right side of the brain showing the areas important for the production of NREM sleep.

neurotransmitter GABA together with neuromodulators somatostatin and cortico-statin to dampen activation in the forebrain directly and indirectly by dampening activity in the ARAS. The cells in the basal forebrain area that perform this function are more active during sleep than during waking.[10] The nucleus of the solitary tract and nearby posterior brainstem areas are a secondary area important for the production of NREMS using their own direct projections to the forebrain.

Another key for NREMS is the change in the influence of the thalamus on the cerebral cortex during NREMS. In contrast to waking, during NREMS, its discharge is relatively slow (less than 1 Hz) and comes in bursts. This pattern of stimulation results in the slow waves and spindles in the cortex characteristic of NREMS. The intricate details of how this process is accomplished at the cellular level, featuring the release of GABA, are known but go beyond the scope of our discussion.

It used to be assumed that activation in the entire cerebral cortex was uniformly depressed during NREMS, however newer brain imaging research, enabling the study of the functioning brain in humans without surgery, shows this is not true. With this neural imaging, there is now a better understanding of the functional organization of the brain during various stages of sleep and how this differs from other states (cf. Maquet, 1999). As expected, your overall brain activity is lower during NREMS compared to waking in the dorsal pons and mesencehpalon, thalamus, and basal forebrain. Surprisingly, there is also a greater reduction in some subareas of the forebrain than in others, including the parietal cortex, anterior cingulate cortex, and the associative areas of the frontal cortex located just above the eyes. The lower activity in the cerebral cortex during SWS is thought to indicate that many parts of the brain are still working together but at a reduced overall level.

Interestingly, other areas, including some cells in the anterior hypothalamus and amygdala, show an increase in firing rates during NREMS over waking.

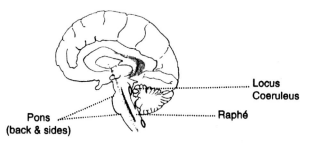

Figure 27. A view of the inside of the right side of the brain showing the areas most important for the production of REM sleep.

REM Sleep

Beginning near the end of the 20th century, Pierre Maquet of the University of Liège in Belgium and his colleagues, like others using functional brain imaging, have found greater overall activation in the brain during REMS than found even during waking. This activation is especially great in the junction of temporal and occipital cortical lobes, the back of the pons and midbrain, the thalamus, and portions of the limbic system including the amygdala, hippocampus, anterior cingulate cortex, and frontal cortex above the eyes (Maquet, 1999). A particularly important finding, as we shall see when considering dreaming later in this book, was much less activity in the associative areas of the upper front portion on the sides of the frontal cortex plus a few other portions of the forebrain. Additionally, there were two patterns of activity noted during REMS not seen during waking. The relationship of the activity in different parts of the visual cortex was the opposite of that seen during waking, and the amygdala seems to influence the temporal cortex.

Studies of the changes in sleep following different brain surgeries in cats located the key brain area for REMS (see Figure 27). When a cut is made just above the pons, cutting off communication with higher parts of the brain (cut A in Figure 28), there are no signs of REMS in the cortex—only wake (shown by waking EEG and eye movements typical of waking) alternating with NREMS (shown by EEG typical of NREMS). Below the level of the cut are signs of REMS (the regular ultradian occurrence of the EEG typical of REMS accompanied by body muscle paralysis and rems). When the cut is made just below the pons (cut B in Figure 28), the brain above the cut shows alternations of wake (shown by waking EEG), NREMS (shown by EEG typical of NREMS), and REMS (shown by EEG typical of REMS). Below the cut, only wake (EEG accompanied by high levels of body muscle tone with heart and respiration rates all characteristic of waking) alternating with NREMS (EEG typical of NREMS accompanied by body muscle tone and slow, regular respiration) can be observed. Conclusion: *the pons is necessary for the production of REMS.*

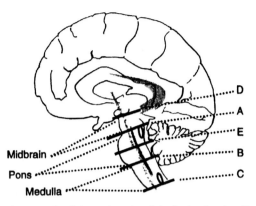

Figure 28. A view of the inside of the right side of the brain showing five different experimental cuts.

Further studies showed that it is only the sides of the pons toward the cerebellum that are responsible for this task. A group of interacting cells, called "REM-on" cells, are located here among other types of cells. Each of these interacting REM-on cells is involved with one or more components of REMS, but none alone is sufficient to trigger REMS. Rather, full-blown REMS requires the cooperation of numbers of them, plus the recruitment of nearby midbrain cells, plus cells in the medulla and the hypothalamus. Some REM-on cells manifest high and steady activity during REMS but are nearly silent otherwise. Collectively, they are the source of the tonic aspects of REMS. Other REM-on cells are located in another area of the pons and show bursts of activity during REMS and seem to be responsible for phasic REMS activity such as PGO waves.[11] The key neurotransmitters for REMS are acetylcholine, glutamate, glycine, and GABA.

The REM-on cells activate other areas of the brain to produce the recognizable qualities of REMS. For example, the paralysis of the muscles of movement occurs because the REM-on cells stimulate parts of the medulla to use glycine to prevent any activation of the nerves that cause muscles to contract. Motor impulses from higher portions of the brain still occur, but any movements they command are blocked in this way. However, muscle twitches may occur when strong impulses break through the inhibition. This happening occurs more in animals and human infants than in adult humans. Damage to or dysfunction of this portion of the medulla or controlling axons to it from the REM-on cells result in the absence of muscle paralysis during REMS. The result is an acting-out of dreams (see Chapter 10).

Additionally, during REMS, the hippocampus is in a different functional state as shown by the presence of high voltage theta waves. During waking, its waves are faster and more irregular except for the occurrence of theta during body movements. The amygdala is the forebrain area very intensely activated in human REMS.

Other cells in the pons, scattered among REM-on cells, and other parts of the brain stem are minimally active during REMS but greatly active during waking and nearly as active during NREMS. Some researchers have found that the activity rate of individual cells in these areas does not change, but the pattern of discharge changes greatly. Either way, the difference is important. These cells are called REM-off cells and are concentrated in the locus coeruleus (using norepinephrine) and the raphé (using serotonin).

The Hobson and McCarley model (Alan Hobson, MD, is professor of psychiatry and director of the Laboratory of Neurophysiology at Harvard Medical School; Robert McCarley, MD is Professor and Chair of the Harvard Department of Psychiatry at the Brockton/West Roxbury VAMC) describes how the interaction of these REM-off and REM-on cells produces the ultradian rhythm of the NREM-REM sleep cycle (see Figure 29). Active REM-off cells inhibit the REM-on cells. REM-off cell activity is influenced by many sources including sensory input, the suprachiasmatic nucleus, and other areas of the forebrain. During NREMS, the activity of REM-off cells gradually weakens and eventually become so weak that they no longer can inhibit the REM-on cells. This occurrence allows the REM-on cells to become active, causing REMS to begin. After some time, the relative activity strengths of the REM-on and REM-off areas quickly reverse, causing REMS to cease and NREMS to return. And so they alternate through the period of sleep, but the REM-off area gets successively weaker as sleep progresses, resulting in longer and longer REMS periods

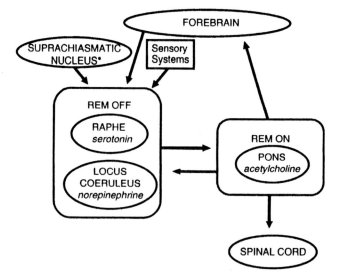

Figure 29. The reciprocal interaction model of REM sleep. After Hobson (1988) and McCarley & Massaquoi (1992).

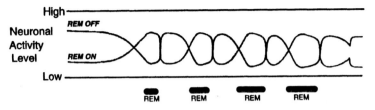

Figure 30. Output of the reciprocal interaction model yielding alternations between NREM sleep and REM sleep. Adapted with permission of the author from J. A. Hobson (1983).

(see Figure 30). The REM-off cells also directly block the areas of the brain involved with the components of REMS, thereby preventing these components from occurring during any state other than REMS. Notice also the decrease of the use of the neurotransmitters norepinephrine, dopamine, serotonin during REMS but the reoccurrence of the use of acetylcholine (see Table 3).

Transitions

Whether we are asleep or awake depends in part on our level of awareness of sensory information coming to and from our body. Cortical response to such stimuli is reduced to 80% during stages 1 and 2 sleep, 65% during SWS, and to over 90% during REMS. Much of this response, especially during NREMS, is due to a decrease in the transfer of such information through the thalamus. Thus, an early event important for sleep onset occurs in the thalamus where there is a reduction of sensory input directed to the cerebral cortex, even though there is no change in the amount of such information arriving at the thalamus. Serotonin from the raphé may facilitate this reduction of input at sleep onset by damping sensory input as it travels through the brainstem and decreasing cerebral cortical activation as well. There is, however, some sensory input that facilitates sleep such as general warmth and fullness after a big meal. During REMS, less information arrives at the thalamus itself because of inhibition at the sensory receptors and their transfer points in the spinal cord and brainstem.

What causes the start of sleep? Recently, sleep and brain researchers in California, Dennis McGinty and Ron Szymusiak (2000), summarized their work and integrated it with the work of others directed at this question. They have found that a very small group of cells in a portion of the anterior hypothalamus called the ventrolateral preoptic nucleus (VLPO) work with other cells very close by to act as an apparent sleep switch for the brain. These cells become very active at sleep onset, their activity is proportional to the depth of sleep, and they are sensitive to sleep deprivation. Lesions in this area and very nearby areas of the brain result in a reduction of sleep. The VLPO is thought to be facilitated by numerous sleep factors (see Chapter 5) and other areas of the brain that promote sleep including nearby warm-sensitive neurons. The VLPO was shown to have inhibitory connections using GABA to the wake promoting areas in the ARAS and posterior hypothalamus. These areas in turn have an inhibitory influence on the VLPO. The levels of activity of the VLPO and wake promoting areas are negatively correlated.[12] Importantly, the SCN feeds into the VLPO, thus coordinating its activity with the circadian clock (see below).

During wakefulness, adenosine accumulates in proportion to the length of waking. It acts in the basal forebrain to inhibit arousal and thus produce sleepiness (Strecher et al., 2000). To a lesser extent, it also disinhibits the anterior hypothalamus and the VLPO, thus promoting NREMS. Additionally, it may block arousal in neurons that use acetylcholine in the ARAS.

Circadian Rhythms

Although it has been known since the 1970s that the suprachiasmatic nucleus (SCN) (see Figure 31) is the location of the circadian clock, only recently have details of how this clock works begun to be understood. If this area is damaged, many circadian rhythms, including that of sleep/wake, cease; sleep becomes essentially randomly distributed throughout the nychthemeron. If a SCN from another animal is subsequently implanted in the brain, the circadian rhythms largely return but with the characteristics of the rhythm, such as the length of the period, of the donor!

The SCN is like a microchip for timekeeping (Moore, 1999). Within the cells of the SCN, the transcription process of several genes with names like "timeless" and "period" are turned on approximately once per day. The result is the synthesis of proteins that subsequently interact to influence the neural activity level of the cell. These proteins also inhibit further transcription by the genes. Gradually, during the course of about a nychthemeron, these proteins are degraded, releasing the genes from inhibition and the transcription process begins again. Each individual cell in the SCN has

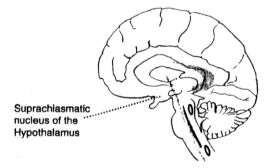

Suprachiasmatic
nucleus of the
Hypothalamus

Figure 31. A view of the inside of the right side of the brain showing the area most important for the production of circadian rhythms.

been shown to have this timing mechanism but may be slightly faster or slower than other SCN cells. In some way not yet understood, when grouped together, the output of these cells is synchronized as the output of the SCN.

Entrainment can, within limits, influence the intrinsic period of the SCN to be somewhat longer or somewhat shorter. Additionally, prior consistent entrainment can have an effect on the intrinsic period of the cells of the SCN that lasts for months after the entrainment stimulus is no longer present. Less consistent zeitgebers can, within limits, temporarily entrain the SCN without having a longterm effect.

The main zeitgeber is light whose influence travels via a pathway from the retina in the eye to the SCN. Information on this pathway has nothing to do with visual perception or visual reflexes, because some animals like the blind mole rat and some, but not all (see Chapter 3), blind humans are able to respond to light as a zeitgeber. The presence of light driven activity on this pathway influences the levels of the neurotransmitter GABA in the SCN that in turn can advance or delay the phase of the circadian rhythm produced by the SCN. But the SCN also responds to regulatory input not involved with light, including from some of the hormones it causes to be released.

The output from the SCN influences other, mainly nearby areas of the brain both via its axons and chemicals it releases. This output affects many rhythmic physiological and hormonal activities in addition to sleep/wake. It may cause these effects directly by itself or indirectly by being a zeitgeber for other local clocks in the body as suggested by the fact that the sleep/wake cycle and body temperatures can become desynchronized during forced desynchrony experiments (see Chapter 2).

Among the glands influenced by the SCN is the pineal gland. It produces melatonin during the subjective night portion of the circadian cycle (see Chapter 2), but can be inhibited by light occurring during this time. Melatonin, in turn, acts as a zeitgeber on the SCN. The SCN also produces arousing signals during the subjective day portion of the circadian rhythm. Output of the SCN is also thought to influence the sleep onset switch of the VLPO.

Chapter 5

The Body during Sleep[14]

If we are going to understand sleep completely, we need to understand what effects sleep has on the body and vice versa. Prior to the latter half of the 20th century, it was assumed that the physiology of the body was the same when asleep as it was when awake. Since it is generally easier to study the body during waking, little attempt was made to investigate its physiology during sleep. As mentioned in earlier chapters, the discovery of REMS prompted scientists to view sleep differently and look for things in it they never thought of looking for earlier. As a result, they soon began to discover that in some ways we are physiologically different during sleep. Some of these changes are large, involving whole organ-systems, but others are subtler. Yet, all of the differences are important. Additionally, contrary to common belief, we do not sleep simply because our body wears out while awake and needs sleep to reverse this effect. It is now realized that changes in any of several physiological processes may either facilitate or impede sleep. Also, what we do and what is done to us while awake can also have an effect on our subsequent sleep.

THE NORMAL PHYSIOLOGY OF SLEEP

Generally, what happens in the body during NREMS is what we all think sleep ought to be. Things are quiet and at a generally low level as it would be for the body to rest and recuperate. The feedback systems of the various organ systems are working well but maintaining steady levels somewhat lower than during quiet resting. Any internal or external disturbances are quietly compensated for by these feedback mechanisms.

In contrast, REMS is everything we would imagine sleep should not be. It is a time of irregular activation of many bodily processes. Local reflexes are operating the organ systems of the body, but their control is frequently being overridden by lower parts of the brain. What's more, the brainstem is controlling this operation with a general lack of feedback about what is going on in the body. As a result, REMS is

97

anything but restful and recuperative. In fact, it can be said that from a physiological standpoint, REMS entails a bit of a risk to the welfare of the body, since things are a bit out of control and can fluctuate wildly.

Central Nervous System

The central nervous system is composed of the entire brain plus the spinal cord. During NREMS, many neurons in the central nervous system have a lower rate of activity than they do during waking, and the overall metabolic rate in the brain is lower than during waking. It is as if the brain is just active enough to keep things going at a basic, low level. It is almost as if it is idling (but as we shall see in Chapters 6 and 12, there is still a lot of mental processing going on). Yet, there are a few areas that are more active than they are during waking. These are the areas that assume control in order to actively produce NREMS.

During tonic REMS, the cells in several of areas in the brain are actually more metabolically active than they are during NREMS or waking. Not only are these areas active because they are causing REMS, but, as we shall see in Chapters 6 and 12, there is quite a lot of mental activity going on in REMS. Additionally, during phasic REMS, the cells in some regions of the brain, especially the visual areas, are sporadically wildly active.

ANS

The autonomic nervous system (ANS) is responsible for controlling many of our internal physiological processes such as the heart, lungs, stomach, intestines, and many glands. The ANS is composed of two parts. One part, the sympathetic nervous system (SNS), prepares our body to deal with emergencies and threats. When awake and faced with a perceived emergency or threat, it will do things like accelerate the heart rate, increase blood pressure, speed and deepen respiration, but diminish digestion. The other part of the ANS, the parasympathetic nervous system (PNS), mostly does the opposite. It functions to conserve and maintain the body resources in the absence of any perceived emergencies or threats by slowing the heart, decreasing blood pressure, slowing respiration, but facilitating digestion. It is important to note that seldom is the SNS or the PNS completely in control. Typically the *entire* SNS is relatively more or less active, while *individual portions* of the PNS are more or less active.

During sleep, the ANS maintains the same control over the internal processes but more related to the stage of sleep than any real or perceived threats or stresses. NREMS is characterized by an active PNS with a relatively quiet and stable SNS. During tonic REMS, the PNS is at the same level as in NREMS, but SNS is operating at an even lower level than during NREMS. However, during phasic REMS, the PNS is more active, but the activity of the SNS has been described as a storm, that is, variable but with intense activity. Hence, as you will see shortly, there are dramatic and irregular surges of activation of many of the internal organs during REMS for no apparent reason.

Cardiovascular

During NREMS heart rate is slower than when awake and, likewise, blood pressure is at a slightly lower level. During tonic REMS, blood pressure and heart rate are like that of NREMS, except they are less responsive to even large changes in blood flow need in the organs of the body. During phasic REMS, heart rate and blood pressure are extremely variable with noticeable surges and pauses in HR. Average blood pressure is generally higher and can peak by as much as 30% over resting level.

When in NREMS, most areas of the brain have relatively less blood flow, but a few areas (the "night shift" actively in control of sleep, see Chapter 4) have an increased blood flow of 4% to 25%. When in tonic REMS, unlike other organs of the body, most brain areas have a 50% increase in blood flow over that during waking, with some getting as much as 200% of waking levels. During phasic REMS, there are even greater transient increases in blood flow in the brain.

Respiration

We breathe for many reasons. Primarily, breathing brings oxygen into the body and expels carbon dioxide. However, we also use our breath to talk and make other sounds, to blow on things, to cough, and so forth. Much of our respiration is under automatic control but can be overridden or captured by conscious control (such as when talking or holding breath to dive underwater) or other automatic control mechanisms (such as when sneezing). There are separate, but partially overlapping mechanisms for automatic and behavioral breathing.

Throughout NREMS the control of breathing is entirely automatic, functioning to mainly maintain the level of carbon dioxide in the blood but at a slightly higher level than when awake and, to a lesser extent, oxygen at a slightly lower level. There is about a 15% decrease in air volume entering and leaving the lungs per minute during NREMS. On the other hand, in the same way as during waking, breathing rate and breath volume are automatically varied as the levels of carbon dioxide or oxygen vary. Overall, breathing, especially during SWS, is regular and slightly deeper. However, airway resistance to air flow doubles, especially in males, resulting in a considerable increase in the effort exerted to breathe.

Breathing during REMS is another story. Breathing rate and depth are very irregular with a rapid and shallow pattern tending to prevail. The average air intake can be about the same or less than that of NREMS. There may even be pauses in breathing. The control is much more behavioral with levels of blood carbon dioxide and oxygen having little, if any, influence. As a result, the level of oxygen in the blood may be about the same or lower as that in NREMS. As in NREMS, there is an increase in upper airway resistance to airflow, but the compensation for this increase is irregular and weak in REMS.

During all sleep, the cough response is suppressed. If the irritation in the air passages is great enough, you will awaken, then cough, but not cough while asleep.

Additionally, because of the changes in breathing regulation, many people, especially the elderly, when falling asleep, alternate several deep breaths with several shallow breaths even to the point of stopping breathing for a few seconds. This pattern continues for 10 or 20 or even 60 minutes until the person is solidly asleep.

Sex Organs

The penis is erect in REMS and sometimes during NREMS in adolescents. The percent of REMS accompanied by erections reaches a peak in mid teen years and declines after that. Vaginal enlargement and lubrication also occur during REMS in females but not to the extent that penis erections do in males.

Body/Brain Temperature

Did you know that 98.6°F is your average body temperature, but it actually varies by about a degree warmer or cooler depending on the time of nychthemeron and whether or not you are sleeping? When you go to sleep at your regular time at night, your body temperature drops to its lowest level of the nychthemeron. It would seem that this occurrence is due to the immobility during sleep, but people who are paralyzed, bed ridden, or just inactive in bed for the entire nychthemeron still have about half of the average body temperature drop during night sleep. Also, people who remain awake and active during their regular night bedtime also experience about half of the average nightly body temperature drop. (Maybe you have noticed becoming cold during the night when you were pulling an all-nighter.) The obvious conclusion from these observations is that the nightly body temperature drop during sleep is due to both a circadian body temperature fluctuation plus a sleep induced body temperature drop.

During NREMS, your body continues to regulate its temperature using the same several methods as it does when you are awake. If you are too warm, more blood is sent to the surface of the body where it can be radiated to the air. If really hot, you will sweat. When you are cool, less blood is sent to the body surface to avoid loosing heat. If really cold, you may shiver. The only difference between sleep and wake is during NREMS when your body temperature set-point (like a thermostat setting) is a bit lower than when awake. When you first fall asleep, blood may be sent to the surface of your body to help bring your temperature down to the sleeping set-point. If you are too warm at sleep onset, you may sweat for a while.

A portion of the hypothalamus functions as a thermostat, receiving temperature input from sensors throughout the body as well as monitoring its own temperature. It has outputs to the parts of the brain that control the temperature regulation mechanisms described above.

Body temperature during REMS is another matter. Your body is still producing heat as it does when in NREMS or awake. It is just not regulating your body temperature. It's the difference between having a room with a thermostat that turns on the heater or air conditioner to keep the room temperature steady versus having an unregulated fireplace with a nice fire going in it. With only the fireplace going when it is warm outside, the room will tend to get warmer, but when it is very cold outside, the room may tend to get cooler. The same thing happens during REMS; if you are in a warm room, your body temperature may go up a bit, but the opposite can happen in a cool room. The body makes little, if any, attempt to regulate its temperature, such as by sweating or shivering during REMS. However, if your body gets too cold or too warm, you will wake up and begin regulating again.

Your brain temperature, like your body temperature, will decline a bit in NREMS, but it tends to warm up during REMS because of the high amount of neuronal activity during that state that burns so much energy. It may even get warmer than it typically is when awake.

The relationship between sleep and body temperature has yet another level of complexity. Our tendency to sleep and to sleep well depends on our body temperature. Under normal conditions our sleep/wake rhythm shows a phase relationship with our circadian temperature rhythm. We have a propensity to sleep when body temperature is low or dropping but to be awake when body temperature is high or rising. Typically, sleep onset is 6 hours before our core body temperature nadir, about 6 a.m. in the average young adult, and sleep offset follows about 2 hours after the nadir when body temperature is rising.

When we try to sleep during a different phase of our temperature rhythm, we may encounter difficulties. If we go to bed later than typical, we can fall asleep easily but may awaken too early or find our sleep fragmented as our body temperature does its typical rise. There is a bit of a mid-afternoon drop in body temperature corresponding to the mid-afternoon dip described in Chapter 2 during which a brief nap can be beneficial. However, if we try to get all of our nychthemeral sleep during the day when our body temperature is high, we may find that we have trouble falling asleep, remaining satisfactorily asleep, or getting enough sleep.

Finally, REMS and rems are more likely when body temperature is low and less likely when it is high. Thus, we have more REMS in the early morning hours.

Room temperature also affects both sleep quantity and quality (Parmeggiani, 2000). REMS is generally more sensitive to room temperature than NREMS. As a rule of thumb, people sleep best when the room is about 29°C (84°F) but without covers or clothes. When protected by pajamas and covers, a lower room temperature is best. Sleep is still quite good when the room temperature is slightly above the ideal to several degrees below the ideal. However, the further room temperature gets from this range, the more sleep deteriorates. Also, people show long term adaptation to air temperature, so, during the winter, a lower room temperature would be best compared to the summer.

If your room temperature is above 75 degrees or below 54 degrees, your sleep can noticeably deteriorate. When too cold, waking increases, sleep time decreases, time to get to sleep decreases, and movements during sleep increase. Also, there is a decrease in REMS and stage 2 sleep. When the room is too hot, waking increases, there is more fragmentation of sleep (see Chapter 3), and both REMS and NREMS decrease. Generally, too hot of a room is worse than too cold. On the other hand, the more you are sleep deprived, the less room temperature is going to affect your sleep.

The temperature of your body when you begin sleep also has an effect on your sleep. Consider the following experiment, which is actually a combination of several research projects done by Jim Horne and colleagues in the mid 1980s. You and some of your physically fit friends show up at the sleep research lab during the evening. Some of your friends have to run hard on a treadmill in a warm room with little air movement until their body temperature increases 2°C. Others of your friends are luckier, because while they have to run as long as the first group, they can have a fan blowing on them, and they only gain 1°C of body temperature. But you and a few others are luckiest of all, because you get to soak in a hot tub until your temperature goes up 2 °C. Finally, another group of friends get in a different hot tub only to discover that the water is not hot. They have to stay in it as long as you stay in yours.

After a bit, all of you are prepared for a night of sleep recording in the lab. Before going to sleep, all of you are asked how sleepy you feel. The results are that you and the other hot hot tubbers and the hot exercisers felt sleepier, slept a bit longer, and got more SWS than the cool exercisers and cool tubbers. The next week, you all come in during the day for the same exercise or tub experience. Then you return later that night to sleep in the lab. This time by the time you go to bed, there are no differences in sleepiness or actual sleep.

In related experiments, it was found that taking an aspirin, which tends to lower elevated body temperature, following the exercise or hot tub also results in no differences in sleepiness or actual sleep. Yet, if your body temperature were increased during the last half of sleep, then the amount of NREMS increases. Of course, there is also the relationship between room temperature and both your body temperature and your body's efforts to control its temperature.

Box 13

Effects of Sleep Deprivation on the Body

Eve Van Cauter, PhD, research associate and professor at the Department of Medicine of the University of Chicago, and her colleagues have shown the negative physiological effects of chronic sleep deprivation on the physiology of the body. Prior to her work, it was shown that the release of growth hormone is severely reduced during sleep deprivation but rebounds when sleep is subsequently obtained. Her studies looked at sleep deprivation effects involving other hormones, especially insulin.

In one study (Spiegel, Leproult, & Van Cauter, 1999), 11 young adult males were allowed to sleep for only 4 hours per night for six nights, and then as much as they wanted while in bed for 12 hours for the subsequent six nights. Naps were not allowed. They found that during the sleep deprivation, it took 40% longer to regulate blood sugar levels after a high-carbohydrate meal, a 30% decrease in insulin secretion ability, and 30% drop in ability to respond to insulin—all characteristics of early diabetes. Since similar changes are found during normal, non-sleep deprived aging, Van Cauter and colleagues concluded from these and other observations that sleep deprivation mimics human aging and can speed it up.

Van Cauter's studies of people who maintained that they had adapted to chronic shortened sleep again showed a 40% decrease in insulin sensitivity, unusual cortisol release, a decrease in leptin (a hormone that reduces hunger), and greater sympathetic nervous system activity. There is also an increase in insulin secretion causing more storage of fat that then causes more secretion of insulin that causes more storage of fat and on and on. Chronic shortening of sleep also results in elevated evening cortisol levels and increases sympathetic nervous system activity. The long-term results of chronic partial sleep deprivation are obesity, high blood pressure, diabetes, and memory impairments.

Hormones[15]

Generally speaking, there is a two-directional effect between hormones and sleep. Sleep can affect the release of many hormones, and many hormones can affect sleep. The levels of most hormones are influenced by sleep and a few are influenced by specific sleep stages. As we shall see, some are more related to process C and others more related to process S (see Chapter 2). Those hormones more tied to process S tend to follow sleep when taken at an unusual time. Those hormones that are more tied to process C less easily follow sleep to an unusual time. That is, they tend to occur at the same circadian time. On the other hand, some hormones can make sleep more likely and others make it less likely, or they may affect the amounts of REMS, NREMS, or SWS.

Growth Hormone

The nychthemeral release of growth hormone occurs primarily during the first SWS period. This release occurs even if sleep is taken at an unusual time and does not occur if sleep is deprived. But this process is qualified. It is most true for the average young adult male. It has been found that for women, there are more pulses of growth hormones released throughout the day, and the night pulse may not account for even the majority of growth hormone released each nychthemeron. Adolescents have growth hormone released during subsequent SWS stages and even during the day. After adolescence, the release of growth hormone gradually declines such that in the elderly there is little or no release of it even during the first SWS period. Finally, there is also a weak circadian influence on the release of growth hormone such that more is released when sleep is taken at its typical time. Growth hormone is reduced by sleep deprivation, but there is compensation later such that the total released per nychthemeron is unchanged. However, note that these data and data on what happens to cortisol levels following sleep deprivation (see below) show that the nychthemeron following sleep deprivation is not normal.

The hormone from the pituitary gland that causes growth hormone to be released, Growth Hormone Releasing Hormone, is sleep promoting and increases SWS when present at bedtime. However, growth hormone itself seems to increase REMS indirectly, probably because it stimulates the release of the hormone somatostatin that directly increases REMS. Somatostatin, in turn, generally works against sleep promotion in the elderly.

Sex Hormones

In pre-pubescent and pubescent teens, some of the sex hormones are released during sleep. Luteinizing hormone is released at sleep onset and inhibited by wakefulness (but not in adults). Follicle-stimulating hormone is released during sleep but inhibited by wakefulness. The level of testosterone is highest during sleep until old age. As indicated in Chapter 3, progesterone promotes sleepiness and sleep. Specifically, it reduces sleep onset time, promotes NREMS, decreases waking during sleep, and causes the first REMS period to occur earlier. Estrogen promotes REMS by reducing the time to the first REMS period and increasing the amount of REMS time.

Estrogen replacement therapy decreases sleep onset time, reduces waking during sleep, and increases total sleep time. Although there appears to be no effect on sleep of starting oral contraceptives, which contain various combinations of estrogen and progesterone, when they are discontinued, some women complain of increased sleepiness and increased time sleeping.

Prolactin

The release of prolactin is stimulated by sleep, mainly SWS, regardless of when it is taken, but more is released if taken during the individual's normal sleep time and some release occurs at this time even if the individual stays awake, especially in women. Thus, prolactin release is strongly influenced by process S and weakly affected by process C. There is a rise in the release of prolactin from puberty to old age in both males and females beginning 30 to 90 minutes after sleep onset and peaking near the middle or end of sleep. Little of this hormone is released if sleep is skipped but will be released if sleep occurs at a different time. More of it is also secreted during naps. Its release seems to be most related to SWS, but there is also a weak circadian influence. Prolactin, in turn, seems to promote sleep and is thought to increase REMS.

Cortisol

Cortisol and its controlling hormones promote wakefulness. In doing so, they make sleep less efficient, reduce both REMS and NREMS, and shorten sleep time. Cortisol release primarily follows a circadian rhythm with highest levels right before or after typical time of awakening and a long period of low levels during waking and into early sleep. This pattern takes several days to follow an abrupt change in the timing of sleep. Sleep, especially SWS, does seem to have an attenuating effect on its release, because when sleep is delayed a bit, the nadir of cortisol release is also delayed a bit and the peak level mildly attenuated. Also, the peak of its release seems to depend on the intended time of awakening determined before sleep onset (Born et al., 1999). Additionally, there is an increase in the release of cortisol in the evening just prior to sleep, following a night of sleep deprivation (Leproult et al., 1997).

Melatonin

Melatonin facilitates sleep and has been shown to act as a mild zeitgeber (see Chapter 2). It is released about 14 hours after awakening, which is normally 2 hours before sleep onset, by the pineal gland located in the middle of the brain. It reaches its peak near the middle of the sleep period, returning to its low waking levels by the end of sleep. Its release is strongly controlled by process C with apparently no effect of process S. However, light striking the eyes inhibits its release (see Chapter 4). If there is an advance or delay in the schedule of light and dark, it will take several days before the release of melatonin follows.

Melatonin has been shown to cause sleepiness, speed sleep onset, and facilitate sleep maintenance. When ingested in pill form, it may have noticeable sleep promoting effects depending on the time of day. Given during the day or several hours before typical sleep time, it promotes sleep, however if given near or during the typical time of nocturnal sleep, it seems to have little effect on sleep in normal sleepers, perhaps because the pineal gland is already releasing it. Also depending on time of day, melatonin ingestion may increase REMS or decrease NREMS.

There are melatonin receptors in the suprachiasmatic nucleus by which it has its mild zeitgeber properties and can cause phase changes of the circadian rhythm for sleep/wake (see Chapter 4). However, it has a weaker effect than light as a zeitgeber. (See the cautions in Chapter 10 about using melatonin as a sleeping pill or to reset the circadian clock because of jet lag or shift work.)

Thyrotropin

Thyrotropin is a hormone that stimulates the thyroid gland to release thyroxin. It reaches a peak of output in the evening prior to typical sleep time, reaches its peak at sleep onset, and then declines as sleep progresses. The timing of its release is controlled by circadian influences, but SWS tends to inhibit its release. Thus, the release of thyrotropin is influenced by both process C and process S. When sleep is deprived, thyrotropin is still released at the typical time, but total release in increased. Sleep taken at other than typical times has little effect on thyrotropin release. Thyrotropin increases SWS.

Insulin

Insulin release appears to be influenced by both process C and process S. Insulin levels are elevated during sleep. An attenuated elevation is seen even when awake during the typical sleep period, and there is an elevation of insulin when sleep occurs during the typical waking period.

Other Hormones

Several other hormones are also involved with sleep. The levels of both aldosterone and parathyroid hormone increase during sleep. Rennin release is correlated with SWS. Vasoactive intestinal peptide increases the amount of REMS and lengthens the NREM-REMS cycle. Sleep deprivation or sleep fragmentation diminish levels of leptin and cortisol, which regulate hunger resulting in greater appetite (Spiegel, Leproult, & Van Cauter, 1999). Similarly, thyroid stimulating hormone is reduced by sleep deprivation.

Age Changes

As we age, there appear to be two phases during which the relationship between sleep and hormones changes. The gradual decline of SWS correlates with the decline in growth hormone through about 50 years of age. After age 50, correlated with what some researchers see as a decline in REMS, cortisol levels increase. These changes in endocrinology with age may be the cause of some aging effects such as memory impairments and insulin response.

GI Tract

Generally, digestive processes are slower during sleep. Gastric acid production is decreased later in sleep except in those with duodenal ulcers. They produce 3 to 20 times the levels of gastric acid produced in people without ulcers. Swallowing rate decreases in sleep, and the swallowing reflex is absent. Saliva is not produced during sleep. Generally, there is a decrease in the speed at which food and waste move through the GI tract during sleep, but some of this process may be circadian rather than a direct sleep effect.

Renal

Smaller quantities of urine are produced during NREMS, but it is more concentrated. Production is further decreased and concentration further increased during

REMS. Rennin, a hormone produced by the kidneys, is higher during NREMS and closely follows NREM–REMS cycles.

Endogenous Sleep Factors

In addition to substantial evidence for several substances in the body that influence sleep that we have already discussed such as cytokines (see below) and adenosine and some peptides (see Chapter 4), there are other substances that affect sleep. Some of these substances are found primarily in the cerebral-spinal fluid, while others can be found in the blood. This idea is derivative of a very old "hypnotoxin" notion about what causes sleep. It holds that during wakefulness some chemical builds up that eventually poisons the brain, resulting in sleep. During sleep, this chemical is degraded or eliminated allowing the return of waking.

Some of the earliest experiments in the 20th century on sleep involved removing cerebral-spinal fluid from a sleepy animal and injecting it into the ventricles of an awake animal. The recipient appeared to fall asleep. However, relatively little research attention was directed toward such substances until the last two decades of the 20th century. It turned out to be not all that easy to do. Often, when techniques were available to isolate components of the fluid from the donor and inject only that into the ventricles of the recipient, the result was not genuine sleep but a kind of coma. However, some substances did seem to produce genuine sleep, yet none seemed to be necessary and sufficient for sleep. Rather, they appear to be one of many things that facilitate sleep.

Many of these substances were peptides. One of the first peptides isolated was **delta sleep inducing peptide (DSIP)**, which often caused the recipient to enter into prolonged SWS. Eventually, DSIP was synthesized and found to be effective in many animals. However, some researchers have reported negative results. The sleep caused by DSIP occurs within an hour of injection and lasts several hours. Several kinds of observations, such as the brain waves and the fact that the animals can be aroused by strong stimulation, suggest it is normal sleep.

More recently, other peptides have been shown to influence sleep. One of these is alpha-melanocyte-stimulating hormone that is found in the cerebral-spinal fluid of brains and increases SWS following injection into the ventricles. Another peptide naturally occurring in the cerebral-spinal fluid somatostatin and its relative cortistatin can induce the production of delta waves in the cortex when injected into the cerebral-spinal fluid.

Many blood-borne factors have also been shown to have an influence on waking and sleeping, including epinephrine (waking), histamine (sleep), and insulin (SWS). Cholecystokinin (CCK) is a hormone that is released into the blood by the gut following substantial food intake. It has long been known that it helps regulate the flow of food through the digestive tract. More recently, it has been found also to reduce hunger and promote rest and SWS. Bombesin is also released by the digestive tract after eating and increases SWS. These and other substances may promote sleepiness following eating.

Prostaglandin D_2 is another substance found in the cerebrospinal fluid that induces sleep (Urade & Hayasihi, 1999). The concentration of prostaglandin D_2 is higher during sleep and further increases during sleep deprivation just as sleepiness increases.

Genetic

Since the 1980s, evidence has been accumulating that there is a genetic basis for normal and abnormal (see Chapter 10) sleep. Questionnaire studies of twins show the more closely they are related, the more similar their sleep patterns, even if not raised together. Identical twins have more similar bedtimes, total sleep time, and sleep quality than non-identical twins. However, these same studies also show that environment plays a large role in some sleep/wake variables. Morningness/eveningness questionnaire scores are closer when the genetic relationship of twins is closer. Polysomnographic studies of twins generally have supported these findings. They also show that in addition to sleep efficiency and total sleep time, NREMS characteristics are more genetically determined than are REMS characteristics. The more the genetic similarity, the greater the similarity of alpha, beta, delta, and theta waves.

More extensive genetic studies of sleep in animals reinforce these findings. Species-specific sleep patterns have been shown to be highly stable, strongly suggesting a genetic basis. Some studies have included using genetically similar vs. dissimilar animals and other studies used selective breeding techniques to show a genetic basis for sleep characteristics, especially total sleep, total REMS, and aspects of circadian rhythms of sleep/wake. Studies in rats show that the amounts of SWS and REMS are inherited via different genes, as are characteristics of the circadian rhythms. Noteworthy are long-sleep and short-sleep strains of mice that were developed by selective breeding. Another noteworthy line of research involves direct genetic manipulation of certain genes in mice with consequences for sleep/wake.

EFFECTS OF THE BODY ON SLEEP

Health and Illness

No research is needed to confirm that sleep and sleepiness often increase when illness strikes. It has been assumed by mothers and doctors that this increase in sleep is beneficial, but little research has actually been done to confirm this assumption. In contrast, the common belief that sleep deprivation can increase susceptibility to illness has research support. Little research was directed at these questions until the late 1980s, but continuing efforts since then have begun to provide answers.

It is now well established that bacterial infections lead to changes in sleepiness, SWS, REMS, and sleep maintenance. An increase in sleepiness is an early and enduring symptom of infections involving the whole body. SWS time and the amount of delta waves typically increase for a day or two following infection, followed by decreases to below normal levels. In contrast, REMS is decreased for the duration of the infection. Sleep maintenance is disrupted, but other aspects of sleep, such as the NREM–REMS circadian cycles, appear to remain unchanged. The degree and timing of these effects depends on the nature of the bacteria, how it got into the body, and the state of the immune system at the time. For example, drugs that increase or decrease the immune system also change sleep during an infection.

One of the better-understood mechanisms for how bacterial infection alters sleep and sleepiness involves the following chain of events. White blood cells called macrophages attack and digest the bacteria and then excrete chemical components, such as muramyl peptides that were part of the bacteria's cell walls. These substances initiate a cascade of biochemical processes that stimulate immune responses, cause fever, and result in sleep changes. One result of this process is an increase in a group of interconnected biochemicals known as cytokines, including interlukin-1β and tumor necrosis factor α. As the levels of either of these increase, sleepiness and the amount of NREMS increase, but REMS decreases. Yet, the sleep produced is normal, since awakening is possible.

Interestingly, these same substances seem to play a contributing role in normal sleep. They meet all the criteria for influencing sleep: increasing or decreasing levels increase or decrease sleep, they occur naturally in the brain, and they are found in higher concentrations near sleep onset. If special research drugs inhibit their effects, then normal levels of NREMS diminish. Also, sleep deprivation increases them, but if they are inhibited, less sleep rebound occurs. Their source comes from our body constantly fighting off bacteria in our GI tract, resulting in ever-present moderate levels of breakdown products. During illness, their quantities are increased, resulting in exaggerated effects on sleep. Other important related biochemical factors include interferon and prostaglandins.

Fungal, viral, and protozoan-induced illnesses have effects on sleep that are similar to those of bacterial infections. In fact, many of the underlying biochemical mechanisms appear identical, involving cytokines and other substances involved with the immune system.

Whether or not these changes in sleep during illnesses are really beneficial is less well researched, making our knowledge limited. It is likely that extra sleep with more SWS enables the body to devote more resources to healing, to the high metabolic demands that fever causes, and to reduce the possibility of spread of a localized infection. There is one study that directly demonstrates the benefits of sleep during bacterial illness. Linda Toth (Veterinarian, Director of Laboratory Animal Medicine in Springfield, Illinois) and James Krueger (1992) showed that the greater the increase in NREMS shown by rabbits challenged with bacterial infections, the more likely was their survival.

On the other hand, sleep deprivation compromises the immune system. Prolonged sleep deprivation decreases host defenses, such as natural killer cells and interleukins. Levels of interleukin-6 have been found to increase during stage 1–2 and REMS (Redwine et al., 2000). Experiments have also shown that sleep deprivation will increase vulnerability to viral illnesses. Even some lost sleep on one night results in a reduction of natural immune responses (Irwin et al., 1996). Additionally, it has been shown that sleep deprivation significantly decreases the effectiveness of flu vaccine.

Sleep disturbances are a prominent symptom of HIV infection (the agent that causes AIDS) and have been carefully studied. Complaints of daytime fatigue and sleep problems are among the earliest signs of HIV infection and worsen as the disease progresses. Early on, it becomes somewhat more difficult to fall asleep and to stay asleep, and there is a bit of an increase of daytime sleepiness. During this phase, there is an increase in SWS and other changes, but SWS is more evenly distributed during the sleep period. As the infection worsens, the daytime sleepiness gets worse and sleep onset and maintenance problems continue to get worse. SWS now decreases as does sleep efficiency. The NREM-REMS cycles become more and more disorganized. During the advanced stages of the disease, sleep quality is very poor, and fatigue and lethargy are great. SWS is absent or nearly so, and sleep efficiency is very poor. There are no recognizable NREM-REMS cycles. Yet, the need for sleep greatly increases. Those with HIV who show fewer disturbances of SWS survive longer. The exact mechanisms by which HIV causes these sleep changes is unknown but changes in cytokine levels that occur during HIV infection are suspected.

Box 14

Sleep Hygiene

It should be obvious from the material in this chapter that our wake time affects our sleep time just as much as our sleep time affects our wake time. There are things that can be done when we are awake that can make our sleep come easier and be more effective and less of a problem. All of these suggestions are based on research and have been shown to be effective in many if not all people. People who have difficulties with their sleep should pay special attention to these things.

- Try to sleep only when you are drowsy.
- If you are unable to sleep after being in bed for about 20 minutes, get out of bed and go to another room. Return to bed only when you feel drowsy.
- Get up in the morning at the same time every day, even on weekends and holidays. Going to bed at the same time is a good idea, also. Choose these times

so that you get 8 hours of sleep per night (more or less depending on your individual sleep needs—see Chapter 3) and are sleepy when you go to bed but alert after you get up.

- Reserve use of the bed for sleep. Using it for sex is also permissible, but do not use it to watch TV, read, work, or for other non-sleeping activities.
- Avoid excessive napping. A brief (20 minute or so) mid-afternoon nap can be refreshing and natural. More than this amount can cause sleep problems later that night.
- Have a pre-sleep routine that is calming and separates going to sleep from the activities of waking. This routine might include bathing and teeth cleaning, reading, meditating or praying, and the like.
- Avoid rigorous activities and aerobic exercise in the hours prior to bedtime. Regular exercise in the late afternoon may help you sleep later that night.
- Refrain from drinking or eating caffeine for several hours (or more if you are especially sensitive to it) before bedtime.
- Do not drink alcohol prior to bedtime and especially do not use it as a sleep aid.
- Do not smoke for several hours before bedtime. Reduce or stop smoking if you awaken during the night because you need to smoke.
- If you find yourself worrying after you go to bed, tell yourself that you will worry tomorrow and then think of or imagine something else that is calming and relaxing. If worrying in bed occurs, often choose a time earlier in the day to write out potential problems and their possible solutions.
- Arrange the bedroom to make sleeping easier. A comfortable bed in a dark and quiet bedroom with comfortable temperature and humidity can greatly help sleep.

Stress

Stress, whether negative or positive, can affect sleep (Van Reeth et al., 2000). You, like everybody else, have probably noticed this effect at one time or another, although some people are more susceptible to stress. Both acute and chronic stress can be sleep disrupting, fragment sleep, and change the amounts of some of the stages. Following the stress, there are often rebound effects with more REMS and NREMS. Stress causes an increase of several hormones including adrenal cortical tropic hormone and cortisol that can disrupt sleep continuity and stages. Stress also affects the immune system that, as we have seen, also impacts sleep. Animal studies show that recovery from acute stress includes an increase in both NREM and REMS.

Drugs

Some drugs prescribed for non-sleep related problems, especially those that act on the brain, affect sleep/wake in one way or another. Some drugs may cause insomnia and other problems with sleeping. Others may cause sleepiness, sedation, and/or fatigue. Some drugs prescribed for specific sleep or wake problems may have effects that carry over into the succeeding wake or sleep period, respectively. Other drugs may affect sleep/wake for a period of time after they have been discontinued. Although there are many kinds of drugs that cause some or all of these effects, those drugs used to treat depression, schizophrenia, anxiety, breathing disorders, cardiovascular problems, or those drugs that manipulate histamine or steroid production or response more commonly have significant effects on sleep/wake. Some over-the-counter drugs (including nasal decongestants, pain relievers with caffeine, and antihistamines) can affect daytime sleepiness and/or nighttime sleep.

Pain and Other Sensory Stimuli

In addition to the effects of room temperature on sleep, it is well known that other sensory stimuli can also affect sleep. Pain, either sudden or chronic, affects sleep, and sleep affects pain. Laboratory studies have confirmed that people in pain may find it more difficult to get to sleep and/or not sleep as well, have less SWS, and experience more awakenings. Not sleeping well can make pain worse.

Stimuli such as loud or disturbing noise, including stimulating or annoying music, can make it more difficult to get to sleep and even disturb sleep. Soft and soothing noises or music may facilitate getting to sleep. Likewise, bright or changing light can disrupt sleep onset as can irregular bumping and jarring of the body, such as when riding in a car on poor roads. Some people report that some smells can cause problems with sleep, while other smells facilitate it. Indigestion, too, can cause fragmentation of sleep.

Exercise

It is not possible to make a blanket statement about the effects of exercise on sleep. Exercise can mean too many different things to different people—aerobic or non-aerobic, mild to intense, and so forth. Also fitness level and age make a difference in the effects of exercise on sleep. While most exercise is generally recognized as beneficial to the body, it can also cause injury, which in turn can affect sleep. These considerations not withstanding, the overall experimental evidence shows that *regular* exercise can increase total sleep time, slightly delay REMS onset, increase SWS, and slightly reduce REMS (Driver & Taylor, 2000). However, whether exercise promotes sleep in people with and without sleep problems has not yet been determined. The best time to do aerobic exercise in order to benefit sleep is the late afternoon. Many sleep specialists caution against exercise in the evening prior to bedtime, because it may be too arousing, making falling asleep difficult, while beneficial effects of exercise done in the morning seem to be gone by bedtime.

Sexual Activity

Many men report that orgasm aids them in falling asleep. In contrast, sexual activity and orgasm are arousing, not relaxing, for many women. Not only can this difference affect sleeping, it can also affect relationships. Women need to realize that men fall asleep after sex because of biological based tendencies, not insensitivity. Men need to be sensitive to the fact that women do not share the same tendencies and like loving attention, not sleep, following sexual activity.

Nutrition

Throughout recorded history, sleepiness has been thought to be a consequence of eating a big meal. Not only how much you eat, but also what you eat has been thought to contribute to sleepiness and influence subsequent sleep. Scientific research has confirmed some, but not all, of these relationships.

Survey research has found that many, but not all, people report having felt sleepy after eating. Some report that this feeling occurs only after eating an especially large meal. The greatest sleepiness is felt to occur about $1\frac{1}{2}$ to 2 hours later. However, when lipids are consumed, subjective sleepiness is maximal 3 to $3\frac{1}{2}$ hours later.

In a related study, Orr and colleagues (1997) investigated sleep onset times following different types of meals. They had 10 male subjects take five polysomnographically recorded naps over a period of 4+ hours. Between the first and second nap, they ate a meal that was either high-fat, or high-carbohydrate, or a mixture of the two. For another group of 10 males, the meals were either solid, liquid, or an equivalent amount of water. There were no significant differences in sleep latencies as a result of consuming the high-fat, high-carbohydrate, or mixed meals, but the solid meals, unlike the liquid meal, resulted in shorter sleep onset times than the water.

Other research has shown that greater sleepiness occurs if the meal is high in carbohydrates compared to proteins or a balance of carbohydrates and proteins. Comparisons of high-fat plus low-carbohydrate to low-fat plus high-carbohydrate meals show that the former, but not the latter, increases subjective sleepiness more than 3 hours later. Yet, both increase MSLT sleep latency scores $1\frac{1}{2}$ hours later. Studies using all night polysomnography have shown that a meal of low carbohydrate plus high fat increases REMS time, whereas one of high carbohydrate plus low fat increases SWS time. Meals of proteins also increase REMS time. The amount of energy contained in a meal regardless of its source does not affect subjective sleepiness or polysomnographically measured variables.

Size of the meal has an effect, also. Studies in animals show that larger meals result in longer SWS and REMS periods. Excess food intake increases muramyl peptides (see above) and hence sleepiness because of increased absorption of bacteria and bacteria products into the blood.

Weight loss as a result of malnutrition or dieting has the opposite effect on sleep than weight gain. When losing weight, there is an increase in the time it takes to get to sleep, less time spent asleep, and a decrease in SWS. Additionally, there is more fragmentation of sleep when losing weight. During the time a person is gaining weight, total sleep time increases because of increases in both SWS and REMS as well as less fragmentation of sleep. Skipping a single meal or several meals prior to bedtime increases the amount of SWS but also increases sleep fragmentation. A light snack such as cereal and milk, yogurt, or crackers prior to bedtime tends to increase sleep duration and reduce the amount of wake time during the sleep period. However, a large meal or eating something that results in indigestion before bedtime may disturb sleep.

In some very interesting studies, Iraki and associates (see for example Iraki et al., 1997) has found that Moslems experience decreases in daytime alertness resulting from changes in sleep habits during the month of Ramadan, when they give up eating and drinking between sunrise and sunset.

Although sleep is typically a long period of fasting, glucose levels in the blood do not decrease. They do decrease during a similar period of fasting while quietly lying down awake. This difference occurs because glucose is used more slowly during night sleep. A minimum of glucose usage occurs during mid-sleep but begins to increase as morning approaches. Two-thirds of the decrease in glucose usage occurs because of the lower metabolic rate of SWS, but other factors also play a role, such as a decrease in muscle tone and changes in hormone levels during sleep. The gradual increase later in sleep occurs because of less SWS during that time.

There are many ideas about which specific foods influence sleep, but there has, with several important exceptions, been little research done to verify them. To my knowledge, there have been no studies of the sleep/wake effects of specific foods like carrots, spinach, hamburgers, rice, and so forth. (Many of us have also looked in vain for a sleep study confirming the benefits of eating oatmeal raison cookies!) Most studied have been the effects of caffeine, alcohol, nicotine, and tryptophan in food.

Caffeine

Caffeine has been confirmed to combat the effects of sleep deprivation but also to disrupt sleep. It works by reducing the effects of adenosine in the brain (see Chapter 4). Although it has little effect on people who are not sleep deprived or not dependent on it, caffeine can increase arousal and decrease sleepiness in sleep-deprived people. It can make performance more efficient and more accurate in people who are sleep-deprived. The degree of the effects depends upon the amount of caffeine consumed. Generally, good effects are seen with 100 mg, individual sensitivity, the type of task, and the level of sleepiness. Consumption of caffeine every few hours has improved alertness and performance over that of a placebo for 40 to 48 continuous hours without sleep. (Notice carefully what this statement says; caffeine did not

Table 4. Amount of Caffeine in Some Common Foods

Coffee, brewed	100–150 mg
Tea, cup	60–75 mg
Cola soft drinks, 12 oz	40–75 mg
Chocolate, 1 oz	36–47 mg
Pain medicines, over the counter	32–65 mg
Cold remedies	15–60 mg
Stimulants, OTC	100–200 mg

restore alertness and performance to the level it would have been with normal sleep, but it did make things better.)

Caffeine consumed before bed, even several hours before bed in some people, will disrupt sleep. This disruption can occur even in people who have no awareness of the effects caffeine is having on them. It increases the time it takes to get to sleep, sleep fragmentation, and the frequency and duration of wakefulness during the sleep period.

Considerable caffeine is found in many popular drinks but is also in many foods and medicines (see Table 4). It reaches its peak concentration in the body about $\frac{1}{4}$ to 1 hour after consumption, with half still present after an additional 2 to 6 hours, but may not be totally cleared out for 8 to 14 hours. In some individuals, children, pregnant women, and the elderly, it stays active even longer, sometimes much longer. Regular consumption of caffeine can lead to tolerance and dependence. That is, it becomes less effective, yet the person experiences negative withdrawal effects such as lethargy, sleepiness, fatigue, and performance decreases without it. Some people may continue to consume caffeine to avoid these withdrawal effects.

Alcohol[16]

Like caffeine, alcohol affects both waking sleepiness and nighttime sleep. During waking, the effects of alcohol can be described as having two phases; it is initially arousing followed by a sedating effect. The higher the alcohol level in the blood, the shorter the MSLT sleep onset times. But its effects on sleepiness also depend on the degree of prior sleep deprivation and the circadian time of the nychthemeron. It has been calculated that 3 drinks (drink = 1 oz of 80 proof liquor, 12 ounces of beer, or 4 ounces of wine) are the equivalent of 6 in a person who has had 5 successive nights of only 5 hours of sleep. In contrast, people who have extra prior sleep are made less sleepy by alcohol than a person who has averaged 8 hours of sleep per night. Alcohol produces a greater sleepiness when consumed during the night or mid to late afternoon ("happy hour") when the body's circadian rhythm for sleepiness is higher. Surprisingly, the sleepiness produced by alcohol has been shown to outlast the presence of alcohol in the blood for several hours or until sleep is obtained. It is as if alcohol flips a sleepiness switch in the brain that stays that way until it is switched off again. Thus, experiments have shown that a sleepy person who has a few drinks during happy hour can be a dangerous driver long after their blood alcohol level returns to zero.

Since alcohol causes relaxation and sleepiness, it is widely used by people to help them sleep at night. Unfortunately, this practice, too, is a problem because of the two-phased effect. After drinking moderate amounts of alcohol that bring the blood concentration to .05 at bedtime, the time to get to sleep is much shorter, and SWS time often is initially increased. However, there is a delay in getting to the first REMS period, and total REMS in the first half of the night is reduced.

By the second half of the night, blood alcohol level is at or close to zero, since the body clears about one drink per hour; at this point there is a rebound effect. Sleep is generally disturbed and restless, there is more wakefulness or stage 1, and REMS is increased. The net effect can be a relatively poor night of sleep. After several consecutive nights of going to bed following moderate drinking, the first-half-of-the-night effects are diminished but not the second-half-of-the-night effects. Subsequently, the night or nights of sleep not preceded by drinking alcohol may contain excessive amounts of REMS.

Nicotine

Nicotine also affects sleep and sleepiness. (OK, it really does not belong in a section labeled nutrition, but it seems to fit in with discussion of caffeine and alcohol.) It increases alertness and reduces sleepiness. Smokers get these benefits during the day, but one-pack-a-day smokers also have more difficulty getting to sleep and have lighter sleep. Although no differences in amounts of REMS and NREMS are seen in smokers, many have more difficulty staying asleep. Quitting smoking results in the improvement of time to fall asleep and an increase in SWS and REMS. Some reports also say there is a decrease in waking during sleep, but other reports say there is an increase in arousals for a number of nights.

Tryptophan

Tryptophan is an amino acid prevalent in foods like dairy products, fowl, beans, some nuts, and bananas. It also is the raw material used in the brain to manufacture the neurotransmitter serotonin. Since early research implicated serotonin with sleep (see Box 11 in Chapter 4) and anecdotes prevail about the sleep inducing properties of things like a warm glass of milk, it was thought that ingestion of tryptophan could promote sleep onset. While research was being conducted to test this hypothesis, many people tried taking easily available, unregulated tryptophan pills during the 1980s as an alternative to other sleeping pills. But a serious side effect, possibly from contaminants in the unregulated tryptophan pills, quickly caused them to be removed from availability in the United States. Meanwhile, the research was equivocal about its ability to promote sleep. It was suggested that some of the research used too low of a dose of tryptophan or that it was tested on normal sleepers in whom it would be hard to show an improvement in sleep. Later studies suggested that it could help about half of insomniacs get and stay asleep if they took doses of one to two grams.

Since there are problems with the pill form of tryptophan, can eating foods rich in it before going to bed help your sleep? The answer is unclear. It is not all that simple for tryptophan in food to get to your brain, and often there simply may not be enough of it that gets there to make a significant difference. It has to go through the digestive process that may be too slow when a lot of other food is also being digested. Also you cannot be sure that the food you eat contains a sufficient amount of tryptophan to make a difference. Finally, it competes with other amino acids to get into the brain; if there are many competitors, then little gets in. At best, it takes about an hour for the brain to manufacture serotonin from newly arrived tryptophan. In the end, it seems that even if all goes well, the effect of consuming tryptophan rich food is a mild one that does not always work. So eat something like milk and bananas an hour or more before bedtime if you like. It might help you sleep, but don't count on it simply because of the extra tryptophan you take in.

Herbs and Supplements

The use of herbs and supplements to obtain better sleep has become very popular with many "experts" offering advice on what is effective. However, the information provided is too often conflicting, actual scientific evidence from well designed research studies to back up the claims is sparse, and sometimes dangerous interactions of these herbs with one another or drugs is becoming apparent. The most frequently mentioned herbs are passionflower for temporary insomnia, the aroma of lavender for calming, and valerian or kava for promoting sleep. Also catnip, camomile, lime flowers, gotu kola, cowslip flowers, hops, lemon balm, lady's slipper, and skullcap have been recommended for sleep disorders. Some of these are to be ingested, others inhaled in steam, and some can be either ingested or inhaled. Supplements recommended for sleep include melatonin for sleep problems, GBL for sleep problems, magnesium for sleep disorders, and serotonin for good sleep.

There has been some good research done on valerian. It has been used for centuries for its reputed relaxing and calming effects and thus to relieve insomnia. For example, Donath and colleagues (2000) had 16 people with insomnia (4 male, 12 female) take valerian extract for 1 day or 14 consecutive days preceded or followed by a look-alike placebo for another 1 day or 14 consecutive days. Neither the subjects nor the researchers knew when the subjects were taking the valerian extract or placebo until the experiment was completed. Polysomnographic recordings were made before and after taking the course of valerian or placebo, and subjective ratings of sleep and daytime performance were also obtained at these times. The one-day dose of valerian extract had no effect on any of the measures. The 14-day use of valerian extract resulted in no difference in sleep efficiency, but a more rapid onset of SWS and an increase in the amount of SWS were seen. Subjects reported they fell asleep more quickly. They also noted few side effects from taking valerian extract. The authors concluded that valerian extract might be useful for the treatment of mild insomnia. However, other studies have not shown such clear-cut or even positive results (Cauffield & Forbes, 1999).

Yet, there are potential problems with available valerian extract in purity and actual strength as well as its stability. A 2001 study (see http://talkaboutsleep.com/news/Valerian.htm as of November, 2001) by an independent lab that evaluates nutrition products and dietary supplements and independently confirmed by a second lab showed that 4 of 17 products claiming to contain valerian actually had none, and another 4 had less than half of what was stated on the label. Cautions about the use of other herbs and supplements have been issued because of preliminary or inconclusive research data on their effectiveness and the potential for bad side effects (Cauffield & Forbes, 1999).

Kava has also received research attention. It has been show to reduce the time to get to sleep and promote deeper sleep. Studies of the long-term effects of taking valerian and kava are needed. There have been no published studies using good scientific methods on the other herbs.

Other folk and natural remedies for improved sleep have included rubbing garlic on your soles, putting a cut raw onion under your pillow, or sleeping on a small pillow filled with hops flowers. There are suggestions to avoid foods with a lot of tyramine (the raw material the brain uses to make norepinephrine) before bedtime. This list includes cheese, sauerkraut, wine, cured meats, eggplant, spinach, and tomatoes. There appears to be no scientific research to back up the use of any of these remedies.

Weather

Outside of the effect of air temperature (see above), there has been little research done on the effects of weather on sleep. It is thought that weather extremes or obvious changes in the weather can have effects, generally negative, on sleep. But there is also some evidence that more subtle differences in things like barometric pressure, ionic fields, lunar phase, solar disturbances, and so forth also affect sleep.

Box 15

Awakening without an Alarm (Part 2)

In a Box 7 in Chapter 3, I reviewed my research on the ability of people to awaken at their desired time without using an alarm clock. Jan Born and colleagues (1999) at the University of Lübeck in Germany wondered if the expectation of awakening at a certain time influences the secretion of adrenal cortical tropic hormone (which tells the adrenal glands to release cortisol). They monitored 15 people during three nights of sleep starting at midnight. For one of the nights, these people were told they could sleep till 6 a.m. For the other two nights, they were told they could sleep until 9 a.m., but on one of those nights were surprised by being awakened earlier at 6 a.m. The amount of adrenal cortical tropic hormone in the blood was sampled frequently during their sleep. It began to rise sharply the hour before the early-expected awakening time but not in those expecting the later awakening time. Born and colleagues conclude that the increase in adrenal cortical tropic hormone is a part of the preparation by the body for awakening early. Still unanswered is how the brain keeps track of time during sleep to be able to cause this release of adrenal cortical tropic hormone prior to the anticipated time of awakening. For example, polysomnographic study of their sleep revealed no difference, including their brief arousals, in any of the three conditions.

Part III

Dreams and Dreaming

Humans have been curious about dreams throughout recorded history and, we can speculate, well before then. Typical questions include:

- What are they about?
- Where do they come from?
- What are their functions?
- How can people use them?

To which there have been a variety of answers.

Part of the problem with finding answers is that dreams are so very private. All of us have our own dreams while asleep, and we are the only ones who can experience them. People have endeavored to share their dreams with others when awake by describing their recall of them verbally or, less often, by drawing them, acting them, or dancing them. Sometimes this recall occurs the next morning but often hours, days, or even years later. And almost always people report that they cannot completely and adequately do justice to their dream experiences in their dream reports.

Also, there is not much that can be done to influence the content of recalled dreams (Domhoff, 1996). This difficulty severely limits the experimental possibilities for manipulating dreams to see what they are all about. And it is not possible to independently check the accuracy of the dream recall, which constrains the ability to be certain of our findings about the contents of dreams (Domhoff, 1996).

Additionally, it has always been obvious, just as it must be obvious to you, that dreams are not easily recalled. Sometimes we feel that we have recalled a dream perfectly and can describing it fully and accurately. More often, we know that we have related something of the dream but are frustrated that we cannot completely or adequately describe it because our words, or paintbrushes, or movements are insufficient to do the dream complete justice. Other times, we just cannot remember everything about the dream and have to settle for describing the parts we do recall. Then, most frustrating of all, are the times we know we dreamed but just cannot bring any of it into our waking memory. This inability to remember causes a problem of representativeness (Domhoff, 1996). We cannot be sure that the dream recalls we are able to collect for study are an unbiased sample of all dreams in all people.

For centuries, these problems have limited the ability to study and understand what dreams are all about. That limitation did not stop people from trying to study and understand them, but until recently there was only a smattering of scientific research done on dreams and dreaming. The late 19th century marks the beginning of systematic dream research, for this period is when a few psychologists began to write down their own dreams and then to study the nature of these recalls. But it was during the 20th century that there was an increase in interest within the scientific community in dreams. Starting with Freud's *Interpretation of Dreams* published in 1900 (see Chapter 8), there was great psychological interest that continues today.

Just as important, there was another transition point in the mid-1950s, with the discovery of REMS and its apparent association with dreaming, that stimulated broader interest in dreams and the process of dreaming. People sleeping in the lab could be awakened during or right after a period of REMS and immediately asked what was going through their mind before they were awakened. Eighty to ninety percent of the time, they responded with a recalled dream. As a result, it was believed that scientists could get more dream reports and, since they were recalled immediately after they were experienced, much more accurate ones.

This awakened interest in dreams and dreaming led to an explosion of research. Today, people in various academic areas including clinical psychology, cognitive psychology, biopsychology, anthropology, brain research, religious studies, and literary criticism are doing research on dreams and dreaming for the purpose of trying to understand these things themselves (Bulkeley, 1996). Because of these efforts, we now have a greater and better understanding of dreams and the process of dreaming. But, as, we shall see, there is still considerable disagreement about the nature of dreams and dreaming.

DISCOVERY OF REMS

It was one of those discoveries of the serendipitous type that are surprisingly important in the history of science. Graduate student Eugene Aserinsky was working with physiologist and pioneer sleep researcher Nathaniel Kleitman's in the sleep laboratory at the University of Chicago looking for slow eye movements throughout sleep like those that had been observed when people fell asleep. But watching the eyes move under the eyelids during the wee hours of the morning was tedious. Therefore, they decided to record them electrically using EOG. To their surprise, they also found periodic occurrences of rapid eye movements during sleep. They then turned their attention to these periods of rapid eye movements and soon found the movements were associated with dreaming.

Shortly thereafter, medical student Bill Dement joined Kleitman's lab and took over the study of these rapid eye movements. The team noted the apparent association of dreaming with rapid eye movement sleep that occurred every 90 to 100 minutes during the course of sleep. While it took several years for these observations to become recognized by the scientific community, once they were, many researchers were waking people up during REMS and recording their dreams for intensive studied.

At first, it was eagerly anticipated that the study of dreaming during REMS would lead to an understanding of the unconscious mind, but that hope has not been borne out. Other research investigated the effects of REMS deprivation, thinking that they were investigating the effects of dream deprivation, which, at that time, was thought to be potentially psychologically devastating. Although it was found that this hypothesis also was wrong, much interest in sleep and dreams and good information about REMS came out of these misdirected experiments.

REMS, NREMS, and Dreaming

Right from the start of research on the relationship between REMS and dreaming, researchers noted that they occasionally could get a dream report from awakenings out of NREMS. Nevertheless, the notion that dreaming only occurs in REMS was maintained then and generally persists today. One of the early explanations was that these NREMS dreams were not really experienced in NREMS but were memories of a dream left over from the recent REMS period. Later, others examined these NREMS dreams and concluded that there was mental content during NREMS, but it was, for the most part, not like REMS dreams. The reports coming out of NREMS were often shorter, blander, more vague, more oriented in the present, and lacking ongoing activity. They were more like a photograph, while REMS dreams were like a movie. But this did not satisfy everyone nor explain all of the data.

Soon it was reported that it was not unusual to get a good dream report from people in the sleep lab who were awakened *before* the first REMS period. Obviously, they were not left over from the prior REMS period, since that was many waking hours ago. Also, when corrected for length, naïve judges were unable to determine which reports were from REMS awakenings or NREMS awakenings. At this point, the equating of dreaming solely with REMS apparently broke down. But not entirely, for REMS awakenings more often resulted in dream recall than did NREMS awakenings.

Nielsen (2000) extensively reviewed 29 REMS and 33 NREMS studies of recall rate. The average REMS recall rate was around 80% compared to an average recall rate for NREMS of around 40%. Also, there was still the qualitative difference; very many of the NREMS awakening recalls were shorter, blander, more vague, and lacking ongoing activity, but REMS awakening recalls were rarely of this type. It was not unusual for subjects never to report a recall following NREMS awakenings in spite of multiple tries over several nights, which is rare following REMS awakenings.

Because of data like these, it seems to some that much of the time something different is going on in NREMS that is different from what is happening in REMS. So the debate continues even today (e.g. Foulkes, 1997; Hobson, Pace-Schott, & Stickgold, 2000; Nielsen, 2000). There is no issue about whether we dream when in REMS, but there is disagreement about what is going on in NREMS.

Lab vs. "Home" Dreams

There is another issue that has emerged. Once it was found to be possible to collect dreams in the lab by awakening people from REMS, the question was asked, "Yes, but what is the effect of the lab on the dreams?" It was noted that images and references to the lab environment were present in 20 to 30% of lab dream recalls. Could the lab have other effects on the content of recalled dreams? Research was undertaken aimed at answering this question.

It was reasoned that the lab dream recalls were sampled, but home dream recalls were selected, which could make a difference in content. That is, lab dream recalls were similar to having you wear a beeper and recording what was happening to you just every time the beeper went off, but home dream recalls were like asking you at the end of the day (or even days later) to describe what you experienced during the day. The beeper technique would probably produce a lot of bland, ordinary stuff, but the asking technique would more likely return the notable or unusual. It was hypothesized that it would be the same with dream recalls. Another hypothesis was that people would feel more inhibited in what they reported in the lab, a more public venue than home.

Research in the 1960s found just the differences predicted by both hypotheses (Domhoff & Schneider, 1999). Lab dream recalls are blander (e.g. less aggression, less sex, fewer misfortunes), and the way the dream recalls were gathered influenced the content. Yet, in other ways, lab and home recalls were very similar in things like types of characters and presence of at least one bizarre element.

Researchers in the 1970s endeavored to make the conditions for dream collection in the lab and at home more similar by using the same procedures in each. For example, in both situations, an alarm clock would randomly awaken people from sleep, then tape record any dream recall. The result was the virtual elimination of the differences in dream recall content from the lab compared to the home. Also, reanalysis of some of the key 1960s data showed that the differences reported earlier were actually quite small in extent except for there being less aggression in the lab dream recalls.

More recently, comparisons have been made of sleep-awakening recalls with what was recalled of the same dreams the next morning. Contrary to expectations, saliency of dream content did not appear to be a factor influencing which dreams were recalled in the morning. However, there was a greater likelihood to (1) recall the dreams from the end of the night, (2) recall those that were longer, and (3) recall those with more emotional intensity (Domhoff, 2003).

Today, it is realized that the setting and methods of dream recall collection can affect dream content, but this difference lessens the more similar the collection conditions are. It can be concluded that while setting and method of collection can have a bit of an effect on what is recalled about the dream, the essential dreaming process is the same. Also, the few effects of the laboratory on dream content appear now to be known. The major advantage of the laboratory has been the ability to sample dreaming across the night and in specific stages. However, newer technology is now allowing this sampling to occur at home, too, so the home versus laboratory issue may fade in the future.

PROBLEMS WITH STUDYING DREAMS

Before we turn to what has been discovered about dreams and dreaming, we need to attend to the fact that dream research is difficult. The main problem is that there is no direct access to dreams. Each one is created by an individual and experienced only by that individual. The *only* way dreams can be studied is to have the dreamer recall the dream after it happened. REMS awakenings are thought to facilitate this process by having the recall as close as possible to the experience and therefore are assumed to produce more accurate recalls.

Yet, even this technique is far from perfect, because the dreamer still needs to awaken to collect the recall that causes a change in the functional organization of the brain (see Chapter 5). Also, dreams are experienced primarily visually, but the typical dream report is verbal. Verbally describing a visual experience is imperfect and incomplete at best. Furthermore, studies have shown that the gender, age, status, and so forth of the person who obtains the recall and whether it is written down, taperecorded, or whatever affect the content of the recall. In addition, my research has shown that our memories of dreams are highly labile (see Box 17 in Chapter 6). Additionally, people usually report more about what *happened* in a dream than how intense or detailed these experiences were (Strauch & Meier, 1996).

In spite of these difficulties, it is still beneficial to study dream recall, because it gives us insights into the nature of dreams and dreaming and the recall itself can be useful for dream recall interpretation. Nevertheless, the constraints these difficulties pose need to be kept in mind.

DEFINITION OF A DREAM

An even more basic problem is defining just what a dream is. Even among professionals who study and work with dreams, it has not been possible to reach agreement about what a dream is—and what it is not (Pagel et al., 2001). Part of the problem comes from the wide range of backgrounds (psychological, medical, anthropological, literary, philosophical, physiological) among those who study dreams. For some researchers, dreams are only created during sleep and have a narrative quality but with hallucinatory and bizarre elements. For others, dreams may also occur when awake, such as during meditation, drug influenced states, daydreaming, hallucinating, and during drifting waking thought.

As a follow-up study, Jim Pagel, a sleep disorders physician and dream researcher in Colorado, asked college students, sleep disorder patients, and medical professionals with an interest in dreams to select what they thought was the best definition of a dream from a list of widely differing definitions (Pagel, personal communication, July, 2002). The most commonly selected definition was "a report of mental activity occurring during sleep," but this definition was chosen by only slightly less than one-third of the participants. The selections also differed by group. For example, college students most often (one in three) selected "any non-conscious thought, feeling, or emotion," but this choice was the least selected by the medical professionals (less than 1 in 20).

Since the focus of this textbook is on sleep and dreaming, I will use a more restricted definition of a dream. I exclude what may occur during waking and any mental content during sleep that is not story-like. (I will continue this discussion in Chapter 6.) This topic is an important issue, though. Science means precision, and a part of being precise is to define its terms carefully. Without doing so, there is a very real danger that misunderstandings and miscommunications will occur, because people are not talking about the same thing, resulting in a muddled understanding of natural phenomena. Without precision of definition, the data collected and labeled as dreams may be quite different in different studies, making the conclusions unable to be compared.

Chapter 6 describes what is known about the content of dreams based on the study of people's recall of their dreams. Chapter 7 looks at the process of dreaming. Chapter 8 summarizes many of the major theories about dreams and dreaming.

Chapter 6

Dreams[17]

In this chapter, we will focus on the characteristics and content of dreams as gleaned from the study of what people recall of their dreams, but first I have to clarify the focus of this endeavor.

DREAMING IN NREMS?

Much of the controversy over whether dreams occur in NREMS is over what should be included as a dream and what should not be included. Part of the problem is, as discussed in the introduction to this section, there is no universally agreed upon definition of a dream. If any kind of mental activity is accepted as a dream, then around 60% of NREMS awakenings yield dream reports. However, as the criteria for a dream becomes more stringent, the percent of awakenings from NREMS that yield dream reports drops. Using the strictest definition of a dream, which is the one I prefer—a holistic mental experience (some would say hallucination) while asleep consisting of characters interacting over a period of time in a succession of several organized and apparently real, although often bizarre, vivid images or scenes—then reports of dreams following NREMS awakenings occur less than 10% of the time.

There is no doubt that some mental processes are occurring during much of NREMS, but using the stricter criteria, the experiences cannot be called dreaming. While a small percent of NREMS mentation fits these dream criteria, most of the rest are shorter, not as dramatic, not as vivid, not as emotional, not as elaborated, not progressive, and contain less activity. Most of what is recalled from NREMS is more like a photograph, often not clearly in focus, compared to a clear movie such as experienced in REMS. It has also been described as more thought-like. Such mental activity during NREMS should be called **NREMS MENTATION** to distinguish it from dreaming.

If REMS dreaming and NREMS mentation are truly different but mixed together, then our research and understanding of dreaming and other mental processes becomes muddled, just as if we were to say that apples and bananas are really the same and mixed them in a bowl to study their attributes. On the other hand, if we treat REMS dreams and NREMS mentation as separate, but later discover that, as some now maintain (c.f. Foulkes, 1978), they really are results of the same mental processes, it would be easy to combine our knowledge and understanding of them into a unified theory. So, for the rest of this book, we will consider them as separate. (For a more complete analysis of the data leading to the strong conclusion that REMS dreams are indeed different from NREMS mentation, see Hobson, Pace-Schott, & Stickgold, 2000). Furthermore, we will assume that when we are in REMS, we are dreaming, and the memory of the dream is "lost" during the 10 to 20% of the time that there is no dream recall when awakened from REMS. In contrast, there may be mentation occurring only in a portion of our NREMS.

Reinforcing this view are studies of brain activity during sleep (see Chapter 4). They suggest that much of the cerebral cortex during REMS shows activity levels comparable to that of waking. During NREMS, however, the activity patterns in much of the brain, including the cerebral cortex, is much less than that of waking. Assuming that the cortex needs to be active to engage in the mental processes necessary to put dreams together, we can conclude that, while some mentation can occur during NREMS, it is not of sufficient quality to be called dreaming.

Some studies have looked at the EEG response to meaningful sensory stimuli. They find indicators of cognitive processing during REMS that are diminished or absent in NREMS. Tore Nielsen, a Canadian brain and sleep researcher in Montreal, maintains that those recalls from NREMS that meet the definition of a dream may occur because the brain processes that produce dreams in REMS are partially activated (Nielsen, 2000). He finds some support for this hypothesis in the facts that (1) computer analysis shows the EEG during NREMS from which dreams are reported is different from other NREMS EEG, and (2) more NREMS dreaming is reported when NREMS occurs close to a REMS period. In contrast, New York cognitive psychologist John Antrobus (1983) maintains that the generation of REMS dreams and NREMS mentation is identical, but retrieval of the content is more difficult from NREMS than from REMS because of the state of the cortex.

About one-third to three-fourths of awakenings shortly after sleep onset result in reports of NREMS mentation. These reports are short, but otherwise have all the elements of REMS dreams (Strauch & Meier, 1996). However, they lack a narrative structure, and the occurrences of the dreamer being an active character is unusually low. Additionally, the content of these "sleep onset dreams" does not relate to what the sleeper was thinking about prior to sleep.

There are differences in the nature of recalls from different kinds and times of sleep. There is more episodic memory present in sleep onset dream recalls and more thinking than in REMS recalls, with NREMS recalls intermediate between them. There is considerably more hallucinative content in REMS recalls than in sleep onset dream recalls, with NREMS recalls intermediate between these two (Stickgold et al., 2001).

Sleep onset recalled mentation is more related to the dreamer's immediate and recent past and more resembles waking fantasy than does REMS dream recall.

I should note that it has become standard to ask subjects, "What was going through your mind?" rather than "What were you dreaming about?" Some people may not consider NREMS mentation or fragments of REMS dreams to be dreaming and fail to report them when asked to recall a dream. A loss of valuable data is less likely to occur when asking the more general question about what was going through the person's mind when asleep.

WHO DREAMS AND HOW OFTEN

Everybody dreams every night. We know this fact because of being able to awaken people in the sleep lab and immediately asking them what was going through their mind just before being awakened. Typically, when any of the 6% of people who adamantly profess they never dream were awakened during REMS, they frequently, in a groggy manner, would begin describing the dream they were just experiencing. Then they would suddenly pause with this look of surprise on their face, when they realized that they do dream. So we conclude that everybody dreams every night, but some people do not remember doing so.

This information brings up a related question. Why is there no recall following 10 to 20% of REMS awakenings? One possibility is that there was no dreaming going on then. While there is no direct evidence to refute this statement, there are some indirect indicators. Dreams are not always easy to recall. Most of us have had the experience of being able to recall only a fragment of a dream or of knowing that we dreamed but were unable to recall anything about it. On other occasions, something we experience later in the day may trigger recall of a recent dream previously unrecalled. From these common experiences, it can be inferred that it is likely that we all dream during every REMS period, but sometimes recall of the dream is lost in the transition to waking.

Box 16

Dreams of People who are Blind

I am often asked about the dreams of people who are blind. Since dreams are so visual, do blind people have dreams? If so, what do they dream about? The answers to these questions, as so often happens, are not simple but in this case very understandable. They are summarized by Hurovitz, Dunn, Domhoff, and Fiss (1999).

Blind people dream. Their dream reports are as complex as those of the sighted. Whether or not there is a visual aspect to their recalled dreams depends on when they became blind. If totally blind since birth, they never report visual images in their dreams. If they became totally blind before the age of five, they seldom report visual images in their dreams. Those people who lost their sight after the age of seven continue to report visual aspects to their dreams, but often the clarity and frequency of them diminish with time. Those who lost their sight between the ages of 5 and 7 may or may not report some visual imagery in their dreams. When visual images are absent in the dream recalls of people who are blind, they are replaced by more taste, smell, touch, and sound.

In other respects, with a few exceptions, their dream report content is much like that of sighted persons. Two notable exceptions involve aggression and moving from one place to another. People who are blind report having more dreams with at least one incidence of aggression. They also have higher numbers of dream recalls involving moving about, either under their own power or by some means of transportation. These transportation dreams are often linked to misfortune for the dreamer. Uniquely, two women who were blind had an unusually high number of dogs in their dream recalls, mostly their guide dogs.

CHARACTERISTICS OF DREAMS

How Much are Dreams Like Waking Experiences?

How do dreams compare to our waking visual experiences? In a clever experiment, Rechtschaffen and Buchignani (1983) prepared 129 variations of a single photograph. They varied the degree of fuzziness in the foreground and in the background, the brightness, the color intensity, and so forth. They then awaked 22 subjects from REMS and asked them to choose the photograph that best matched the visual quality of their dream. Four out of 10 times, they selected the photo that was most like typical waking visual experience. The rest of the time, there was less intense color and/or fuzzy background. Early in the night, the selected photos were least like that of typical waking perception.

Antrobus and colleagues (1987) did a similar experiment but found that images experienced in dreams were at best three-fourths as bright as those experienced during waking, while the clarity was close to that of waking. Yet, some dreams were experienced as having little color and poor clarity. Interestingly, they also found that the clearer the details perceived in a dream, the more likely that they were strange in some way, such as being too large.

When looked at from a waking perspective, dreams are often bizarre (Hobson, Pace-Schott, & Stickgold, 2000). The most common kind of bizarreness in dreams is sudden discontinuities between sequences. These perceptions are often marked by the dreamer's words, "All of a sudden ..." But dreams often contain other kinds of bizarreness, such as characters in our dream may be a composite of two or more real people, have something about them that is highly irregular, or may physically change during the course of the dream. The same things can happen with settings, objects, and even time.

Yet, just as it does when awake, our mind attempts to explain and integrate all the experienced elements of our dreams. However, unlike when we are awake, dreaming accomplishes this task by creating a story line attempting to meld everything into a single confabulatory narrative from which self-reflection and critical evaluation are missing. Dreams have been called "single minded" by Alan Rechtschaffen, a research psychologist and long-time sleep and dream researcher at the University of Chicago (Rechtschaffen, 1978). By this term, he meant that while dreaming, the mind is wholly focused on the dream and less interrupted by other thoughts and images. It does not reflect on the fact that it is dreaming, what it is dreaming about, or that it is actually lying in bed. Likewise, it is little influenced by external and internal stimuli. This experience contrasts greatly from waking where our attention easily shifts from our thoughts to salient internal or external stimuli and back again, we reflect on our mental processes and current state, and we evaluate our experiences.

What People Typically Dream About

Leaving interpretations aside, just what kinds of things do people describe dreaming about? Common folklore and Freud's writings leave the impression that dreams are full of sex and violence, but this assumption only appears to be the case, because people remember and tell others more of these types of dreams. It turns out that simply asking or surveying people about what they typically dream about does not provide very accurate data when compared to the content of actual dream reports from REMS awakenings, dream diaries, or having people write out their most recent dream.

The best research with such dream reports often uses what is called content analysis developed by two psychologists, Calvin Hall and Robert Van de Castle. Essentially, this method first categorizes things like the characters, settings, objects, activities, social interactions, and so forth that are found in a dream and then counting the number of instances in each category. For example, characters might be grouped according to sex and age (such as male adult, female child, or indeterminate elderly). The categories are carefully developed so that different researchers working with the same dreams will produce nearly the same results. An excellent resource to learn more about the technique of content analysis and how to use it is dreamresearch.net.

Results from such objective studies of the content of dream recall show that rather than being filled with sex and aggression with lots of emotion, recalled dreams are mostly mundane and ordinary but with some bizarre elements or happenings.

But neither do dreams precisely reproduce memories and typical waking experiences. For example, there is a noticeable absence of things like writing, reading, keyboarding, or calculating. People mostly dream about people, things, pets, and so forth that directly influence and interest them during their waking lives. The typical dream is best described as a set of novel creations with a theme, using mostly the common and ordinary from the dreamer's waking experiences. They are most akin to a short fiction story or TV program.

Dreams are primarily experienced as perceptions. Unless a person is blind, all dreams are visual. Sounds are noted in about two-thirds of dream recalls, touch is a distant third at 8%, while the rest of the senses are reported in less than 4% of dream recalls. Pain sensation is extremely rare. However, over 40% of dream report content is more like thinking. The thinking is simple with no complex relations or reflections on questions from multiple points of view. Nor is there any puzzling at length over a problem. Often dreamers are unable to confirm that they actually heard talking or just knew that it occurred even during subsequent questioning about this experience.

Emotions or moods are experienced in about three-fourths of dreams but are not mentioned in dream reports unless dreamers are specifically prompted to do so. However, when asked, dreamers may report experiencing emotions in the dream that differ from what others might infer was present from the rest of the dream report. This emotion is almost always what the dreamers said they would have experienced had they been awake. Contrary to what people think they dream about, negative emotions are actually experienced far more often than positive emotions in dreams. Moderate emotions are experienced much more often than either extremely strong or very weak emotions.

Box 17

Memory for Dreams

There is no denying that dreams are difficult to remember. Almost everyone can report having difficulty completely recalling a dream they had or even remembering anything at all of a dream they know they recently had. But when people report their recall of a dream, whether following a sleep awakening, the next morning or days, weeks, or even years later, it is tacitly accepted as being a faithful reproduction of that dream as it actually occurred. After finding very little experimental research in the literature about this issue, a number of my students and I set out to test this assumption.

We awakened 17 sleepers during an early morning REMS period and tape-recorded their dream recall. Upon the participants' final awakening later in the morning, we also tape-recorded their recall of this same dream. We also obtained recalls a week later and a month later. We had complete data from 14 of the sleepers that we analyzed. Each recall was transcribed and parsed into its "storyboard" components (= any aspect of the dream that was a piece that could be removed or inserted as a unit such as "he played his harmonica for the people in line"). Then we compared the recalls with one another to see how many components were deleted or added.

We found that the average recall of a dream contained only half the number of the composite of components reported for it. There was no difference in the total *number* of components included in any of the four recalls, although many specific components were different. Likewise, each of the subsequent recalls were missing more than half of the components that were present in the REMS awakening recall but also contained 22% new components. Yet, the changes did not distort the gist of the dream, because several people who had nothing to do with the experiment could accurately sort all the recalls into their respective dreams.

In a follow-up study, we awakened 15 sleepers during an early morning REMS period and immediately showed them a 6-minute dream-like video taken from a 20 year-old movie they had not seen before. We then proceeded as if this video segment were a dream to be recalled. The advantages with this procedure was that all subjects had the same "dream" that made comparisons between subjects easier and we knew the exact content of the "dream" and could tell what was included, left out, and added. We had complete recall data from 11 of the sleepers for analysis.

The data were analyzed just as they were in the first experiment, and the results paralleled those of the first experiment except that recall was slightly better for the synthetic dream and, for some measures, the morning recall was slightly better than subsequent recalls when comparison was made to the REMS awakening recall.

Additional analysis was possible, since we knew the components that were in the "dream" itself. We found that the average recall contained only about one-third of the storyboard components from the entire synthetic dream. We were quite liberal in our comparisons such that, if the recall contained a component that even partially resembled a component in the "dream," we counted it. However, we also found that about 10% of the recalled components were *not* actually present in the original "dream." When we excluded the REMS awakening recall done immediately after viewing the video, the average recall contained over 20% of components not present in the original "dream."

In a third experiment, we looked for any rehearsal effect that may have improved subsequent recalls. Again using the synthetic dream technique, we always obtained an immediate recall but only one subsequent recall per subject, either next morning, next week, *or* next month, but not all three. There were 10 subjects per group. The results showed a slight, but not significant, drop off in the number of components recalled with the passage of time. Thus, we did not see much of a rehearsal effect.

We conclude from these experiments that although the gist of the dream is present in each recall, many of the components vary depending on the time of recall with many components of the actual dream never recalled, some components only sometimes recalled, and other components added that were never part of the original dream.

Furthermore, there is no indication in these data that the REMS awakening recall or the next morning recall is greatly superior to any subsequent recall. These results imply that what we know of dreams and dreaming from the study of dream recall may be imperfect due to the imperfections of recall. Nevertheless, the study of dreams and dreaming (as well as dream interpretation—see Chapters 8 and 9) utilizing dream recalls is the best we can do and is worthy of our efforts as long as we realize that actual dreams may be somewhat different.

Content

The characteristics of the content of recalled dreams are more similar than different across cultures in things like the percent of male and female characters, more aggression than friendliness, more misfortune than good fortune, and more negative emotions than positive emotions.

The content of dream recall is most likely to vary in the nature of aggressive content. There are noticeable differences in aggression in dream recall between males and females, people from different cultures, home and lab dreams, and people of different ages (Domhoff, 2003). Less aggression is found in the dream recalls obtained in the sleep lab than at home. Typically, men manifest higher aggression in their dream recalls than females except for the percent of victimization. Aggressive content in recalled dreams is highest in the United States of all industrialized nations. But it is even higher in small or tribal groups, with the exception of Hopi Indian males. Furthermore, aggression seems to increase gradually with age in the recalled dreams of children and begins a slight decline during adulthood. Overall, people show the most aggression in dreams toward those with whom they most clash during their waking lives.

Strauch and Meier (1996), in reviewing 500 REMS awakening dreams from 18 males and 26 females, found only a few differences in the content of dream recall by males compared to females, and these differences were more a difference in emphasis rather than sharp contrasts. There were no gender differences found in things like friendliness, whether unfriendly actions were physical or verbal, degree of participation of the dreamer, specific emotions, intensity of feelings, and the ratio of everyday events to leisure events. Female dream recalls contain a greater array of events. Males showed a tendency to have more male-only dreams. Females demonstrated a bit of an edge in familiar characters in distinction to being alone or among strangers. Male recalls contained a bit less aggressiveness and friendliness and were a bit more realistic. However, in male dream recall, males were more frequently the perpetrators rather than the recipients of aggression—just the opposite of female dream recalls. Female dream recalls had relatively more negative emotions. There also was evidence that what people dream about reflects their understanding of their sex role.

Frequently, the recalled dreams of college students are used for content norms, probably because they are the most accessible population for dream researchers. Bill Domhoff, a psychologist and sociologist at the University of California Santa Clara, has been carrying on the Hall-Van de Castle tradition. He summarized the accumulated norms, which have not changed in the last 50 years, in his book *Finding Meaning in Dreams: A Quantitative Approach* (1996). Additionally, Austrian dream researchers, Inge Strauch and Barbara Meier, summarized their findings on 500 REMS awakening reports supplemented by morning follow-up questions from 44 young adult, self-reported good dreamers in their book, *In Search of Dreams: Results of Experimental Dream Research* (1996). Here we will sum up the norms gleaned from both of these sources with a special focus on characters, social interactions, activities, misfortunes, emotions, and settings, since it is possible only to discuss the main characteristics of what people dream about in the space available here. You may want to consult the references and additional sources for more details.

Characters.   The nature of the characters in recalled dreams shows some interesting features.

- It is extremely rare for there to be no characters at all in a recalled dream.
- Most often dreamers are a character in their own recalled dreams (in 89% of recalls) and most often as an active character (71%) rather than a passive observer (11%).
- One of the more striking findings is that males populate their recalled dreams with two-thirds males, but females average a nearly equal number of males and females.
- Most remembered dreams have a mixture of both familiar and unfamiliar characters.
- Thirty-one percent of the characters in the recalled dreams of males are recognized as friends compared to 37% in dreams recalled by females.
- Acquaintances and colleagues are more common than are family members in the recalls of both men and women, but women recall dreaming more about babies and children.
- Males have a higher percent (28%) of unfamiliar male characters in their recalled dreams than do females (15%), but the number of unfamiliar females is nearly equal in the remembered dreams of males (10%) and females (11%).
- Among the familiar characters, both males and females have nearly equal numbers of familiar males in their recalled dreams (25 and 23% respectively), but female recalls have more familiar females (29%) than do male recalls (16%).
- Most characters are adults, and more of them are from our present life rather than from childhood.
- Sometimes strangers are in our dream recalls by virtue of their role or function such as firemen or teachers.

- Males identify more characters on the basis of their occupation.
- Seldom do we populate our remembered recalled dreams with characters from fiction or with prominent persons.
- Animals are not nearly as common as people.

Social Interactions. Characters in recalled dreams frequently have neutral interactions with other characters.

- Dreamers are as likely to be initiaents as recipients of social interactions.
- While percent of social interactions that are aggressive is almost equal in the remembered dreams of males (47%) and females (44%), the aggression is more physical in the dream recalls of males (50%) compared to the recalls of females (34%). In both cases, the dreamer is involved in about 80% of the aggression, most often as a victim.
- Thirty-eight percent of the interactions in dreams recalled by males are friendly compared to 42% in dreams recalled by females.
- Aggressive or friendly interactions are mainly via words and gestures rather than physical contacts.
- When the dreamer of either sex is attacked in a recalled dream, the attacker twice as often is a male, usually unfamiliar in the dreams remembered by males but familiar as often as not in dreams remembered by females.
- Women's recalled dreams contain more friendly acts than do the recalled dreams of males, but the recipient of friendliness is more likely to be a female in the recalled dreams of both males and females.
- Most conversations focus on everyday practical things with few occasions of professional, political, or impersonal topics reported. Nor is there much superficial conversation, such as talking about the weather or sports, or much social ritual (e.g. asking, "How are you?").
- Interactions that are sexual are surprisingly low at 12% for males and 4% for females, but the dreamer as a character has sexual interactions with familiar characters more often in female recalls than in male recalls. The sex that is reported in the recalled dreams of males is often with attractive women who are strangers. The recalled sex dreams of females have a more romantic quality, whereas the recalled sex dreams of males are more in the nature of conquests.

Activities. Characters usually engage in a multiple activities in any one dream.

- Overall, males are more active as characters in their recalled dreams, but the activity that women display as characters is generally more verbal than physical.
- Movement and talking contribute to around three-fourths of the activities in the dream reports of both males and females.
- Conversations occur in two-thirds of remembered dreams.
- Characters often move under their own power but also move in vehicles.

Misfortunes.

- Thirty-six percent of male recalled dreams have misfortune compared to 33% in the recalled dreams of females.
- Good fortune, however, is in only 6% of the remembered dreams of both males and females.

Emotions.   Contrary to common belief, many dreams are emotionally neutral.

- Spontaneous reports of emotions in dreams are surprisingly low in both male and female dream recalls, with females reporting more than males.
- However, of the emotions reported, about 80% are negative with apprehension and confusion the most frequent emotions experienced.
- The experience of pain in remembered dreams is extremely rare.

Settings.   Most dream reports contained a setting.

- Unknown settings are most common (44%), followed by familiar (26%), then vague and non-specific (19%) and distorted (11%) in the dreams of both males and females.
- Familiar settings are more common in the recalls by females.
- Females report more indoor settings (61%) than do males (48%).
- In 25% of the recalls of both males and females, the setting was changed before the end of the dream.

Objects.   There are two key differences in the recall of objects in dreams.

- Males recall more dreams involving automobiles and weapons, while females recalled dreams contain more household objects.
- Women also recall how their dream characters looked, including what they wore and how their hair was styled, more than do males.

Other elements.

- Seventy-two percent of the situations recalled in dreams are from everyday life, with domestic/routine daily occurring more often than professional. Another 22% are from leisure time, but only 1% are fictional or fantasy.
- Overall, over one-half of the reports combine realistic with fictional elements with another one-fourth having only realistic elements. Entirely fictional or fantastic situations account for only one-fifth of all recalls. However, some individuals consistently have more fictional or fantastic elements than do other individuals.

- Dream reports contain few crimes and little illness or injury. Likewise war, national catastrophes, severe losses, or deprivation are rare as are outstanding good fortune, unexpected success, and distinctions.
- Some of the things typically reported in dream dictionaries such as transmogrification of objects, losing teeth, flying, and falling are actually not very common.

Bizarreness.   One of the striking features about dream recalls is bizarreness.

- It is extremely rare for everything in the dream report to be bizarre, but some bizarreness is present in about three out of four remembered dreams, present in only one minor element in 4 out of 10 recalls, and strongly present in about 1 out of 3.
- The bizarreness, when present, is found more often in the elements of the dream report (almost 50%) than in the form of the entire recalled dream (less than 10%) with bizarreness in both form and content in less than 20%.
- Content bizarreness occurs in actions 43% of the time and characters 27%, with settings at 18%, objects at 13.7%, experiences at 10.3%, and speech at 3.4%. However, these percents simply parallel the percents of all occurrences of these contents, so bizarreness seems to be equally spread around.

Generally, these findings show that recalled dream experiences are as multifaceted as waking experiences and seem as essentially integrated and as real as waking experiences, but perhaps with more awareness of strangers or unrecognizable people and more unknown settings than we experience while awake. Yet, our dreams as we recall them are not exact reproductions of the real world; rather, they have been described as "inventive realism" or "realistic-fictional." They are more akin to creative short stories than to factual histories. At the same time, our dreams as remembered seem to be self-governing and out of our control.

The events recalled in dreams, with their actions and interactions, are most often the focus of dreams. The setting is usually secondary to the events. Our recalled dream characters sometimes react to what occurs in our dreams much like when awake, with two very key exceptions—thinking and emotions. Thought processes during remembered dreams are simpler than those when we are awake, and we seem to recall uncritically accepting what occurs during our dreams no matter how bizarre. Dreamers are personally included, usually in an active manner, in most of their recalled dreams, yet the dreamer is usually not the central focus. Our self as a character in our dream reports focuses almost entirely on the moment to the exclusion of concern for the past or future. We do not wonder who we are or how we are impressing others.

Those who are more interested in dream interpretation in order to get at the true or real meaning of the dream (see Chapter 9) have a different view of what people typically dream about. For example, San Francisco psychologist Gayle Delaney talks about the following commonly recalled elements in dreams in her book, *All About Dreams* (1998): being chased, losing teeth, appearing in public naked, unable to run, sex with an unexpected partner, loss of purse or wallet, finding new rooms in a house, taking exams, dreams of flying, famous actors or actresses, dictators, automobile breakdown, drugs (or cigarettes or alcohol), clothing, family or another close relative's home, a certain town (or state or country), cats, and snakes. However, as already mentioned, many of the things that people say they typically dream about in surveys rarely show up in more objective content analysis of dream reports with the exception of being inappropriately dressed in public and flying (Domhoff, 1996). Yet, some things, while not generally common, may be more frequent at certain times in a person's life, such as recalls of dreaming of a deceased loved one months or years after the person died.

Others have maintained that we cannot lump all dreams as recalled together and then try to discern their essential nature. They maintain there are different categories of dreams including those extremely important, pivotal recalled dreams that do not happen very often. Literature, novels, essays, and poems are usually not mixed together for study, but each category is studied in its own right. For example, Don Kuiken, a psychologist at the University of Alberta, Canada, obtained recalls from 26 women and 10 men of (1) a recent impactful dream which he defines as a dream that influenced how they felt or what they did during subsequent waking, and (2) the first dream that they had after at least 4 days had transpired from the impactful dream (Busink & Kuiken, 1996). The subjects also filled out questionnaires about features of these remembered dreams. Both the recalled dream content and the questionnaire data were then statistically analyzed for clusters, such as feelings of discouragement, being weak or unable to move, vivid sounds, and amazement. Five cluster patterns emerged that they labeled Existential Dreams, Anxiety Dreams, Transcendent Dreams, Mundane Dreams, and Alienation Dreams. The characteristics of each of these are elaborate and need not concern us here (see Busink & Kuiken, 1996 for these details). Such categorizing of qualitatively different kinds of dream reports may lead to more fruitful ways to study dream recalls in the future.

Box 18

Some Popular Myths about Dreams

1. *People only dream in black and white.* One study found that when awakened from REMS in the lab and asked immediately about the presence of color, the response is affirmative over two-thirds of the time. However, if the color question follows other questions and/or the complete recall of the dream, then this ratio drops to one-third. In other studies, 75% to over 80% of dream reports collected following REMS awakenings contained color. It thus appears that much, if not all, dreaming is done in color, but this detail, like many other dream details, is easily forgotten.

2. *Eating spicy or exotic foods will cause us to dream more.* Anything that causes indigestion, such as spicy or exotic foods are more likely to do, will cause us to awaken more frequently from sleep. The more we awaken, the more we are likely to *recall* the dreaming that has been going on regardless of what we have eaten.

3. *The eye movements of REMS are following or causing the activity of the dream.* When dreaming of looking up at the Eiffel Tower, for example, there would be vertical eye movements, whereas, when watching a tennis match, there would be many horizontal eye movements. This intuitive hypothesis has occasionally been explored for over 30 years with generally negative results, mainly because the nature of the eye movements differs from those that occur when awake (Hobson et al., 2000), and correlations between reported dream content and recorded eye movements is not always present. Also, rapid eye movements occur in human fetuses, cats with no cortex, and people blind from birth. None of these examples has visual experiences, so it is unlikely that they are scanning visual images in their dreams. Nevertheless, some recent findings find support for this hypothesis (e.g. Hong et al., 1997).

4. *If you dream that you are falling and you hit the ground, then you are really dead.* Whenever I hear this one, I ask the question, "How were the data for this conclusion collected?" Also, there are people who have awakened quite alive from a dream in which they report they were falling and hit the ground.

5. *Sleeptalking and hypnosis can be used to find out what people dream about.* These experiences have been tested several times but with very little success.

AGE

The data on common elements in recalled dreams presented above is for young adults. As we saw in Chapter 1, sleep changes with age. Does what people dream about likewise change with age?

Children

Psychologist and dream researcher, David Foulkes (1982, 1999), did the most extensive studies of recalled dreams in children. For the first study, he sampled the remembered dreams of the same two groups of children, starting at 3–4 years of age and 9–10 years of age, from 1968 to 1973 (called a longitudinal method) using sleep awakenings in the sleep lab. To see if being in a study of dreaming for several years influenced the frequency or quality of the dreaming in these children, he added some children in subsequent years but found no essential differences in their dream reports. The age range in the first study was from slightly close to three at the start going to slightly older than 15 at the end. Each of these children spent 9 nights per year in the lab with three awakenings for dream recall collection each night. Some dreams recalled in the morning at home were also collected for comparison, and extensive daytime cognitive and mental testing and assessment of the children was also done. When awakened during the night in the lab, each child was asked to relate what they were dreaming about then questioned further about the dream's details. Content scales similar to those of Hall and Van de Castle plus evaluation of qualitative aspects, such as degree of realism, were used to evaluate and compare the dream reports.

In the mid-1980s, he replicated this study but with a different group of children at each age (a cross sectional method). The follow-up study was otherwise very similar except that each child spent three nights in the sleep lab. There were 10 boys and 10 girls each at ages 5, 6, 7, and 8 for this study.

The most surprising result of these studies was with the 3–5 year olds. They reported dreaming after only 15% of the wake-ups, and what they recalled was poorly developed, stagnant, and emotionless. Even with these few reports, Foulkes had reasons to be uncertain if they were really dream recalls or confabulations or statements of what the child was experiencing at the time of questioning. The reports obtained were very short, averaging a bit more than a dozen words, with no story line, and they seldom contained any movement. More of the recalls were of animal characters than people. These animals were like those found in children's stories or fairytales but not family pets or exotic animals. They were described as being engaged in a simple activity, such as eating. Beyond this content, there was a paucity of movements or social interactions among the characters. If the dreamer was present as a character in the dream recall, most often it was not as an active participant. Rather, most commonly the character was asleep! Contrary to popular beliefs about children's dreams, there was no emotion in the vast majority of their recalls. Yet, in other ways, these dream recalls were similar to those at any age in that they put things together in unusual yet mostly plausible ways.

Big changes in the content of dream recalls were noted during the ages of 5–9. Genuine dreams seemed to have emerged. From ages 5 to 7, there was an increase in social interaction. One-fourth of this interaction was aggressive in form, but primarily involving characters other than the dreamer. There were still a lot of animals present, but they were no longer the central focus. Although watching TV and being occupied by schoolwork take a lot of waking time for children at these ages, very little of what was on TV at the time or in their schoolwork could be seen in their dream recalls. Rather, play activities, events, and settings became prominent. Although there was no distortion, especially unfamiliar characters and settings, dreams were seldom reported to be frightening.

By 7 years of age recalled dreams became three times longer, but no more frequent. Social interaction became common, as did general movement, interaction, and event sequencing. Yet, the dreamer was seldom an active participant. A few months later, the frequency of dream recall began to increase, and the recalled dreams were more complex. Also, the dreamer became a more active character in the dream. Emotions began to be present.

Between 7 and 8 years of age, there was a big jump in the quality of the narrative of the dream recall reports. They became more and more story-like.

Overall, between ages of 7 and 9, the rate of dream recall continued to increase, now averaging a recall from 43% of awakenings, as did the number of words per recall, now averaging 72. As the dreamer became more of an active character in the remembered dream, most often in a friendly manner, the number of animal characters began to decline. The emotions, which were now reported, were more of happiness than fear and anger.

The content of dreams became relatively mature by age 9. Between 9 and 11 years of age, percent of recall following REMS awakenings almost reached adult levels at near 80% and stayed stable thereafter. Their length also reached that of adults. The level of the dreamers' participation as a character in the activity of the dream equaled that of other participants. The dreamers' social interactions were more positive than negative. Boys' dream reports now contained more aspects of assertiveness, aggression, venture-someness, self-reliance, and success orientation. The remembered dreams of girls now showed more social awareness, interpersonal orientation, munificence, and openness. At the same time, the number of animal characters continued to drop.

From age 11 to 13, there was an increase in the number of vague settings or no setting at all. There was also a reduction in specific descriptions of physical activities such as manual labor or moving from one place to another. Social interaction dropped a bit, too, and there were more unknown or unfamiliar characters and settings. There was a noticeable decline in the locomotor activity of the dreamer as a character as well their initiations of positive social activity. In contrast, all of the dream characters manifested more cognition, found in one-fourth of the reports, than seen at younger ages, but emotional contents contained in the recalls decreased a bit.

The content of the children's dream reports was unlike that reported by adults until they were 13–15 years old and exhibited low levels of aggression, misfortune, and negative emotion. Gender differences in dream recall were not apparent until late childhood.

Others who have studied dreaming by children and teenagers using different methods (Domhoff, 1996; Strauch & Meier, 1962)—some with only home dream, morning reports, others with different methods for analyzing sleep awakening, dream report contents—often agree with the findings of Foulkes, but some are quite critical of them (c.f. Resnick et al., 1994). There is general agreement that the length of dream reports increases as children get older—although there is disagreement on the cause of this occurrence—and that children's recall of dreams contains more animal characters, especially when younger.

Domhoff (1996) summarizes the studies relying on Hall-Van de Castle content analysis of home dream recalls of children.

- Generally boys report more boys than girls in their recalled dreams (69% to 31%), while girls report equal numbers of boys and girls in their dreams.

- Children more often report dreams with misfortune. They also report more aggression per character with the dreamer often being the victim, especially of aggression by an animal.
- Although more study of teenager's recalled dreams is needed, there are suggestions that when compared to males, female teens report more friendliness but are more likely to be victims of aggression. However, a smaller percent of this aggression is physical. Male teenagers report more aggression than do female teenagers, and a higher percent of it is physical.
- Children report content that is relatively realistic, featuring settings of the home or recreation areas.
- Recalled characters are mostly family members and other known persons.
- Recall reports from girls are longer and contained more people.
- Like men, boys report more about implements but less about clothing.
- The most common emotion reported is apprehension, at twice the frequency reported by adults.

Hobson and colleagues (Resnick et al., 1994) collected dream recalls from children sleeping at home. They had the parents tape record whatever dream recall occurred at the time of morning awakening and after a few mid-sleep awakenings. The parents were also instructed to prompt the child considerably for details. Key differences from the results of Foulkes include the following.

- They found a level of dream reporting in 4 to 5 year olds (56%) that is nearly the same as that of 8 to 10 year olds (57%), however mid-sleep awakening reports were only 12% compared to morning reports at 65%.
- The reports were long and detailed with many of the same characteristics of adult reports following prompting, which added 250% to the length of the recalls from the younger children and 70% to that from the older children.
- The dreamer was reported to be an active character in well over 80% of the dream recalls at both ages.
- About 40% of the dream recalls of the 4 to 5 year olds contained bizarre elements with an apparently even greater, though not statistically different, percent in the 8 to 10 year olds.
- Thirty percent of the characters recalled were family members.
- More settings were recalled compared to the findings of Foulkes.

These results of Resnick and colleagues (1994) have to be considered with caution because of the very real possibility, not withstanding the authors' insistence to the contrary, that the children confabulated a good deal of the time to please their parents. Nevertheless, these findings are important because they at least reflect what parents and others are likely to hear from their children when they report their dreams.

Box 19

Do Animals Dream?

If you have been around dogs or cats much, you probably have noticed that they sometimes twitch their feet or face when asleep, and dogs even make sounds. If you are like most people, you probably assumed they were dreaming. Yet, knowing for sure that animals dream is difficult to establish directly. We cannot ask them if they are dreaming like we can people. Reflexes and not dream content may cause the movements and sounds they make. Yet, there are many indications that they probably do dream.

The strongest arguments in favor of the presence of dreams in animals, at least in other mammals, include the following:

(1) There is great similarity in brain structure and functioning, especially among mammals, which includes the areas known to be involved in sleep and dreaming.

(2) Animals also show signs that they have mental processes similar to those of humans such as those involving emotions, sensory perceptions, and even cognitions—the very processes that are a part of dreaming.

(3) Cats with damage in the brainstem area that causes muscle paralysis during REMS are completely normal whether asleep or awake except for one thing. They move while in REMS in ways that strongly suggest they are reacting to and interacting with something they are experiencing in a dream. Some even walk and seem to be searching or looking at something imaginary, yet they do not react to real stimuli. Similar behaviors occur in humans with damage to this area, and they report having had dream content that matches well with the behaviors they were doing while in REMS (see Chapter 10).

(4) A gorilla that was taught to communicate to its handlers in sign language spontaneously combined the signs for "sleep" and "pictures."

Arguments against the notion that animals dream include the fact that we cannot ask directly or indirectly what they were dreaming about so that we can make qualitative comparisons of their dreams to the dreams of humans. Until we have direct access to the content of animal dreams, we simply have no way of knowing for sure if they dream. From a more philosophical point of view, it is argued that only humans can do the symbolic mental processing necessary to dream (Foulkes, 1999).

Adults

The recalled dreams of adults show remarkable stability with reactive change. Throughout the long period of adulthood, Domhoff (1996) finds much consistency in the major categories of what people report they dream about at home. That is, on the whole, when averaged over many people, the types of characters, social interactions, objects, and activities really change little during the extent of the adult years except for possibly a reduction in aggression and negative emotions. He also finds remarkable consistency in what U. S. college students almost 50 years apart recall dreaming about when the studies are properly done. These data are in spite of much social and political change during that time. Especially noteworthy is the consistency in the differences in recalled dream content between males and females in spite of the great change in the role of women. Additionally, the recalled dreams of older people show no more references to the past than do recalls of younger people.

Yet, Domhoff notes, there are changes in what individuals recall dreaming about that are consistent with changes in their individual lives, such as career upsets, marital changes, and so forth. For example, working women have more masculine types of dream imagery, featuring more aggression and anxiety, than do women who are homemakers. At all ages, remembered dreams tend to focus on the present. Still, studies of long series of dream recalls from individuals of typically more than a hundred samples sometimes spanning decades show basic consistencies within recalls of individuals, but differences in the recalls between individuals.

More clinically orientated studies of what people report dreaming about as they age (Cartwright, 1979) show young people report that they dream more about guilt and morality, middle aged people report dreaming more about sexuality and aggression, and elderly persons report dreaming more about death and illness. These reflect the changing concerns that typically accompany aging in the United States.

DREAMS THROUGH THE NIGHT

In the lab, it is possible to awaken a dreamer several times during the night (usually near the end of each REMS period) and collect a dream recall each time. The natural question to ask about these series of dream recalls is if they are related like chapters in a book or weekly segments of a TV series. The answer seems to be "It depends." Based on uninterpreted content alone, the answer is no. The content of what you recall dreaming about during one REMS period and the next (or NREMS periods for that matter) appears unrelated. We seem to jump from one theme and setting, one set of characters and activities, and so forth in one dream to entirely different ones in the next. It is rather like watching a sequence of different half hour programs on TV on a particular night.

Cartwright's (1978) research leads to some different conclusions. In addition to noting that when awakening subjects after the same duration of REMS, the first REMS period yields only 50% recall which increases to 99% by the last REMS period, she also observed that as the night goes on, there is more emotion, less distortion, and more drama in the dream recalls. Even reports of NREMS mentation become more dreamlike as the night wears on. Additionally, she, like some other psychologists and psychiatrists, finds that the dream recalls obtained by REMS awakenings during a single night are related when looking below the surface content to see what the dream purportedly really means.

Cartwright sees three phases in the dreams of a single night as the typical pattern. The dream during the first REMS period sets the theme on an emotional level (such as threat to self-esteem) for the dreams of a night. During the second and third REMS periods, past experiences related to that theme are brought to bear. Then during the fourth and fifth REMS periods, possibilities for the future relating to the theme are explored. The result is a progression, often beneficial to the dreamer, in this emotional concern. But this sequence may not occur if the dreamer is under a lot or very little stress (Cartwright, 1979). If stress is too high, then the single theme is simply repeated without progression and benefit. If the dreamer's stress is low, then the dreams are not ordered and have many themes.

RECURRENT DREAMS

Fifty to 80% of college students report recalling recurrent dreams over a period of a few months to many decades. They may occur a couple of times per week or a couple of times per year. Most begin in childhood, others in adolescence, and a few during the adult years. About two-thirds of the dreams feature negative affect. Most frequently, the main character in the remembered dream is the dreamer who is being attacked or chased by living things or by natural forces such as fires, floods, or storms. For many people, recurrent dreams eventually cease but not for everyone. (For more on nightmares, see Chapter 9.)

LUCID DREAMING

Lucid dreaming means being aware that you are dreaming while you are dreaming. When people are asked if they have ever experienced a lucid dream, 50% respond positively and 15% say that they experience one more than once a month. Many people also report that while having a lucid dream, they have the ability to modify the dream in minor to major ways. For example, a high school student who competed on the track team once told me he dreamed that he came in third in a race. When he realized he was dreaming, he had everyone run backwards to the starting line, then race again, only this time he arranged it so that he came in first.

The legitimacy of lucid dreaming has been scientifically verified in a number of experiments using similar methods. Self-avowed lucid dreamers are given an instruction before going to sleep in a sleep lab to give a prearranged signal when they are having a lucid dream. Signals used have included a specific sequence of eye movements, an unusual pattern of breathing, or even twitching a finger a number of times. The sleepers may be awakened right after giving the signal, a few minutes later, or at the end of the REMS period for a dream report. Upon awakening, the sleepers verified that they had experienced a lucid dream. Furthermore, the time between the signal and the moment of awakening closely corresponded to the time that the events recalled in the dream would be expected to take if they had occurred in real life.

Some dream researchers maintain that anyone can learn to become a lucid dreamer, but others believe that this ability ranges from easy to hard to acquire. Other dream researchers have cautioned that it may not be advisable to control many of your dreams, because dreams seem to have their own agenda (see Chapter 7) and controlling them may upset their natural function (see Chapter 12).

CREATIVITY IN DREAMS

Every night each of us composes, directs, stages, and usually acts in what is the equivalent of several TV programs, a highly creative endeavor. But we can be creative in other ways in our dreams, creative in the sense that we bring something novel yet useful back to our waking lives. There are numerous historical examples to illustrate this ability.

Ellias Howe had spent years trying to invent a mechanical sewing machine. He was successful only when he had a dream of "natives" throwing spears at him. These spears had holes just below the sharp point at the front and they kept bouncing in and out of the ground. Upon awakening, he realized that he first needed to move the hole for the thread from the blunt end, where it is on a typical hand-sewing needle, to the sharp end. Second the entire needle should not pass through the cloth, but just the sharp end penetrate then withdraw over and over again. With these changes suggested to him by the dream, he successfully developed the sewing machine.

James Watt was familiar with how to make lead pellets to be used as shot for the guns of his time. A block of lead was cut into pieces and formed into nearly spherical shapes by hand. However, the shot was not always formed into a perfect sphere, having a negative effect on how it performed. Howe dreamed on three different occasions that he was caught in a rainstorm of molten lead. After the third dream, he realized that this image was the key to making perfect shot, because drops of hot lead, just like drops of water, assume the shape of near perfect spheres while falling. He constructed the first shot tower—a tall structure from which splattered molten lead was dropped. As the drops fell, they assumed a spherical shape and cooled before hitting bottom. The result was nearly perfectly shaped shot.

Notice what happened in both of these examples. Each time, the dreamers were very involved with a problem in their waking life. It was personally important to them, and they were very familiar with it. These facts probably caused them to have the dream but certainly caused them to attend to the dream and recognize the creative solution to the problem.

There are numerous examples of creative solutions coming from dreams in areas beyond technology. Kekule made the scientific discovery of the nature of the benzene ring when he dreamed of snakes each biting their own tail. Writer Robert Lewis Stevenson got the idea for his famous story of "Dr. Jekyl and Mr. Hyde" from a dream. Composer and violinist Tartini heard the devil playing a beautiful tune on his violin. Upon awakening, Tartini reproduced, as best he could, what he heard in his dream, resulting in his greatest composition, "The Devil's Trill Sonata." Paul McCartney says he got the tune for his song "Yesterday" in a dream that he wrote down upon waking. These examples are not unusual. You, or somebody you know, probably has had some creative insight that came from a dream, even if it was less spectacular than these examples.

Dream researcher, Deirdre Barrett (1993), asked students to try for a week to incubate (see Chapter 7) a dream about a problem that was of personal importance to them and to seek a solution in their dreams. Later, the submitted dream reports were scored independently as to their relevance to the problem and whether or not the dream presented a reasonable solution. The results showed that about one-half of the recalled dreams were about the problem and one-fourth also contained an apparent solution.

Box 20

How to Recall Dreams Better

Often people are frustrated because they cannot remember their dreams and they want to know how they can remember more of them. It has been estimated that less than 10% of dreams are recalled (Domhoff, 1996) and that most people recall about two dreams per week with fewer people recalling either more or less. Research has shown that how often people recall their dreams has very little relationship to their personality except for somewhat greater recall frequently in people with "thin boundaries" (see Chapter 9), high creativity, a positive approach towards dreams (Blagrove & Akehurst, 2000), and openness to experiences. People with better visual memories when awake recall more dreams as do people with greater waking creativity and fantasy (Schredl, 2001). Also, people who awaken easily report recalling more dreams. Mood and stress also affect dream recall frequency (Domhoff, 1996).

Recall is facilitated by a brief arousal of the brain following the dream or a period of quiet upon awakening. Habitual short-duration sleepers recall fewer dreams (Hicks, Lucero, & Mistry, 1991) but shortening REMS intensifies dreaming (Fiss, 1991). Women tend to remember more dreams than men, and it seems like the most vivid and emotional dreams are the most recalled (Strauch & Meier, 1996).

While there is no magic formula that works for all, the following have helped many people increase their dream recall:

1. Tell yourself that dreams are important and that you want to remember them. People who take their dreams seriously and attend to them usually remember more dreams.

2. Have a tape-recorder or notebook at your bedside, so you can record the dream recall as soon as you awaken. Memory of dreams tends to fade quickly, so the sooner you get it down, the better.
3. Before you go to sleep, tell yourself several times, "I will remember a dream tonight."
4. If all else fails, set your alarm clock to awaken you during the early morning, or, better yet, have someone else set it to a time you are not aware of, or have someone else awaken you. REMS is more likely to be occurring then, and you are more likely to remember a dream when waking from REMS.
5. To improve what you do recall, right after you awaken, stay in bed and concentrate on what you were dreaming about from beginning to end.
6. If nothing comes, force yourself to write or dictate into the tape recorder a sentence about the first thing that came into your mind when you awoke. This practice gets you into the habit of concentrating on what is mentally occurring to you at awakening. Often, after a week or two of practice, the dream recalls start coming.
7. Get enough sleep. People who awaken sleepy may not be awake enough to recall their dreams.
8. Finally, be aware that alcohol and some drugs may make the recall of dreams more difficult. Make adjustments accordingly.

Chapter 7

Dreaming[18]

In Chapter 6 we reviewed the knowledge of what people dream about, in other words exploring dreams as objects. We now turn to examining the source of those dreams, that is, dreaming as activity. We will need two chapters to do this. In Chapter 8, we will explore first the theories of dreaming from the early 20th century, then more recent theories. In this chapter, we will review various elements of dreaming that are not comprehensive enough to be called a theory but nevertheless offer some understanding of the process of creating dreams. We will start by focusing on a few things that have been learned about the process of dreaming in the last 50 years, then overview how people in various cultures throughout recorded history have viewed the process of dreaming emphasizing current Western views.

THE PROCESS OF DREAMING

There was a time that it was believed that dreams occurred instantaneously, often at the time of awakening. Much of this belief can be attributed to a dream report by Alfred Maury, a 19th century dream researcher. He had a dream that he was in Paris at the time of the French revolution. He recalled being led to the guillotine and his head placed in it; a procedure that would have taken some time in real life. He awakened just as the blade struck his neck only to find that the headboard on his bed had fallen on this exact location! He reasoned that the entire dream must have been instantly fabricated from the sensation on his neck caused by fallen headboard.

The notion that dream formation is instantaneous was contradicted by 20th century research that found a correlation of the apparent time that had elapsed in the dream recall story with the amount of time the person had been in REMS before being awakened. However, this research used a small sample size, and replication has not been attempted (Domhoff & Schneider, 1999). Other research using incorporation was more conclusive. Incorporation occurs when a sound (or, less often, some other sensory stimulus) heard by a dreamer is woven into the dream rather than being ignored or causing awakening. (Many of you have had this experience, for you would raise your hand if asked, "Have you ever slept through your alarm clock, because it became a part of your dream?") A mist of water sprayed on the dreamer's face is often effective for producing incorporation. When in REMS, people were misted and then awakened at different times, such as 1, 3, or 7 minutes later, they generally reported events that would have taken an equivalent amount of time after the "cloudburst," "being splashed," "feeling a bird dump on their nose." Also, Maury did not write this dream down until 10 years after he recalled having it, which causes questions about its veracity. Conclusion: we probably dream in real time, although we may at times speed the process up.

Brain Organization

The functional organization of the brain is different during sleep than during waking, especially during REMS (see Chapter 4). The cortex is virtually isolated from sensory input and motor output during REMS. While much of the cortex is active during REMS, the prefrontal area, important for making critical assessments of perceptions and conceptions, is not active then. Thus, brain areas important for cognitive processes are active during REMS but some key components are not. This fact is consistent with the nature of recalled dream content, namely the bizarre, illogical, and non-volitional aspects of dreams.

Additionally

There may be multiple dreams per REMS period, especially for the longer bouts of REM, somewhat like watching a single channel on TV during a sequence of different half hour shows. However, since the boundaries between dreams are not always clearly defined, it is not possible to say for certain just how many different dreams are typical per night.

HISTORICAL/CULTURAL VIEWS ON THE SOURCES OF DREAMS

People from different cultures and different historical periods have varying opinions about just what dreams are. These beliefs can be sorted into the following four categories (from Webb, 1992):

- During the dream the dreamer exists in a different world.
- Dreams are omens and other indicators of the future.
- Dreams are meaningless artifacts of brain activity.
- Dreamer creates dream using things from their waking life.

Different World

Various peoples isolated in different parts of the world have independently had some form of the notion that when we dream our *self* (what we would call soul or spirit) leaves our body in this world and travels to another world where it exists for awhile. The dream is an awareness of this other existence. For some peoples, this other existence is totally separate from the waking world. For others, the two are related.

The Pantani Malay people and the unrelated Eskimos of Hudson Bay are two examples of peoples who understand dreaming as existence in a totally separate world. The Tajal of Luzon so strongly believe this idea that it is taboo to awaken a person who is asleep for fear that the person's self that is off in another world will be unable to rejoin the body in this world.

For other people, the dream world and the waking world are connected. People, such as those of the Kamchatka, Zulu, Borneo, and Kurdish cultures, believe that a favor received in a dream requires a return favor when awake. Likewise, if the dreamer insults someone in a dream, then an apology must soon be issued when awake. A crime committed in a dream is just as bad as one committed when awake. And so on. Other cultures seek to carry useful messages from the dream world back to the waking world. In many cultures, recalled dreams are used in collective decision making involving things like war and choosing political leaders.

Another variation of this category comes from some of the ancient Greeks who did not believe that persons went somewhere in their dreams; rather they were visited by dreams. Hypnos, the god of sleep, had a son, Morpheus, who was the god of dreams who oversaw this process.

Box 21

Senoi Dream Theory

During the 1960s, the Senoi dream theory became very popular and influential. This theory is said to derive from a small tribal group by that name who lived in the mountains of what is now central Malaysia. The Senoi were reported by Kilton R. Stewart, most notably in his widely reprinted 1951 journal article (Stewart, 1951), based on visits to them beginning in 1934, to greatly value dreams which in turn gave them better creativity, superior mental health, and a peaceful, cooperative culture.

Stewart reported that the Senoi had exemplary health and happiness. Mental illness was unknown among the Senoi and violence among them was nonexistent. All these traits were true, Stewart claimed, because the Senoi daily shared and discussed their dreams with others in their communities, encouraged and guided their children in sharing and using their dreams, and even were able to control and shape their dreams. Furthermore, they acted upon what happened in their dreams. For example, he reported that if a Senoi man dreamed that he hurt another person in a dream, then the dreamer would try to be especially friendly to that person during subsequent waking life. Or if another person injured the dreamer in a dream, then the dreamer should inform that person when awake in order to reverse the effects in a friendly manner.

Additionally, the Senoi were said to shape their dreams. They would meet threats in their dreams head-on, confronting them and attacking them if necessary. They would continually attempt to allow, and even work toward, the most pleasurable experiences in their dreams. They endeavored to have positive outcomes to their dreams and to bring to their waking life a message or gift from each dream.

Stewart's reports of Senoi dream theory led a number of people in the United States in the 1960s to try to emulate the Senoi in order to obtain the same kinds of benefits from working with their own dreams. Groups shared and discussed their dreams, and individuals made efforts to control their dreams for better outcomes. Reports of the benefits of the Senoi theory were given at psychological, anthropological, and sleep society meetings. Articles were written and published in both the academic journals and popular magazines. In short, the Senoi dream theory was taken seriously and became popular in the United States.

The Stewart study of the Senoi was seriously challenged by psychologist and sociologist William Domhoff in 1985. He had done his Ph.D. thesis on dreams a couple of decades earlier and had published a number of articles after that. For his 1985 book, he gathered and read what Stewart had written, some of it unpublished, about the Senoi, especially things Stewart had written prior to his pivotal 1951 article. He also interviewed or corresponded with colleagues and family of Stewart, who was dead by this time, and read accounts by others who had studied the Senoi. His conclusion was that Stewart had over time infused his own notions about the benefits of dream sharing and dream control into his idealized notions of Senoi society. The Senoi, by all other accounts, were not as happy, peaceful, and mentally healthy as Stewart described them in 1951. Nor was the sharing and controlling of their dreams a dominant aspect of their daily lives. In fact, the Senoi thought about and used dreams no more than any other native culture. Nothing special was going on. Domhoff speculated that Stewart wrote about the Senoi and their supposed dreaming practices based on Stewart's personality, but this opinion need not concern us here.

Domhoff goes on to say that regardless of the veracity of Stewart's claims regarding the Senoi, there may be benefits of dream sharing and control. Yet, the research evidence covering the application of Senoi dream theory in the United States is not very encouraging. It has not been possible to demonstrate many positive benefits of the type Stewart and contemporary Senoi dream theory practitioners have claimed.

Dreams as Omens

The notion that dreams are a means to guide or forecast the future also has its origins in the ancient world. For example, dreams play an important role in the *Odyssey* offering guidance and providing omens. Vestiges of this notion remain today in the Western World often joined with other understandings of the psychic role of dreams, such as clairvoyance and telepathy.

Numerous cultures have designated certain individuals to aid people in understanding what their dreams are telling them about the future. Typically these priests, priestesses, elders, and the like were held in high esteem and were often very powerful and influential. The Greeks had hundreds of temples where people could go in order to have dreams of guidance, with the priests interpreting the meanings for them.

The Judeo-Christian world is familiar with this concept, because of the many prophetic dreams found in the Bible, especially those of Jacob's ladder, the dreams of Pharaoh that required interpretation by the Hebrew slave Joseph, and the dreams Joseph had about Mary being pregnant with Jesus as reported in the Christian New Testament. These stories reflect the prevalent understanding of the source of dreams at the time the Bible was written and the serious regard that people had for them then.

While this idea can no longer be considered to be the dominant understanding of the source of dreams in the Western world, the idea that dreams have predictive capabilities is nevertheless prevalent. People still consult dictionary-like books in which they can look up an object or action from a dream to see what it "really means," including indicators for the future. (Great caution should be exercised when using such books. They have never been shown to have any accuracy or validity. Many draw heavily from the *Oneirocritica* written by the Roman physician Artemidorus in about 150 A.D., using the writer's personal experience and imagination or surveys. None of these books demonstrates any attempt at objective verification. It is better to consider them entertainment rather then taking what they say seriously.)

Psychic dreams, a variation of this category, is given serious consideration in the Western world today. Reports of dreams that are telepathic (= thought transfer), precognitive (= seeing the future), and clairvoyant (= perception of current events beyond sensory awareness) are taken seriously by many. This idea is present even at the annual meetings of the Association for the Study of Dreams in the United States where organized attempts at group dreaming and thought transfer via dreams are interleaved among the scientific sessions.

A number of attempts at scientific verification of such psychic dreams has occurred in the 20th century and still continue today. However, none of these experiments is found to be satisfactory when critically scrutinized. In some cases, the designs of the experiments contain flaws or lack appropriate controls. In other cases, minimal effects are exaggeratedly viewed as being significant.

For example, in one experiment (Ullman, Krippner, & Vaughan, 1989), pairs of friends participated. One slept in a typical sleep lab, while the other spent the night concentrating on a famous painting randomly selected from a group of 12. During each REMS period, the sleeping friend was awakened for a dream report. Any kind of a similarity between some aspect of the selected painting and any portion of any of the dreams were considered evidence of telepathy. Additionally, the next morning the sleeper was shown the 12 paintings and was asked to rank in order how similar each was to dreams from the night. If the painting selected for the night viewing was in the top six picked out by the sleeper, this result was considered additional evidence for telepathy. Both of these criteria for success are extremely weak. Directly dreaming about the entire painting and then being able to emphatically pick the painting out from among the 12 would be far more convincing. Additionally, appropriate controls should have been used, such as repeating the experiment with exactly the same procedure except never letting the awake friend view any of the pictures.

Other research has produced decidedly negative results. For example, in the 1930s when the baby of the world-famous flyer Charles Lindberg was kidnapped, Murray and Wheeler (1937) placed ads in newspapers asking people to submit their dreams of the location and fate of the baby. Thirteen hundred dream reports were received. Later, after the baby's body was found buried, the dream reports were compared to what actually happened. Only 7 contained content that even partially resembled the truth. Most contained false speculations that were widely reported in the newspapers. This study concluded that there was no support for psychic dreaming.

Box 22

Comments on the Apparent Psychic Sources of Dreams

Why, you might ask, have people in various cultures at various times believed that there may be psychic sources of dreams? Why do some people today still hold these views? The answer is simple, while the reasons for rejecting these views are more complex yet more valid. The simple answer is that this psychic phenomenon is what people experience. Some people have had "out-of-body" dream experiences. Others have dreamed something that later seemed to come true. Still others dreamed that something was wrong with a distant loved-one only to find out that the individual had been in an accident or had died. Such experiences can be very compelling and seem to offer proof of the psychic source of dreams, or at least some dreams. Yet experience is not proof. Here is where the more complex reasons for rejecting these views enter in.

Our experiencing of the world depends on our brain putting together information from our senses of vision, hearing, touching, and so forth in a meaningful way (see Chapter 8). It usually does a quite good job, but not always. We can and do perceive things that are really not there. Visual illusions are a good example. We can perceive things that appear quite real yet are physically impossible. Movies are another good example. We perceive continuous action when we view a movie, yet all we really are seeing is a series of still images; the portions of our brain responsible for perception smoothes things over so we do not perceive jerky transitions between the individual images. Numerous psychological and brain studies have led to a detailed understanding of how our brain/mind does much of this task.

The brain does the same thing when we are sleeping. It endeavors to make the best perceptions of the sensory information available to it (see Chapter 8). However, little of the sensory information available to the brain while we are sleeping actually originates in our sensory receptors such as our eyes, ears, and skin (see Chapter 4). Rather, it is generated from the areas of the brain that normally receive and process the information from our sensory receptors (see Chapter 8). Perceptions, such as being outside of one's body, often seem as real and as vivid as when we are awake, but they are no more real than are our waking illusions. They have not occurred in a real world sense.

Apparent telepathic, clairvoyant, and precognitive dreams can likewise be explained using scientifically verified knowledge about the workings of the brain/mind, albeit complex, without having to resort to simpler yet hypothetical powers and energies. The experience of some persons that their dreams have been telepathic, clairvoyant, or precognitive, necessarily rely on recall of the contents of these dreams. However, as we have seen in chapter 6, our memories of our dreams are far from accurate and are subject to change over time. Experiments with waking memories for events likewise show that they can be influenced by what was experienced later (see almost any introductory psychology textbook for more on this topic). For example, the memory of a witness to an automobile accident can easily be changed by later seeing a similar accident or even similar vehicles. Thus, it is entirely likely that the memory of a dream that later seemed to come true may have been altered by the later, actual event, giving the strong impression that the dream foretold the future.

An example I have used before (Moorcroft, 1993) comes from one of my students. The event:

> We were at Grandpa's farm. I went for a walk by myself toward the hill that was part of the pasture. I had new white nail polish on. It was a beautiful spring day. Suddenly, Gramp's new white puppy ran over the hill toward me and wanted to play.

The related dream report:

> It was just like the dream I had the week before. In the dream, I was in my backyard putting white polish on my nails. I was sitting on the ground on a bright, warm, sunny day. I looked up and there was a hill covered with wildflowers extending from our backyard, and there was a white puppy running down the hill toward me. It came up to me and playfully kissed me.

Both the event—and recall of the dream—occurred several days after the dream. It is probable that the event influenced the dream report, especially in its details. It may seem that the dream foretold the event, but it is far more likely that the event altered the memory of the prior dream.

Additionally we tend to focus more on the dreams that seem to be psychic and ignore all the rest. In the example above, had the event not occurred after the dream, it is doubtful that the student would have paid as much attention to the dream later. Or if there was no dream related to the event, it is likely that the event would have received little attention. It is only in those startling cases where the event seems to relate to a prior dream that we focus on this connection and may attribute it to being a psychic dream.

Other explanations include the fact that we perceive more than we can consciously attend to when we are awake. Sometimes these perceptions become part of a dream that appears to be psychic. For example, we may have subconsciously noticed that a railing is loose and it may be incorporated into a dream. Shortly thereafter, somebody has an accident because the railing broke, making it look like the dream was psychic.

Yet, for the most part, science can never prove the nature of things and especially cannot prove that something cannot happen. All science can do is to show that something is more or less probable. It can show that apparently psychic dreams are much more likely due to known behavioral and brain mechanisms than to highly improbable hypotheticals. Another way of putting it is that the supposed psychic phenomena in dreams suffer from a low fact to assumption ratio. There is just no hard data to back them up. Nevertheless, it is possible, but remote, that scientists do not yet have the tools with which to discover the facts of psychic phenomena. We need to leave the lid open just a crack on the possibility of psychic dreams.

Dreams as Meaningless

There are people, including many brain scientists, who during the 20th century continuing through today view dreams as meaningless. "Träume sind Schäume" (= German for "Dreams are foam," just like that fluffy stuff on the top of the real thing, the beer) was what many of Freud's contemporaries said. Dreams are meaningless accompaniments of activity of the brain during sleep (see Chapter 12), are accidental fabrications of the brain during the period of transition from the state of sleep to the state of wakefulness (see Chapter 4), or are merely responses of our brain to occasional external stimulation, such as a noise or internal stimulation, such as indigestion, In any case, dreams are seen as essentially meaningless whether at an unconscious level or at the level of full awareness. One theory (Crick & Mitchison, 1983) even maintains that dreams are the result of the mind clearing out useless memories and that, if we try to recall and analyze our dreams, we are undermining this process. Others, even non-scientists, simply reject dreams as not being relevant and important to their own waking lives. To them, it is a waste of time to pay any attention to dreams.

Dreams as Related to Dreamer's Waking Life

Each of us conceives of, writes, directs, casts, creates the scenery, and usually stars in several dreams every night, seven days a week, that are comparable to TV programs for which we are the sole audience. This experience is a tremendous creative endeavor well beyond what most of us think we are capable of when awake. These dreams most resemble TV soap operas with a prevalence of negative emotions involving many familiar characters and settings, yet others contain content of things strange and new. Our dreams tend to focus around things that are of personal importance to us especially at an emotional level. Just as with TV soap operas, our dreams focus on key components of the story rather than include each mundane detail. Aspects may be distorted for emphasis or symbolic in order to bring more meaning. But always they are ours and important to us.

This idea is the most prevalent notion in the Western world today about the source of dreams. Individuals are the source of their own dreams, and their dreams reflect their personal concerns and experiences, self-view, worldview, and waking situations. People in the United States mostly dream about houses and cars, and their dreams are populated with people dressed like their neighbors. The dreams of people in small primitive societies contain huts or tents, yaks or oxen, and people dressed far differently than people in the United States. Preference seems to be given to more recent waking events, thoughts, and emotions. These dreams are not exact reflections of the waking world but rather are more like dramas that portray things in such a way to be useful and meaningful to the dreamer. The elements of the dream are put together according to dreamers' typical ways of organizing their perceptions and knowledge and emotional overlay. These elements and organization may differ considerably from one individual to another.

While never very popular until the 20th century, this view of the source of dreams has ancient roots. Aristotle saw dreams as perceptions similar but not identical to waking perceptions. Many of our waking perceptions are based on sensing physical stimuli, but we can still perceive these things by imagining them in our minds when the stimuli are not present. In the same way, we can imagine things in our minds when asleep. Yet, when asleep, the perceptions may be distorted since the "intellect" is not working as it does when we are awake. This phenomenon is like "eddies in a great river ... (that are often) broken into other forms by collisions with other objects" (Aristotle as quoted in Borbély, 1986). Additionally, to Aristotle, dream content is distorted and exaggerated by our emotions left over from waking experiences.

The great popularity today of this notion about the source of dreams can be attributed to Freud. In his classic book, *The Interpretation of Dreams*, published in 1900, he stressed that dreams are the creation of the dreamer's mind originating in "wish-fulfillment." Although Freud maintained that these wishes are disguised from our awareness, they nevertheless emanate from our own minds and waking lives. And they are of great benefit for the dreamer, for they relieve the pressure coming from unfulfilled unconscious desires of waking life (see Chapter 8). While many of those who followed in Freud's footsteps later rejected the concept that we are not aware and cannot easily be aware of the meaning of our dreams, they nevertheless accepted the basic idea that our dreams are a product of our mind formed out of our waking experiences, needs and concerns.

The contemporary version of this approach toward the source of dreams draws on the understanding of how the brain works. Within the brain/mind of each of us are networks of memories from acquired knowledge and experiences, many in the form of images. There are also networks of stored information about our individual personalities as well our dominant modes of perceiving, thinking, and reacting. Also included are our individual world-views, our hopes and fears, and our current as well as enduring concerns. Various components of these networks are linked with one another such that when one component is accessed, it is easier to access the other linked components. Thus, a particular emotion may be linked to specific experiences, both recent and remote, that evoked that emotion during past wakefulness or in past dreams, for that matter. Some of the components form the core of the linkages while others have varying degrees of remoteness. When a core component is accessed it is more likely that the components linked to it will also be accessed. This linkage can also happen, but is less likely, when a more remotely linked component is the first to be accessed. On the other hand, research by Robert Stickgold in Hobson's dream research lab at Harvard suggests that linkages *to* more remote components are more favored during REMS (see Chapter 12). Others say that even some previously non-associated, or at least not obviously associated, elements are brought into the dream.

When something, especially an emotion, is experienced during the day, it is more likely to form the core of dream content during the next, or perhaps a subsequent, night because various brain cell processes favor reactivating recently activated connections between cells. These core components link to other components to form much of the content of the dream. It is not unusual for what is linked to be to components, such as people, events, settings, and so forth, from the dreamer's past. However, dreams are not simply replays of what happened during the day or the past, but they draw upon these things and use them in ways for, seemingly, their own purposes.

Mid 20th century psychologist and dream researcher, Calvin Hall, stated in his 1966 book *The Meaning of Dreams*, that dreams seldom focus on current events such as elections, war, athletic events, happenings from newspapers. These things may be common topics of conversation, but seldom topics of our dreams. Kelley Bulkeley, who has a Ph.D. in religious studies and a strong professional interest in dreams, has investigated the implications of Hall's statement. He agrees that political themes are relatively rare in recalled dreams, but when they are present, they add to the understanding of the source of dreams. They show how dreams can help dreamers with their personal internal world by relating them to things happening around them that are important to them or that may have personal consequences.

Bulkeley began by studying detailed dream diaries of 12 people during the 2 weeks straddling the presidential election in the United States in 1992. This election contest, mainly between sitting Republican president George Bush senior,

Democratic challenger Bill Clinton, and independent candidate Ross Perot, was exciting and passionately waged and dominated the print as well as electronic media for weeks. Six of the 12 subjects reported at least one dream with some content about the election and of the total of 113 dream reports, 10 contained such content. As Bulkeley concludes, since many people during this election "felt that the political state of the United States was confusing, strange, and frightening" (p. 188), it should not be surprising that some people occasionally dreamed about it.

Additional data from that presidential election and the next one four years later, Bulkeley (personal communication, 2001) find three kinds of dreams related to politics: political cartoons of the mind, new political perspectives, and personal symbols.

Political Cartoons of the Mind

There are dreams expressing in succinct and sometimes very humorous ways the dreamer's waking life political perspective. Here's an example from a 36-year old man from Florida:

> I'm playing golf with Bill Clinton. I've heard people say he cheats, and I understand what they mean, because he frequently improves the lie of his ball. But he encourages the people he's playing with to do the same. He says, "It's just a game, and just for fun!"

This dreamer voted enthusiastically for Clinton in 1992, but in 1996, when he had this dream, he was not sure if he would vote for Clinton in the upcoming election. The dreamer saw the golf imagery of his dream as an expression of his concern that President Clinton is a "cheater" who frequently "improves his lies" and then tries to smooth-talk other people into letting him get away with it.

Personal Symbols

There are dreams using the figures of politicians as "personal symbols" to express strong emotions that the dreamer is feeling toward some matter in his or her waking life. Here's an example from a 55-year old woman from New Mexico:

> I'm back in college, in one of the classrooms, and Bill Clinton is one of the students. Then he's the teacher, and he asks me how alcohol manufacturers get us to drink so much. I say I haven't given the question much thought.

This dreamer had long struggled with alcoholism, and, in her dream, she sees the President as the voice of "executive authority" within her, a voice that is prompting her to think more carefully about why she drinks.

New Political Perspectives

There are dreams directly calling into question the dreamer's waking life political attitudes, leading the dreamer to think anew about his or her accustomed beliefs about a politician or a political issue. This example comes from a 44-year old man from New York:

> I'm on a camping trip with the President and his party in a heavily wooded area. Suddenly, Clinton darts up a hill into the woods. He sees a bear approaching the camping area. None of us moves, as the President confronts the bear; Clinton is very expert and competent as he does this, not wild or frightened. He manages to drive the huge bear, the size of a Grizzly, into a snare set for him. The FBI in the entourage are angry at the close call, but the President seems unperturbed.

This dreamer said that from the start he had been skeptical of Bill Clinton's leadership qualities, but he awoke from this dream surprised by Clinton's swift, assertive, and fearless response to the threat of the huge bear. As a result of his dream, this man reconsidered his generally dim view of Clinton's executive abilities, wondering if he had been overlooking the President's skills as a fighter.

The two of these types of political dreams are helping the politically concerned dreamers understand and sort out their feelings about current political events. The third type uses political characters currently in the news as convenient characters in dreams to help the dreamers better understand themselves.

HOW DREAMS ARE PRODUCTS OF OUR MINDS

There is considerable evidence that dreams are the product of the dreamer's mind. People report dreaming about things familiar to them, and such things must come from their own memory pool. This familiarity includes the person's knowledge, experiences, life-situation, and world-view. Recalled dream content is more related to the dreamer's current concerns, that is, goals that are emotionally important, than other types of themes (Nikles et al., 1998). Additionally, those things most recently experienced or thought about are more likely to be present in dreams. Yet, there are also common elements in what neighbors, friends, and relatives report dreaming about, showing that our culture also influences dream content.

Kramer and Roth (1979) found a correlation of 0.49 in the content of recalled dreams on successive nights. According to standard statistical procedures, this number shows that 24% of what determined recalled dream content on a given night also influenced what was in the recalled dream content of the next night. This finding still leaves over three-fourths of the source of the subsequent night's recalled dream content unaccounted for, which Kramer and Roth believe comes out of the experiences of the intervening day.

In a subsequent study, these same researchers plus additional colleagues (Kramer et al., 1981) compared the content of thinking just before and just after sleep to the recalled dream content during sleep. They found that one-half of the content categories studied showed significant correlations (of which 14 were positive) from which they concluded that what people report dreaming about is largely continuous with what they think about during their waking life. Yet, over half of the categories did not yield positive correlations, suggesting that there are additional factors that influence dream content. What people dream about seems to have many sources, including, but not limited to, what people are thinking about when awake.

While the idea that the psychological state and the personality of a person contribute to dream generation can be found in ancient through contemporary writings, there is only a small correlation between what personality tests reveal about persons and the nature of their dreams. Anxious persons report more anxious dreams, and relaxation training that reduces anxiety in these persons results in an increase in the reported pleasantness in their dreams. Also, people successfully treated for their phobias report experiencing a reduction in phobic objects in their dreams. The dreams of depressed people contain more masochism, dependency, helplessness, and hopelessness, which is like their waking thoughts (Weiss, 1986). Furthermore, age and gender have been shown to cause great individual differences in recalled dream content, but social class, structure of the family, and health also can have an influence.

Based on his studies of dream recall development in children (see Chapter 6), David Foulkes (c.f. 1999) maintains that the ability to dream gradually develops during childhood beginning at about 5 years of age, becomes well formed by age 9, but continues developing through age 12–13. Foulkes sees this development in the ability to dream as depending on the development of visual-spatial abilities in the brain, as measured by various tests during waking.

Others interpret Foulkes's data differently (c.f. Hobson et al., 2000). For example, the low quality and quantity of dream recall at early ages could just as well be due to the fact that language ability is not sufficient to describe the dream experiences that children may actually be having.

PRESLEEP EXPERIENCES

Attempts to manipulate dream content by exposing people to specific experiences prior to sleep have had only mild success. Among the things that have been tried are social isolation, vigorous exercise, difficult or stressful mental tasks, subliminal stimulation, and wearing tinted goggles. Likewise, films with graphic, emotion-arousing scenes, such as a difficult birth, amputation, ritual circumcision, hard core pornography, compared to films with comparatively neutral images, have only occasional influence on dream content. However, some studies suggest the influence of such experiences on dream content may not occur until several nights later.

The best success in this area was obtained by Roffwarg and colleagues (1978). They had nine people wear red tinted goggles for 5 days when awake. During this time, their dream recalls went from containing a normal spectrum of colors to primarily only reds. Overall, there was a three-fold increase in the color red in the dream reports even among those told to expect more green, the complimentary color to red. Furthermore, the amount of red reported in dreams increased from the first through the third days of the experiment.

Actually, it turns out that the waking experience most likely to influence dream content is the sleep lab itself. It is not unusual for someone sleeping in a sleep lab, whether a part of this type of experiment or not, to report dreaming of people in lab coats, a room full of strange electrical machinery, things glued to the head, long wires, and so forth. This experience occurs about one-third of the time.

Dream Incubation

Some who specialize in dream interpretation maintain that people can learn to "incubate" dream content. While little published research has been done on the validity of dream incubation, Delaney (1998) reports that several studies show high success rates. Better results occur when dreamers are given help interpreting the meaning of the metaphorical content of the recalled dream showing how it related to their incubation efforts. Additionally, Nikles and colleagues (1998) found that people are more likely to incubate dreams when directed to dream about things related to their personal current concerns than if directed to dream about other things or given no directive. They also found that suggested topics related to personal concerns frequently became the central topic of a reported dream. (See Box 23 for Delaney's method of dream incubation.)

All in all, dreams it seems are semi-autonomous. They seem to have their own agenda of what to focus on, but sometimes this content can be influenced.

Box 23

Dream Incubation: Delaney's Method

Gayle Delaney, Ph.D., is a dream psychologist who has devoted her career to working with dreaming. In her books *Living Your Dreams* (1996) and *All about Dreams* (1998) she describes in detail her method for successfully incubating dreams. The crucial step in her method is to write down and then repeat what you want to dream about over and over again as you are falling asleep. This request could be to dream about something in particular or to answer a question. This task is all accomplished dream incubators need to do. However, neophytes need to do more in order to insure success.

Begin by choosing a night when you are not overly tired and have some time both before bed and upon awakening to work on this technique. In a journal, begin be writing a few lines about what you did and felt during the day. Next, focus on an issue you would like to dream about and write out a thorough discussion of the issue. Be sure to include your feelings on the issue. Now, and this is an important but not always easy step, compose and write a one-line request or question. As you are ready to fall asleep, repeat the request or question over and over. As soon as you awaken from a dream, or at the end of your sleep period, write down your recall of your dream(s) with as much detail as possible. Perhaps the dream obviously fulfills your request or answers your question, but it is more likely that it is metaphorical. In either case, Delaney recommends that you work with the dream to fully understand its meanings. (See Chapter 8 for this technique.)

CULTURE

Even our culture can influence our dreaming. While some things appear to be typical of recalled dreams in all cultures, such as falling, flying, or being unable to move, anthropological studies show that what people report dreaming about and even the amount of dream recall, and thus possibly the amount of dreaming itself, are influenced by the dreamer's language, religious beliefs, social structures, and customs. For example, there are some differences in the dreams of the Japanese and people in three East African societies from those of people in the Western industrialized world (Domhoff, 1996). While Japanese men report two times as many men as women in their dreams, just as do men in the in the Western world, women's reports in Japan differ greatly. Whereas women in the Western world report approximately equal numbers of male and female characters in their dreams, Japanese women recall a 2:1 ratio of women characters compared to male characters. This difference is thought to correspond to the intense gender segregation in Japanese society. Both men and women report much less aggression in their dreams than do their counterparts in the West. The reduction was much larger for the men than the women. Again, the dream differences are thought to relate to differences in Japanese society regarding everyday aggression.

In three male dominated societies of East Africa, the Gusii, the Kipsigis, and the Logoli, the males revealed a greater percent of males vs. females characters in their dreams, whereas the females showed ratios much closer to equal. This finding closely parallels what is found in Western industrialized societies but differs greatly from that found in Japan. Aggression in dreams showed a different pattern. The East African women reported much more physical aggression in their dreams than did Western women or Japanese women. They also reported more non-physical aggression than their male counterparts did. This finding, too, differed from reports from Western and Japanese women. These aggression results are related to a great concern about being victimized among the East African women.

Other things, such as socioeconomic class, can have an effect on dream content. For example, people of lower socioeconomic status have more misfortune in their dreams; people in upper class less death anxiety (Anch et al., 1988).

In spite of notable differences like those found in cross-cultural comparisons of dream report content, most aspects of dreaming and resultant dreams seem to be universal (Domhoff, 1996). This universality includes things like the widely noted higher ratio of aggression compared to friendly interactions and more misfortune than good fortune.

PHYSIOLOGICAL EVENTS OF THE BODY

A common idea expressed in some ancient through contemporary writings is that dreams are generated by internal sensations, such as indigestion after eating an anchovy, onion, and green pepper pizza right before bedtime, or by illness. Some Greek as well as other writers even maintained that dream content could be used to help diagnose physical illnesses. Yet, of the many studies that have tried to relate physiological changes in the body to dream content, the results have been disappointing.

Dramatic thirst caused by 24 hours without fluid intake prior to sleep failed to produce any dream content related to drinking or thirst. However, in another experiment, the subjects not only went without fluid for 24 hours prior to going to sleep, but also ate salty food just before bedtime. Their dream reports contained various references to water, including snow and lakes and more specific thirst-related objects such as pop. Thus, strong internal physiological stimuli may sometimes contribute to what is dreamed about, but only some of the time (Empson, 1993).

Overall, however, extensive studies of the relationship between physiological events including heart rate, muscle activity of the face, and erections of the penis have failed to show consistent relationships to dream content or amount of recall. For example, heart rate does not seem to be related to the emotionality in the dream but changes during strong emotions when awake. One exception is some relationship between recalled dream content and breathing rate at the time of the dream.

EFFECTS OF SENSATIONS ON DREAMING

Although you, like many people, may recall having slept through a buzzing alarm clock, because you incorporated the sound into your dream, laboratory studies show that incorporation is infrequent. Various kinds of stimuli have been used including light, sound, and touch. Of all things tried, spraying water onto the face of sleepers most frequently produces incorporation but only at 42% in one study (Dement & Wolpert, 1958). It is incorporated directly as being squirted or indirectly as a sudden shower or a leak in the roof. Even electric shocks applied to the wrist result in reported incorporation into a dream only one out of five times. It is extremely rare for the stimulus to become a dominant element in the dream. Most often it becomes some minor element in an ongoing dream. Likewise, internal physiological events such as erections of the penis or a full bladder do not regularly influence dream content. Higher rates of incorporation are reported when less literal representations of the stimulus are counted. For example, when the stimulus was jet sounds, dream recall containing sounds of a gas stove that spits was counted as incorporation as was the stimulus of weeping sounds as squeaking footsteps (Strauch & Meier, 1996).

An example of this kind of research was done by Ralph Berger (1963). While his subjects were awake, he determined which names of each one's friends evoked the greatest emotional responses on recordings of their galvanic skin responses—a component frequently used in lie detection. He then spoke one of these names to each subject while asleep. He found evidence of incorporation on about half of the trials, but only in 3 of the 48 instances of incorporation the named individual appear in the recalled dream. Most of the rest were based on assonance such as "Chilean" for "Gillian" and "like" for "Mike."

One interpretation of these data is that the agenda for a dream has a less literal basis such as some general emotional need and that the specific contents of the dream are there only if they in some way contribute to that overriding theme. This phenomenon includes presleep experiences and stimuli experienced during the dream as well as general knowledge and memories. Another interpretation is that dream contents are randomly selected from all that is available and that presleep experiences and sensations during sleep are simply included in this large pool.

Taking another tack, it is reasonable to hypothesize that phasic events of REMS such as rems or surges in heart rate would affect dream content. Specifically it was hypothesized that dreams would be more intense with more perceptions vs. thoughts and more bizarre during such phasic events. However, laboratory tests largely failed to confirm this hypothesis. Likewise, things like k-complexes during NREMS were shown to have little effect on reported mentation. Yet, reported dream content when phasic events are more frequent, such as a high "density" of rems, have been reported to be more emotional, more vivid, contain more activity, and better recalled.

THINGS THAT CHANGE DREAMS FOR INDIVIDUALS

There is a consistency in persons' recalled dreams over their adult lifetime, but significant emotional events can cause changes (Domhoff, 1996). For example, successful psychotherapy can cause changes in recalled dream content (Hunt, 1989), and people who have experienced sexual abuse have more frequent and intense nightmares (Penn, Bootzin, & Wood, 1991). Even better examples come from the study of recalled dreams when a person is undergoing a distinct major life event that has strong emotional implications such as pregnancy, divorce, or psychological trauma.

Dream Changes during Pregnancy

Pregnancy, especially the first one, is a major change in a woman's life. There are emotional as well as physiological changes that influence dream content as the pregnancy takes its course (Maybruck, 1986; Stunkane, 1985). What happens in recalled dreams during the first pregnancy has been studied.

During the first few months of the pregnancy, sometimes beginning even before she knows she is pregnant, the content of a woman's recalled dreams changes. Some of the dreams are obviously related to pregnancy, such as themes related to fertility and reproductive ability, miscarriage, and dangerous or intrusive fetuses. Other themes are thought to be more symbolically related, such as an increase of small animals (representing the fetus) in recalled dreams. More generally, she may recall dreaming more about herself than she had before.

By the middle of the pregnancy, the content of recalled dreams changes. Now there is more critical judgment of herself and her significant other. There are concerns about being an adequate mother that emerge, as well as many of the kinds of things that can go wrong with being a mother. She may typically dream about her relationship with the prospective father as well as that of her own mother and of her comparisons with her mother. Babies rather than small animals are more likely to populate her recalled dreams. It is not uncommon for these babies to be abnormal in some way. Continuing from the earlier phase of the pregnancy are dreams of the baby as some kind of trespasser. By late middle pregnancy, the fetus in her dream recalls often are more appealing, but there are dreams of various general disasters involving not only labor and delivery but also finances, careers, marriage, and the like.

During the last couple months of pregnancy most women report recalling many more dreams than they had previously. This increased recall seems to happen not because of having more dreams but because of waking up more often during this stage of the pregnancy (see chapter 5) and thus being able to recall more of the dreams. Women recall continuing to dream of the things they did during the middle of their pregnancy, such as comparing themselves to their mother and unusual or abnormal babies, but also about changes in their body and how they are the focus of special attention by others. As the pregnancy draws to a close, they begin to recall dreaming of the birthing process itself and of their doctor.

Subsequent pregnancies also affect the dreams of the woman but with some differences. For example, recalled dreams about her ability to be a mother and comparisons with her own mother tend to be replaced by concerns about the relationship of the new child with the existing family members.

It is not entirely clear if these changes in recalled dream content are due to the psychological or physiological changes that accompany pregnancy. However, the situation is clearer when looking at the changes that also occur in the recalled dreams of the prospective father (Siegel, 1983; Stukane, 1985). Since he is much less physiologically involved in the pregnancy, changes in his dream recall must be psychologically based.

After he becomes aware that he initiated a pregnancy in a woman, the prospective father recalls dreaming more about his sexual masculinity and identity. He may recall dreams with more sexual activity in them. A conflict between his machismo and his nurturance may also emerge. During the middle of the pregnancy, the themes of nurturance continue, but dreams about his general identity replace those of overt sex. In his dreams, he may compare himself to his father and to his family when he was a child. At the same time he may dream of being left out of the pregnancy process, or he may even dream about being pregnant himself. He often will dream about his relationship with his pregnant partner. Later in the pregnancy, his recalled dreams about his childhood family diminish, being replaced by content about his current family. He may also recall dreaming about his changes in his partner's body, what his child will be like (more often as a son than a daughter), and, toward the end of the pregnancy, the birthing process.

Note the similarities between the dreams of pregnant women and their partners responsible for the pregnancy. Early on, both focus on themselves and the changes that the pregnancy may bring for them. As the pregnancy progresses, they both begin to recall dreaming more about the pregnancy itself, the baby, and their relationship to one another.

Dreams of Depressed

Rosalind Cartwright (1989; Cartwright, Young, Mercer, & Bears, 1998) has done an extensive series of research studies on the dreams of people undergoing a major and usually emotionally difficult change in their lives, namely divorce. She hypothesized that if we dream about things that are important to us, and especially if these things arouse strong emotions, then the dreams of divorcing people, many of whom are very depressed during the process, should show obvious differences from the dreams of non-divorcing, non-depressed cohorts.

Cartwright found that people who are divorcing and are depressed have their first REMS period earlier, and their REMS periods are more evenly distributed through the night. Additionally, they have noticeably more rems during their REMS. All these symptoms are considered signs of emotional overload. Further, they report recalling dreams that are shorter, more oriented to the past, more masochistic, more repetitive, and blander. Also, the themes of their recalled dreams are often that things are "all my fault." They seem impotent in their recalled dreams in the sense that, as a character, they are unable to do even simple things such as being able to move their arms. Likewise, things do not seem to work, such as drawers not opening. Also, important things like keys to the car are lost. By the end of the night, the negativity in their dreams is increased rather than reduced, and there is no progression from dream to dream through the night. Cartwright also finds that, as the depression abates, these characteristics of their dreams lessen.

Psychological Trauma

Hartmann (1998) points to recalled dreams following traumatic events as the clearest case of showing the source of dreams. These dreams may occur for some months following the trauma but eventually go away. (For dreams that do not fade with time following trauma, see the discussion about PTSD in Chapter 9.) People will dream of the incident but with changes in details. The changes continue as the person dreams again and again of the incident. In spite of these changes, people will say years later that they remember the dreams as being an "exact replay" of the incident. Others will recall dreams about the incident that are more metaphorical, such as dreaming of a tidal wave or great whirlwind about to overtake them. They report feeling terrified and vulnerable during the dream. These descriptions best illustrate how emotions can be the instigating focus of dream content, because it is obvious that the emotion of the traumatic situation is on the person's mind when awake. (Incidentally, he finds that such dreams can be somewhat equivalent to our own internal psychotherapist, because they enable the dreamer to work through the trauma in a "safe place" just as happens when talking to a trained therapist in the safety of the office following a trauma.)

CONCLUSION

Dreams, like sleep, occur between two periods of wakefulness. They are influenced by prior waking and can influence subsequent waking. Today, most dream researchers agree that dreams are constructed by the same mental processes that we use when awake, but the source of material differs (Bulkeley, 1997). They also seem to concur that dreaming plays a role in processing both external and internal information from waking, which helps adaptation to the environment by organizing perceptions, keeping cognitive mechanisms exercised, and integrating new with existing memories. Dream researcher Bill Domhoff (personal communication, July, 2001) sees the contents of dreams as being mostly continuous with our waking lives, generally expressing our conceptions and concerns. Further, studies of series of dreams show there is a lot of repetition in what an individual dreams about (Domhoff, 1996). Dreams contain the "conceptions, concerns, and interests" of the dreamer (Domhoff, 1996, p. 153), but do not necessarily reflect how they behave during their waking lives. Domhoff (1996) does not believe that dreams are compensatory, that is bringing some kind of balance or healing to our waking lives, but other dream researchers think they can sometimes be compensatory. However, this issue is difficult to scientifically assess (Van de Castle, 1994).

Chapter 8

Theories of Dreams and Dreaming

In this chapter, I will review various theories of dreaming for you. Each theory was chosen, because it has been historically important in introducing new ideas about the nature of dreams, because it has significantly modified old theories, or is new and potentially influential. Also, these theories were selected from among many in order to demonstrate the wide range of such theories. It is not possible completely and adequately to present any one of these theories in one short chapter. What follows is an introduction to these theories that attempts to emphasize their key aspects, especially the things that make each distinctive and important. The reader is directed to the references for each of the theories from which deeper and more complete understanding and appreciation of them can be gained.

A major change in the attitude and approach to dreams began with the work of Sigmund Freud at the beginning of the twentieth century, so we will first explore his theories and methods. Freud popularized a whole new way of thinking about how the mind works, with particular emphasis on the unconscious and the role of dreams. Prior to Freud, most people tended to view dreams as coming from a source external to themselves (see Chapter 6) or, like many scientists of his day, as meaningless products of the sleeping brain. Because of Freud, most people in the Western world began to see dreams as being meaningful creations of the dreamer's mind. After Freud, numerous others accepted his basic notion but were critical of some, or even many, of the working details of his theories. Carl Jung, an early contemporary of Freud, broke away and formulated his own theory that saw the unconscious being organized and functioning differently from Freud's understanding of it. Jung also saw dreams as working quite a different way. By the late twentieth century, Jung's theory had become the most popular and influential. Medard Boss, like Freud and Jung, was a clinician who

Portions of this chapter have been adapted from Moorcroft, 1993, with permission of the publisher.

worked with patients, however rejected the notion of the unconscious resulting in a very different view of the nature of dreams. Brief mention will also be made of two Neofreudians theories, those of Adler and French & Fromm, emphasizing how they differed with Freud. Calvin Hall approached dreams and their analysis as a scientific psychologist rather than as a therapist and thus offered new and important insights.

During the second half of the 20th century, theories of dreaming took very different points of view because of the discovery of REMS and the research that followed. Prominent among these theories is the Activation-Synthesis theory emanating from brain studies of sleep in laboratory animals. A theory quite different from that of Activation-Synthesis comes out of the clinical neuropsychological study of patients with various brain dysfunctions by Mark Solms. Other very different theories of dreaming are offered from the perspective of cognitive psychology by Foulkes and then by Hunt. Psychiatrist and empirical dream researcher, Ernest Hartmann, describes what he sees dreaming to be like from his eclectic perspective. Finally, human research psychologist, William Domhoff, addresses dreaming from a strictly empirical basis of the study of the nature of dreams themselves.

THEORIES FROM THE EARLY TWENTIETH CENTURY

Freud[19]

One of the most common types of dream-formation may be described as follows: a train of thoughts has been aroused by the working of the mind in the daytime... During the night this train of thoughts succeeds in finding connections with one of the unconscious tendencies present ever since his childhood in the mind of the dreamer, but ordinarily repressed and excluded from his conscious life. By the borrowed force of this unconscious help, the thoughts, the residue of the day's work, now become active again, and emerge into consciousness in the shape of a dream. (Freud, 1958, p. 265)

Sigmund Freud's ideas are widely recognized in the Western world. Many of the concepts he introduced are now an accepted part of our culture, including the existence of the unconscious. Yet many of his radical ideas, when isolated from the historical context in which Freud wrote, may seem to be bizarre and overly emphasize issues of sexual conflict. Thus, in order to understand Freud's perspective of dreams and dreaming better, we shall begin by taking a brief look at what influenced Freud's theories.

Born in 1856 to Jewish parents, Freud lived and practiced medicine in Vienna during the time of the decline of the Hapsburg Empire and the reemergence of anti-Semitism, with its atmosphere of strict Victorian moral codes. So pervasive were these codes that, for example, tablecloths extended to the floor, hiding the table legs, in order that males not be aroused by the reminder of women's legs! Living in this Victorian society influenced Freud and his thinking, and it is not surprising to find that it also influenced his theories.

Freud developed his psychological theories, including those of dreams, from his experience with his troubled patients and his own life events. In 1900, he published what many regard as his most important work, *The Interpretation of Dreams.* Freud's theory of dreaming has three basic aspects (Hunt, 1989): (1) why dreaming occurs, (2) how dreams are formed, and (3) a method of dream interpretation.

Because his approach was new and unique, Freud ideas were the basis for the theories of many others who followed him, and these other theories also adopted much of his new terminology. Therefore, as we discuss his theories, we will also emphasize the more important terms of this theory.

Freud believed that all behavior, including dreaming, is motivated by powerful, inner, unconscious forces. These unconscious forces are so strong that they may be too disturbing to think about freely when awake, but they determine the content of dreams during sleep. Yet, the pressure of these unconscious forces needs to be released to keep the individual from going crazy. However, there exists a censor that simply will not allow conscious awareness of these forces.[20]

Consider this example: a happily married man may unconsciously desire to have an affair with his neighbor. For him, to think about this idea may indeed be disturbing, so the topic remains on an unconscious level. But it continually exerts pressure for expression. This unconscious desire thus manifests itself in one of the man's dreams as a **wish fulfillment.** But since our married man may recall his dream upon waking from sleep, his mind transforms the dream content so that the dream is a **disguised** version of his true unconscious desire in order to get past the censor. The undisguised, underlying content of the dream Freud called the **latent** (or hidden) content; its disguised version, what is remembered upon awakening, he called the **manifest content.** In the example above, the latent content of desiring to have an affair with his neighbor may result in a dream with a manifest content of the man being a business partner with his neighbor.

Freud considered the transformation from latent to manifest content an important psychological process called **dream work** that has several components. The transformation process of dream work acts as an editor to **censor** the disturbing material by covering it up with a disguise. Also, an important part of dream work is **secondary revision.**[21] This aspect occurs when thoughts and impulses are logically transformed into a visual format and a storyline is added through the process of **dramatization.**

When recalling a dream, we often can recognize some of the events, people, or sights as having recently been a part of our waking experience. Perhaps during the day you saw someone you have not seen for a long time. That night you may dream about her. Or perhaps you ride your bicycle for the first time in months, then dream about a bicycle that night. Freud believed that we use aspects of our recent experiences, which he called **day residue,** to precipitate some of the images of our dreams. These images are combined with memories, including those of childhood, to become the dream during the process of secondary revision.

Two or more unconscious thoughts often merge together into a single image or event in our dreams. When this merging occurs, our sleeping brain has gone through the type of dream work called **condensation.** In turn, many single images or events in our manifest dream may be overdetermined, that is determined by the condensation of numerous latent dream thoughts. This process can be done because much of the manifest content of dreams is **symbolic**, and a symbol is capable of conveying multiple meanings. The process of transforming latent impulses into visual representations, including symbols, is called **representation**.

Another term Freud used to describe dream work was **displacement**. This process is a part of censorship. If an unconscious desire, emotion, or thought is too threatening to the dreamer, it is transformed into an insignificant component of the dream. Freud saw many neutral objects and events in his own and his patients' dreams as displaced sexual thoughts or desires. Hence to Freud, a dream of a box and a knife was actually about a vagina and a penis in a disguised form. Condensation and displacement use archaic, pre-logical thought processes.

Because dreams are protective disguises of unacceptable unconscious/latent thoughts, dreamers themselves cannot understand them fully without the help of an analyst. Freud developed and used the analytic technique of **free association** to uncover the true meaning of dreams. His patients were instructed to talk freely about whatever came to mind when thinking about their dream or elements of it. They were to do talk without judgment, evaluation, or criticism. Freud then used the associations to get back to the dream's latent content. His method also relied heavily on symbol substitution—replacing the symbols in a manifest dream with their fixed latent equivalents. Symbol substitution needs to be done by the therapist. After weeks, months, or years of analysis, the conflicts that generate dreams, which also cause waking psychological problems, would be "worked through" and Freud would close the case.

Freudian analysis of dreams is still practiced today but is not as popular as it once was because of its heavy emphasis on sex[22] and childhood experience and the enormous amount of time it takes. Yet, we owe a big debt of gratitude to Freud for introducing the notion of a dynamic unconscious to the Western world and for linking dreams to the psychology of waking life and starting us on the road to our current understanding of dreams.

Freud has been much criticized for a variety of reasons. His methods are said to be too "arm chair" with little true empirical data. His theories have been called too narrow. He has been labeled as sexist. His ideas are based too much on abnormal patients and himself rather than a good cross section of people. His notions have been called anti-religious. And so forth and so on. There are too many criticisms to detail here, but some of them become apparent in the ideas and theories of those who departed from his footsteps to whom we now turn our attention.

Jung[23]

Dreams, I maintain, are compensatory to the conscious situation of the moment. (Jung, 1974, p. 38)

Carl Jung was a Swiss psychologist and close colleague of Freud for several years. He broke from Freud in 1913 when he realized his dream theories were taking a much different direction than those of his mentor. While Freud was an excellent and very systematic writer, Jung was not. He is not always easy to read and he was more scattered in the topics he wrote about. As a result, it is more difficult to comprehend and describe Jung's theories and methods. This feat becomes obvious when reading several different accounts of them by different authors. Nevertheless, several key points are obvious and commonly mentioned. I shall concentrate on these key points.

To Jung, humans have a built-in mechanism to become psychologically healthy, a process he called **individuation**. Individuation is the integration of the conscious with the unconscious, a kind of unification of the personality. Dreams are an important part of this process. They serve as a communicator between the unconscious and conscious in order to establish a "balance" of emotional well being. This process begins when dreams with a specific meaning arise from our unconscious and attempt to add something to our conscious knowledge. For example, there may be certain events in your conscious life to which you are not paying attention or are repressing. But this doesn't mean they cease to exist—they simply enter your unconscious.

Here is a specific example: A man who is not psychologically whole walks by a ladder on the side of his house. He does not consciously note that this ladder has a broken rung. But this information is taken in and enters his unconscious without him realizing it. That night he dreams that he falls off a ladder and breaks his leg, objectively telling him about the ladder. But it simultaneously contains a subjective truth. It also means that a "rung" of his personality is in need of attention before it causes him to fall. This information was brought to this dream by his unconscious because his conscious had not taken note of these very important bits of information. In this way, dreams can aid the dreamer in maintaining health, be it physical or emotional.

To Jung the unconscious is broader than it is to Freud. In addition to containing repressed feelings, instincts, and personal memories, it also contains those things that can balance the personality. Additionally, it contains things that are a part of every human's unconscious, what Jung calls the **collective unconscious**. The collective unconscious is composed of **archetypes**, which are predispositions, instincts, or elements that all people have inherited from primitive humans, a kind of natural wisdom. They resemble blue prints into which the individual fills in details. They are seen in the similarities of the motives and images in the dreams, fantasies, and myths from the past and present. This concept is a very important part of Jung's theory. He believes that archetypes serve as a bridge for people to be connected back to nature, because we are too often dehumanized in our scientific society. Archetypes form a link between the ways in which we consciously express our thoughts and a more primitive, more colorful, and more imaginative form of expression. Several of the important archetypes include the persona, the shadow, animus and anima, and the self.

The **persona** is like a mask of personality, the image of ourselves that we endeavor to project to others and to ourselves. We "put our best face forward" as it were.

What Jung called the "**shadow**" is the dark, repressed aspects of personality that press for recognition. These are our traits and attitudes that we hide from ourselves and try to hide from the world. They are poorly integrated into our personalities. For example, a respectable but overly puritanical young woman might have a sexually uninhibited, wild female motorcycle gang member who often appears in her dreams chasing her and causing her problems. These aspects of the shadow need to be appropriately integrated into the rest of the person, and it is up to the unconscious to insure that they are.

Two other very common archetypes described by Jung are the animus and the anima. The animus is the male element in the female unconscious and the anima is the female element in the male unconscious. For example, the anima image is innate in each male child and begins to develop from the mother's effect on her son. The more the anima is developed, the softer his macho character and the more sympathetic, warm, moody, and jealous he is. A man must come to terms with this part of his inner being in order to be a complete person. A very masculine man may appear to have nothing feminine about him. But underneath, there are very feminine aspects that are carefully guarded and hidden in order to prevent being described as "feminine." It is because of this attempt to repress as much of this femininity as possible, that the anima accumulates in the unconscious and must be brought out through dreams. For females, the animus provides a similar, but male, side.

The self is the potential to achieve wholeness. It is often expressed by **mandalas** that look like symmetrical, sometime elaborate pictorial designs. They often take the form of flowers, wheels, or crosses. Often they contain four segments.

It is through the symbolic images of our dreams that the unconscious reveals these things, rather than through rational thought, which is more typical of the waking, conscious mind. These symbolic images are not disguises as Freud thought. Rather, they are used by the unconscious to return the emotional energy that has been stripped away in our everyday life. Our conscious ideas are so barren of emotional energy that we do not really respond to them anymore. We state things as accurately as possible and discard all the excess baggage. The dream language used by the unconscious returns some of that psychic energy, forcing us to pay attention to it. It uses symbolic images to bring things to our attention strongly enough to make us change our attitude or behavior. It is through this process that dreams make us whole. They tell us about parts of ourselves that we are ignoring, suppressing, or not using. To Jung, *dreams reveal, not conceal.*

Jung built upon Freud's theories of dreams, expanding and adding to them. Although Jung believed that wish-fulfilling dreams did exist, he did not agree with Freud that wish-fulfillment should be the sole criterion for interpreting a dream. He stated:

> It is certainly true that there are dreams which embody suppressed wishes and fears, but what is there which the dream cannot, on occasion, embody? Dreams may give expression to ineluctable truths, to philosophical pronouncement, illusions, wild fantasies, memories, plans, anticipations, irrational experiences, even telepathic visions, and heaven knows what besides. (Jung, 1933, p. 11)

To Jung, dreams are more positive than they are to Freud. They are based on more than just infantile sex and aggression. We should not endeavor to travel back to the sources of the dream as Freud suggests, but rather endeavor to finish off the revelation process of the dream. Dreams serve as our partner, not our opposer. They exist to reveal inner resources that are necessary to our emotional well-being. They can be very positive and uplifting experiences. Dreams may seem strange to us, not because of a censor that causes obfuscation, but because of the special symbolic language of the unconscious—images, symbols, and metaphors.

Thus, one of the major functions of dreams, to restore our psychological balance, is referred to by Jung as **compensation**. If a balance between the conscious and unconscious is not achieved, Jung believed that psychological disturbance is very likely. Dreams aim at psychological self-healing. But Jung also believed that dreams could provide prospective visions of the future in the sense that they may show potentials for what might be. They are not absolute predictions.

Jung's methods of dream interpretation are not fully and clearly articulated but contain several recognizable components. Rather than focusing on how dream analysis can help neurotic or emotionally disturbed people, as Freud often did, Jung developed theories and techniques of dream interpretation centered on the non-neurotic or "normal" person. He sees dream interpretation as a joint process between the dreamer and the therapist with the goal of finding meaning that helps the dreamer. The most important steps are first to find the context of the dream, then amplify the dream.

Context

Here the dreamer describes their waking life in relation to the dream and the web of associations between them. In order to interpret a dream correctly and allow it to help a person function, we need thorough knowledge of the conscious situation of the dreamer at that moment. Without this knowledge, it is impossible to interpret a dream correctly. We must know the experiences from the conscious life of the dreamer that preceded the dream in order to untangle what the unconscious has composed in the dream. With the encouragement of the analyst, the dreamer needs to provide the relevant context.

Amplification

Amplification is the main technique developed by Jung for use in dream interpretation. This technique refers to the process of elaboration on, or expansion of, the ideas and images present in dreams in order to make the problems of the dreamer stand out more clearly. There are two kinds of amplification, personal and objective.

Personal amplification involves asking the dreamer to explore and describe any and all possible associations (thoughts, feelings, and recollections) that they can make when recalling a dream, being careful to not stray too far from the dream. Each image is discussed to make possible associations to the dreamer's life. Personal amplification is done by the dreamer from their **personal unconscious**. These aspects are things experienced by the individual, but not at the level of awareness. They may have been forgotten, may not have been intense enough, may have been repressed, and so on. They differ from one person to the next, because each person has unique experiences during life. For example, perhaps there was a flowering plant in the dream. The dreamer might talk about how the plant looked, what its shape was, the color, size, and smell of the flowers. The dreamer might then talk about flowers in general, how to grow them, problems with them, and what use they might have. The dreamer should also relate feelings about flowers. These objective associations are also discussed to determine possible explanations for dream images.

The second step is **objective amplification**, a kind of explanation done by the dream analyst. Things which have not been a part of our personal conscious occasionally arise from the unconscious, resulting in the collective unconscious being expressed. The analyst does assist in this process by relating the elements of the dream to what is known to be typically contained in the collective unconscious and represented by archetypes. A great deal of knowledge regarding the nature of the collective unconscious is required by the therapist.

Jung also advised people to meditate on or have "**interior dialogue**" with the characters in the dream. For it is the dreamer who knows his or her dream better than anyone else and, therefore, can interpret it most accurately. Some consider this process Jung's third technique for interpreting dreams.

Interpretation requires working with more than just one dream. An analyst and dreamer working together with a *series of dreams* can provide the best interpretation. Dreams in a series can throw light on one another and possibly show progression of ideas or events. In any such situation, a comfortable and unthreatening relationship must exist between the analyst and the dreamer during the interpretation.

The primary aim of interpreting dreams is to make dream material serve the dreamer. Dreams contain diagnostically valuable facts. A dream from the unconscious has the ability to add something to our conscious knowledge and if it does not, then it has not been interpreted correctly. When interpreting dreams, according to Jung, one must remember that a dream is a product of the total psyche. He means not just the personal psyche, but also everything that has ever been of significance in the life of humanity through archetypes—a "psyche of humankind." The analysis and interpretation of dreams reveal the structure of both the personal psyche and the collective psyche.

Jung suggested that dream analysis is not really a technique that can be learned and applied according to a certain set of rules. If specific rules are used, the individual personality too easily gets lost. The intuition, imagination, and intelligence of both the analyst and the dreamer are very important and must be freely shared. Dream interpretation should come from the dreamer with the help of the analyst. It should come from what exists in the dreamer's psyche, so that it can serve the dreamer in the best way possible.

The main criticism of Jung is that he is close to being mystical in his views and theories. Also, like Freud, his method has been called too "arm chair" and subjective.

Other Psychoanalytic Dream Theories

Certainly Freud and Jung can be considered the most important and influential of those who are called the psychoanalytic dream theorists. The following theorists are also noteworthy, not because they have shown us a new path by which to understand and work with dreams, but they have modified the path of Freud in some significant way that deserves our attention.

Adler[24]

Alfred Adler was an Austrian psychiatrist who was a member of Freud's inner circle until he broke away with his own ideas. The key for Adler was that people strive to achieve superiority and avoid inferiority. Also, he believed that the conscious and unconscious do not oppose one another. His ideas about dreams are consistent with these basic notions, although he did not focus on dreams as much as did Freud, and his ideas are not as well developed and even contain some internal inconsistencies.

To Adler, dreams focus on the dreamer's lifestyle and relate to the dreamer's everyday existence. Therefore, therapists can use persons' dreams to learn of their typical beliefs, behaviors, and attitudes. Dreams attempt to solve the problems of dreamers yet are often ineffectual, because they are "self protective fantasies" created to defend the dreamers' sense of superiority and self-worth. In a sense, dreams are failed adaptations to waking reality and give no real help, but interpretation of them can be helpful to see these failures that are in need of waking work. Dreams anticipate or prepare for the future, yet seldom are specific solutions for interpersonal problems carried from a dream to waking life, so in a sense dreams fail. Rather, a mood is carried from the dream to waking life.

Dream interpretation requires a trained therapist, but the interpretation is more of an art lacking rules other than to stay within the dreamer's unique logic and language. Free association should be used as well as looking at the emotional context of the dream. Contrary to Jung, Adler believes there are no universal symbols in dreams.

French & Fromm[25]

Thomas French and Erika Fromm, both classically trained psychoanalysts, focused on Freud's notion of the ego, hence they are known as ego psychologists. The goal of ego psychology is to strengthen the ego against anxiety and better adapt to the demands of social reality, a more practical approach with a waking life orientation than that of Freud.

To French and Fromm, every dream has a "focal conflict" involving a current life problem. This focal conflict is personal or interpersonal with emotional overtones. The recalled dream reveals what this conflict is and how the dreamer is trying to solve it. In longer dreams, the same conflict in the dreamer's past is also presented to see what did and did not work. Every element in the dream is connected to the conflict in some way.

Dream interpretation, according to French and Fromm, needs to be done by a trained therapist who uses "empathetic imaginations" from a psychoanalytic viewpoint to guide the session. However, the therapist does not simply dictate conclusions to the dreamer, but also carefully checks for evidence that this empathetic imagination is correct. In the process, the therapist moves between the parts of the dream to the whole and back again. Success with the process is determined when there are no inconsistencies with parts of the interpretation, and the dreamer is enthusiastic about feeling the interpretation is insightful.

Boss[26]

Medard Boss was a Swiss psychiatrist who trained and worked with Jung. However, he came to reject the notion of the unconscious and the notion that there are special messages delivered through dreams. Rather, he aligned with existential phenomenalism that believed that we exist solely in relationship to people and things. This "being-in-the-world" occurs in the world of our dreams as well as our waking world, so we must treat our dreams as an experience rather than as containing symbols and metaphors. As such, dreams mirror our present and open future potentials and possibilities. Dream experiences are more restricted and dimmer than waking existence, but they characterize how the dreamer relates to the waking world.

The key to working with dreams, for Boss, is to focus on the experience. We should strive to get the obvious meaning from the dream. His method, called "explication," was not as explicitly outlined as was that of Freud and Jung, but contains the following elements.

First, look at what is in the dream, but also notice what is not in the dream. Then note the relationship of the dreamer to the elements of the dream and how the dreamer responds to them. Make special note of how the dreamer relates emotionally to these elements. As much as possible, one should try to relive the dream. Stay as close to the recalled dream as much as possible while exploring its details and one's reactions to them. Try to get an "increasingly refined account" of it.

It is necessary for the dreamer to have the guidance of a trained and knowledgeable therapist to find the "significances" of the dream to the dreamer's waking life. The therapist does not need to know the client's life history or even the predream life situation. The therapist does not offer interpretations but does comment on the dream as an existential experience and offers "helpful comments and hints" such as, "Is there anything similar to waking life?" The dream means nothing more than what the dreamer can see revealed in it and how it points to the dreamer's individual traits. The dream experience is the focus.

For Boss, dreams can be useful in psychotherapy, because they can point to constrictions in the dreamer's personality, but they can also disclose potentials for growth. They can be transforming experiences. He also emphasizes that we should pay special attention to very unusual dream phenomena.

Hall[27]

> In short, the images of our dreams are pictures of our conceptions. We study dreams in order to find out what people think during sleep. (Hall, 1966, p. 10)

Calvin Hall was a university professor of psychology prior to becoming the Director of the Dream Research Institute in Santa Cruz, California. His dream theory derives from Freud's basic concepts but differs in its details. Hall found many of the details of Freud's and Jung's theories turgid, unscientific, and impractical. He derived his notions by applying the scientific method to the study of dreams in order to determine precisely *what* people dream about (see Chapter 6). He first published the results of his efforts in *The Meaning of Dreams* in 1953. The following discussion is from a subsequent edition of that book (Hall, 1966).

Unlike Freud and Jung, who used patients' or clients' dreams as the basis of their theories, Hall derived his ideas from the study of thousands of dreams collected from hundreds of normal people—people just like you. Yet, it is interesting to note that, in the end, he concluded that Freud was essentially correct about the nature of dreams, for Hall's normal subjects dreamed in the same way as Freud's disturbed patients. For example, Hall's male subjects often revealed the Oedipal complex in their dreams, just like Freud's male patients. The basic nature of dreams, Hall concluded, appears to be the same in all people, regardless of their psychological health. The details of the content and focus may differ between patients and a nonclinical population, but the basic underlying processes are the same.

To Hall, a dream is "a succession of images, predominantly visual in quality, which are experienced during sleep" (Hall, 1966, pp. 2–3). These images represent the ideas or conceptions of the dreamer that are typically found below the level of consciousness. They are a projective representation of the content of the mind in pictorial form. He even called them hallucinations, since they typically occur in the absence of any immediate real world stimulus. He did recognize that external, sensory stimuli sometimes generate dream content, but he said that they are neither responsible for the generation of the dream, nor are they typically accurately portrayed. For example, a ringing telephone may become a fire alarm in a dream. These, he said, are akin to waking illusions where a real stimulus is misperceived. Real world stimuli may become a part of dreams in another way, according to Hall. People, things, or events of our recent waking experience may show up later in our dreams. Freud called this experience day residue, although Hall did not use that term. For Hall, dreams are an embodiment of a person's thoughts that are *continuous* with the person's waking personality and thoughts.

Hall believed that people dream only of things that are of personal importance to them but not current events, even catastrophic ones. For example, none of the hundreds of dreams he collected from many U.S. citizens shortly after the first atomic bomb was dropped on Japan contained any reference to that event. Neither do people dream about other impersonal things. They do not dream about politics or economics. Nor do they dream about sports. They do not even dream very much about business or work. Rather, dreams are very personal—a *"letter to oneself"* about things that are important to the dreamer.

Dreams particularly reveal what dreamers really think of themselves by getting behind the waking self-facades. Dreams are like a magic mirror that show what is below the surface of the dreamer. In this regard, Hall pointed out that each aspect of the dreamer's personality is often symbolized by a different character in a dream. People also dream about how they view other people and what they really feel about them. Rather than objective picture of others, dreams present the personal subjective portrayal of others as found deep in the minds of dreamers.

Dreamers may have more that one conception of themselves and others. Some of these conceptions may even be contradictory, since logic is not important in dreaming. For example, a dreamer may simultaneously conceive of their mother as warm, intelligent, and productive yet also aloof, absentminded, and disorganized. These various conceptions may all manifest themselves within one dream or some in one dream and others in another dream. Dreamers are perfectly free to say whatever they feel in their dreams.

The contents of dreams reflect a person's worldview such as whether other people are generally kind and generous versus being generally nasty and aggressive. Dreams also show how dreamers view the space that they live in, or how it affects them. This subjective world is never an exact replica of the "real" world, and two different people will certainly have two different views of the same "real" world.

Additionally, dreams are not generated by our impulses; rather they show our attitudes toward our impulses. When asleep, our mind is free of external controls and free to indulge in impulse gratification. The conflict between conscience and impulse is better seen in dreams than anywhere else. For example, does the dreamer see sex as fun or evil? Would he like to have sex with his spouse in a variety of exotic ways, or is he attracted to other men or women? Does she constrain herself sexually because of moral conscience or because of fears of inadequacy? These, or any number of other possibilities, may reveal themselves in dreams.

Nightmares are more extreme examples, according to Hall. "The nightmare is the price [the dreamer] pays for doing something wrong" (Hall, 1966, p. 16). That is, nightmares picture what penalties dreamers will incur if their conscience is ignored. For example, following yielding to temptation that results in a sexual indiscretion, a person may dream of being horribly maimed. Again, note here that Hall is saying that it is not the impulse (in our example, the sexual impulse) that triggers the dream, but the person's attitude toward the impulse.

Finally, and most importantly, dreams show the dreamer's conflicts and problems. Most of the information gained from dreams comes from this source. Hall defined conflicts as opposing conceptions that are constantly struggling and fighting with one another within a person. In dreams, the real, authentic problems, rather than the delusions and pretensions of waking life surface.

Since the dreamers create their own dreams, they determine who is in them and what things become a part of them. Furthermore, everything in a dream is there for a purpose and is important. How these things are included and combined is usually very clever. The dream is a very creative product, but it comes out of our unawareness. We do not consciously create our dreams.

Symbols are an important aspect of dreams. Hall believed that they serve the same function in dreams that they do in waking life. He called symbols "pictorial metaphors", and he emphasized that they are intended not to obscure, but to clarify. They come from the ideas in the mind of the dreamer. They express the dreamer's thoughts better and they convey meaning more precisely and economically. They are a form of thinking used especially in dreaming. Symbols are an efficient and concise way of presenting complex and hard to understand ideas. They can often make visible things that are otherwise invisible, such as feelings.

But the presence of symbols in dreams does make it more difficult to assess the meaning in dreams, thus the need for dream analysis or interpretation. Interpretation of a dream means to turn the symbols back into ideas. Since dreamers are the ones who created the dreams and chose what symbols to use, the dreamers themselves should be an important part of the interpretation process. Most interpretation should be easy, because dreams are relatively transparent. If a dream does not make sense on the face of it as some do, then the dreamer must work with its parts and symbols to get at its meanings. If that approach is not successful, then the dreamer should try free associating to each symbol.

Unlike Freud, Hall believed that you need not have a psychologist, psychiatrist, or analyst present to free associate. Anyone who is clear thinking and is willing to let go without suppressing or controlling or trying to edit can free associate. "Anyone who can look at a picture and say what it means ought to be able to look at his dream pictures and say what they mean" (Hall, 1966, p. 85). The dreamer is the best person to do this because the dream is a product of the dreamer's mind. Hall also advised against reading some theory *into* a dream; rather he advocated reading the meaning *out* of the dream. The goal of dream interpretation is to convert images into verbal ideas.

Hall believed that you should not work with only a portion of a dream. A dream is "an organic whole" and should be analyzed that way. Moreover, he recommended looking at a series of dreams rather than each dream separately. Each dream is like a chapter in a book. While each chapter may contain a lot of information, only by reading the whole book can you understand what the author is saying. Similarly, Hall believed you should consider the interpretation of one dream only as a hunch until verified by the interpretation of other dreams. If it does not agree with other dreams, then consider it wrong. In this way, interpreting dreams is like fitting together the pieces of a jigsaw puzzle. Try various combinations of dreams to see how they fit together until a meaningful whole emerges. Try to take small steps from the simple to the complex. Each dream supplements and complements the others of the series. What is not forthcoming in one dream may be revealed in another.

Hall also recognized the occasional occurrence of "spotlight" or "bareface" dreams whose meanings are obvious, and thus need little interpretation. If such a dream is available, use this one first, then work with other, more complex dreams in the series.

Hall, like Jung, broadened the scope of Freudian dream interpretation by emphasizing the importance of working with a series of dreams and the personal, contemporary nature of dream content. He also eliminated the need for a trained analyst to interpret dreams, believing instead that each of us is best capable of interpreting our own dreams.

Comment

The theories reviewed to this point are from the early 20th century. Except for Hall's theory, they can be considered to be "arm chair" theories based on insights and intuitions gained from working with patients as opposed to being based on objective data. Furthermore, they are in most cases very difficult or impossible to test. While this does not necessarily mean they are wrong, the likelihood of their being wrong is greater than a data based theory no matter how intuitively correct they seem to be. Unlike what is in much of the rest of the book, they are included not because they are correct and have stood up to objective testing over time, but because they are of historical and intellectual interest. Calvin Hall was the exception during this era. He was not a clinician, and he based his ideas on scientific analysis of everyday dreams he collected from non-patient populations.

We now turn to the dream theories of the latter half of the 20th century and beginning of the 21st. These theories were developed in the era of intense scientific study of sleeping and dreaming that resulted from the discovery of REMS and as a result are very much different from the psychoanalytic based theories. We begin with an influential theory that uses knowledge of brain functioning as its starting point.

Box 24

Dream Interpretation[28]

All methods of dream interpretation are based on the interpreter's theory of dreams. Sometimes the theory is described in great detail, but in other cases it is just loosely mentioned or implied. Some methods are strongly intertwined with one theory of dreaming, especially the psychoanalytic, others are eclectic, and still others have a few basic assumptions about dreaming but are essentially pragmatic. Taking a look from the other direction, it should also be noted that some proponents of theories of dreaming are indifferent about dream interpretation, believe it is a waste of time, or even believe it is counterproductive.

It is a good idea when considering a dream interpretation method to begin by asking the following questions:

1. How do the theoretical assumptions behind the method influence the interpretations?
2. What are the roles of the dreamer and the interpreter? Can both roles be played by anyone, or does the interpreter need to be highly trained?

The answers can tell a lot about how narrow or broad the method is and whether you want to invest a lot of time in it.

The following are six of types of methods most frequently used by experts and amateurs alike. They can be used individually but often can and are used in combination.

1. Cultural-Formula

In the Cultural-Formula method, components of the dream are translated into their meaning for the dreamer. This method requires special knowledge possessed by a trained interpreter or written in a book usually organized like a dictionary. It is among the oldest approaches to dream interpretation and, to varying degrees, some or most of the meanings of the components may be tied to a particular culture. This method is recognizable in Jungian and New Age dream interpretation. The assumption is that the culture implicitly agrees upon the meaning of certain objects and actions, but it takes someone who has carefully studied these meanings or been schooled in them to see them in the dreamer's dream or write them down in a book.

2. Psychotheoretical-Formula

With the Psychotheoretical-Formula, a trained analyst interprets the themes and images of the dream for the dreamer. The analyst uses a specific psychological theory to match particular images with interpretations. Freudian analysis is the prime example of this method, but Jungian analysis fits here also. The ordinary person cannot do the interpretation, because it requires working knowledge of the theory and considerable experience working with patients from its perspective.

3. Associative

In the Associative method, the dreamer gives associations (semantic and in many cases also emotional) to components in the dream. It was Freud who first espoused using the associations of the dreamer to help with the interpretation. Later, others believed that Freud allowed dreamers to follow a train of associations too far from the dream itself, and they encouraged dreamers to stay closer to the dream with their associations. An example is Jung's personal amplification technique. In another example, the contemporary Dream Interview Method of Gayle Delaney asks the dreamer to describe components of the dream as if talking to someone from another planet who knows little of the planet earth. The dreamer is to give literal definitions as well as emotional feeling about the component. The underlying idea is that each of us may see the same thing differently and feel differently about it. Since we create our dreams based on our personal meanings and feelings, it is helpful to garner these individual meanings and feelings to understand the meaning of the dream.

4. Emotion-Focusing

The emphasis of the Emotion-Focusing method is for the dreamer to assume the role of an image in the dream and act it out. The image to be acted out is not limited to people but can be animals, plants, or even inanimate objects. The dreamer may alternate between two images as they carry on a dialog. Or in a group setting, others in the group may be asked to assume the role of some of the other images and interact with the image that the dreamer assumes. The idea here is to have the dreamer get to the often intense feelings associated with the images of the dream, and the best way to get to these feelings is to experience them. The Gestalt approach of Fritz Perls champions this method.

5. Personal-Projection

Personal-Projection involves someone other than the dreamer projecting a mixture of cultural associations, psychotheoretical associations, personal associations, and emotional responses onto the dreamers' dream. This method has been around for eons. The method of Ullman and Zimmerman (1979) is a modern version. In it, a small group of people discuss the dream of one other group member as if it is their own, projecting their feelings and associations onto its components. At this point, the dreamer is only to listen. Then the dreamer tells if any of the projections help to interpret the meaning of the dream. The idea is that sometimes other people can see the meanings in our dreams that we are unable to see until others point them out.

6. Phenomenological

The object of the Phenomenological approach is to get the dreamer to fully re-experience the images and feelings of the dream from an individual perspective. The dreamer is to describe in as much detail as possible precisely what happened in the dream as the dream is being re-experienced. There is no presumptuous or restrictive dream theory allowed to get in the way of experiencing the dream just as it was dreamed. Simply re-experiencing the dream well can enlighten the dreamer about new attitudes and feelings and even new ways of being. Medard Boss is credited with championing this method. Delaney's Dream Interview Method also loosely fits in this category; after the dreamer defines the components of the dream, the dreamer is asked if the components remind him or her of anything from waking life

Some Additional Techniques[29]

The following are additional, sometimes useful techniques for interpreting dreams.

- Consider working with a partner or *group.*
- *Automatic writing* involves writing all feelings, thoughts, and associations that come to mind about the contents of the dream. Do this as quickly as you can without pausing to think, censor, or revise.
- To use *dialogue,* write how two characters or other components of a dream would converse with one another. It can be done in the form of a script for a play. Write as quickly as you are able without worrying about grammar or spelling. Just get the ideas down as they come. You may want to think of a few questions to get the dialog going and also imagine the dream scene where the characters or components appeared.
- *Retelling* starts with telling the dream in the present tense a couple of times. Simultaneously, focus on your feelings, body sensations, and associations. Now tell the dream again from a different perspective, usually that of another character. Do it again from yet another perspective. As you do so, note the changes in emotions. Compare the various tellings to your written account of the dream to see what was left out, changed, or embellished.
- To look at the dream another way, try *drawing* it. Perhaps you could make a series of drawings like a cartoon strip. Do not worry about lack of artistic ability. Attend to colors and feelings as well as objects, characters, and events.
- Ask *Questions* of the Dream. List questions you have about the dream and its parts. Then choose one or two of the most central questions and answer them.
- Decipher the *Symbols* of the dream by first selecting an image from the dream. Then let the dream come alive and focus on the symbol. Next, describe/define it to someone from another planet including how you feel about it, what it is doing in this dream, and what it reminds you of.
- Whatever method you use, *finish* by taking a few minutes to reflect on what new insights, possibilities, healing, peace, etc. you have gained. Then write them down.

Note: This description of the various approaches to dream interpretation is intended only for a basic understanding of what has been and can be done. It is virtually impossible to do actual dream interpretation from such brief descriptions. The reader who would like to try dream interpretation is directed to consult one or more books that detail one or more of these methods.

THEORIES FROM THE LAST HALF OF
THE TWENTIETH CENTURY

Activation-Synthesis

In the late 1970s, Alan Hobson and Robert McCarley of the Department of Psychiatry at Harvard Medical School first described their "activation-synthesis" model of dreaming (Hobson & McCarley, 1977) as an extension of their reciprocal interaction model for the control of NREM/REMS cycling (see Chapter 2). The theory has undergone revisions since then to incorporate new data and the neural network model of brain functioning. Also, the synthesis part of the theory has been more defined. I shall present the essence of the latest version here (c.f. Hobson et al., 2000) without specifying the many of its brain anatomy details.

In this model, Hobson and McCarley described a functional organization of the brain that is unique to sleep. REMS is a result of activation of the "REM-ON" area located in the pontine reticular formation, which in turn causes the phenomena of REMS to be produced, including the characteristic EEG, body muscle paralysis, bursts of eye movements, and other "tonic" and "phasic" phenomena. This REM-ON area also cuts off most sensory stimuli from the brain. In other words, in the absence of motor output and sensory input, the brain is virtually isolated during REMS.

According to the activation-synthesis model, dreaming is another result of the REM-ON area by configuring the functioning of the brain differently by *activating* several forebrain systems while a few others are deactivated. The result is a very different configuration of the brain during NREMS with some parts as active as when awake but others less active. The activated areas include those for awareness, eye movements, instincts, vestibular sensations (sense of body position and acceleration), memory consolidation, and emotions. Areas involved in the production of various motor movements and the secondary processing of sensory information are also activated, but the motor output to the muscles for body movement are blocked. Simultaneously, the areas involved in the primary reception of most sensory information are not activated. Importantly, the dorsal lateral prefrontal cortex, that is approximately just inside the front of your temples, is deactivated. As a result of this area of the brain not being online, dreams have their illogical, out of volitional control, and unquestioned bizarreness qualities, and working (or short term) memory is lacking.

The random information from the activated areas is then *synthesized* into a unified, perceptual whole. The result is the experience of a dream isolated from reality but that seems real at the time with heavy emphasis on emotional and sensory content. It includes much that is familiar to you but also includes bizarre elements. It is important to note that the areas of the cerebral cortex that are activated are also responsible for the storage of *your* pre-existing memories, *your* typical emotional responses, and *your* typical way of synthesizing this information. In this way, the aspects of your life and personality become part of your dreams. Thus, the contents of your dreams are very meaningful to you. This important aspect of the activation-synthesis model has frequently been ignored or missed by its critics.

The process of synthesis during dreaming is no different from what occurs when you are awake. All of us constantly synthesize the currently available sensory and motor information with our present affective state and then draw upon our memory banks of similar experiences and meanings in order to try to make it coherent.

Seligman and Yellen (1987) describe a classroom demonstration that illustrates synthesis. The instructor crumples a string of sequentially blinking, miniature, Christmas tree lights into a loose ball. The lights now appear to blink randomly. The instructor then turns on a tape of Beatles' music. Soon most students report that the lights appear to blink in synchrony with the song. When the instructor turns the music off, the randomness of the blinking again becomes apparent to the students. This demonstration shows how a pattern is imposed on something unpatterned. It's irresistible. We cannot help but do it, because our brain does it automatically when awake and when dreaming.

When awake, our sensory information is usually very much related to our motor information and seems "normal." For example, when we stroke a furry cat, we see and feel our hand moving across the fur at the same time that we sense the muscles of our arm producing the stroking movements. Also sensory events are usually sequentially continuous when we are awake. For example, when we watch a baseball game, we see the pitcher wind-up and throw, then the batter swings, next the ball is rocketing toward the left field bleachers, the batter is running the bases, the scoreboard changes the score, and so on. In contrast, discontinuities are more common in dreams. The pitcher winds-up, the batter swings, and starts to run, but is now running up an escalator at an airport in a frustrating effort to get to class. The reason for discontinuities is that when asleep, the activation of the various components is random and varies in strength. Thus, at any time, the activated components may not be so well related; yet the brain synthesizes them as best it can into a single entity. The result is often the bizarreness we perceive in our dreams. For instance, the sensory part of our brain may be activated to produce the image of a wall, while the muscle command area of the brain is sending out signals to produce walking, so we dream of walking through a wall. For similar reasons we may experience abrupt, bizarre scene shifts. We are in a boat at one instant and in class the next. The difference between dreaming and being awake, then, is not the process of activation and synthesis, but the source of the activation: more external (and sequential) when awake, almost entirely internal and random when in REM. It has been said that wakefulness is but a dream that is determined by constraints from specific sensory inputs (Llinas & Pare, 1991).

Originally, the activation-synthesis theory was developed to explain REMS dreaming. Later, the same mechanisms were extended to explain stage 2 dream-like mentation that is frequent toward the end of the sleep period (Hobson et al., 2000). This process is thought to result from an "admixture" of REMS and stage 2 sleep. The length, strength, and closeness of the REMS periods to stage 2 sleep without intervening SWS cause some components of REMS to occur during stage 2 sleep in a weaker intensity insufficient to trigger REMS but sufficient to cause mentation. (Nielsen (2000) describes a similar, more elaborated, and data based theory of "covert REMS" to explain NREMS mentation.)

Since the original formulation of the activation-synthesis hypothesis, data from neurophysiology, cognitive neuroscience, dream recall content, and postmodern literary theory has added to the specification of the synthesis component (Stickgold, unpublished manuscript). The bizarreness in dreams has been found to be not entirely random. Rather, there are rules that restrain the transformation of objects into other objects and determine the degree of plot continuity. Analysis of dream content shows that people tend to morph into other living things but not inanimate objects and vice versa. Furthermore, people are more likely to morph into other people than into animals, rocks into chairs than into flowers. Also, the memories that are sequentially activated during dreaming tend to be associated, resulting in immediate plot coherence, but the memories non-sequentially activated during dreaming are not so associated, resulting in strange twists and turns in the plot when the dream is viewed in its entirety. The result is like a meandering social conversation that twists and turns as the most recent topic leads to the next association, and soon people are talking about things far different from what they were discussing just a few minutes ago. This experience is in distinction to a good lecture where remote, as well as recent topics are very tightly related even after an hour or more. A good lecture, unlike a social conversation or dream, has a specific goal in mind from the very start.

Dream construction, dream experience, and dream interpretation are all worthy topics of study but are independent of each other (Stickgold, unpublished manuscript). The construction of the dream is done from randomly stimulated elements without any intent of specific meaning or plot. While experiencing the dream, the dreamer's mind links its parts together as best it can to form a coherent plot. During interpretation, meaning for the dreamer, that can be very useful, is sought from the elements and the plot. This linkage can be done because the components of the dream, and the way they are jointed to form a plot, come out of the dreamers own mind and are thus meaningful to them. For example, if you have exaggerated concerns about your personal safety, then your descriptions of your waking and dreaming life will be filled with threats to your physical well being. Thus your dreams may contain information that is relevant to you and revealing about you. Such information can be useful in psychotherapy, however, the results of the interpretation cannot be used to infer an intended plot or any intention for the elements whether symbolic or otherwise. There is no need for dreams to have intent in order to have meaning. Experiential meaning and interpreted meaning cannot legitimately be projected backwards to infer intent.

It is important to note that, from the start, Hobson and McCarley are very careful in how they describe the relationship between the physiology and the psychology of dreaming. They specifically state that the activation-synthesis physiology does not cause the dream to be experienced. That is, dreaming cannot be reduced to brain cell activity. Rather, they state that the neural activity is paralleled by the experience of the dream or, when a dream is experienced, there is a correspondent activation of certain brain areas. Neither the physiology nor the psychology is primary to the other; rather they occur simultaneously. The same relationship is known to occur between the physiology and psychology of our senses. For example, when something touches our body, the frequency of discharge of neurons involved in our sense of touch corresponds to the intensity of touch that we perceive. In another example, when you identify a particular sound, there is a parallel and unique pattern of neuronal impulses in the auditory system of your brain. The psychology in these examples is nothing more than a different conceptualization of the physiology. So, too, with dreams.

Criticisms of the activation-synthesis theory have been many and varied over its more than a quarter of a century history. Here is a sampling. (1) It is too neurological or too narrowly scientific to describe what dreaming is really about. (2) It is based on animal brain research that may not apply to a mental function in humans. (3) Evidence suggests the instigation for dreaming occurs in the cerebral cortex not the brainstem. (4) There are people who have REMS and do not dream, and there are people who dream but do not have REMS. (5) Lucid dreaming is said to disavow the notion that higher mental functions of the forebrain play only a secondary role in dreaming, for many lucid dreamers can control the dream. And (6) objective analysis of dreams shows that only a small portion of their content is bizarre, but the activation-synthesis hypothesis only describes how bizarreness occurs.

As an extension of the activation-synthesis model, Hobson has developed a general model of the brain-mind called AIM (c.f. Hobson et al., 2000). It purports to model the nature of mental processes in sleep, waking, and some abnormal states. AIM stands for the three factors in the model. $\underline{A}$ is activation that depends on the level of activation in the ascending reticular activating system. $\underline{I}$ is input source or the ratio of external relative to internal strength of sensory stimuli. $\underline{M}$ is the information processing mode that is related to the relative level of aminergic modulation of the cerebral cortex. The interaction of these three factors determines the instantaneous state of the mental processes in the brain and the mind whether awake, asleep, dreaming, or in an abnormal mode.

Solms (1997, 2000)

In the early 1990s, Mark Solms, a clinical neuropsychologist in London, England, asked every one of the 434 patients referred to him for evaluation of brain damage or brain dysfunction the same set of questions about the quantity, quality, and character of their dreams. He was able to obtain usable data from 361 of these patients, the vast majority of whom did report some significant change in their dreaming. Twenty-nine were eventually found to be free of brain disorders and served as a control group who, like the rest, were admitted to the hospital and tested for possible brain injury. He published his results in *The Neuropsychology of Dreams* in 1997.

A study of the patients with brain malfunctions, but no changes in their dreaming, suggested which parts of the brain were not involved with dreaming. Other patients showed deficits of dreaming, mostly loss of visual aspects of dreaming or loss of dreaming entirely, while some patients showed excesses of dreams or nightmares. He applied classical clinico-neuroanatomical research methods to these data and found that the changes in dreaming were related to dysfunction in one or a combination of five specific brain areas. He compared his findings with 73 studies about dream changes and brain dysfunction from articles published during the last 100 years in neurological journals. Last, he related all these data to the contemporary understanding of brain functioning. The result was the formulation of an entirely new and original "model of the normal dream process." Interestingly, about the same time he was conducting this study, others were gaining information about the brain during sleep using recently developed functional brain imaging techniques. Solms's data and the functional neuroimaging data turn out to be remarkably consistent.

According to Solms's theory, dreams originate in the middle of the forebrain when certain brain systems that use the neurotransmitter dopamine are activated. These mechanisms can be activated during REMS by acetylcholine, but they also sometimes are activated during NREMS by various triggers. Thus, that portion of NREMS mentation that is indistinguishable from REMS dreams is generated by identical forebrain mechanisms that generate REMS dreams. The rest of NREMS mentation is another story that he does not deal with.

For Solms, dreams occur because of a functional reorganization of the higher portions of the brain. When awake, sensory stimuli coming primarily from external sources activate the sensory areas of the cortex that in turn activate nearby perceptual and stored memory areas of the cerebral cortex. These, in their turn, activate the limbic areas that are considered important for goal seeking, appetitive, and volitional activities, and that influence the motor output system. When awake, this flow of information is directed by frontal-limbic mechanisms of attention as well as being constrained by external sensory information. However, during sleep, some of these areas function differently, resulting in a different flow of information. At the same time that volitional activity of the motor output system is blocked, the functioning of the primary sensory areas in the cortex that are responsive to external stimuli are attenuated by the frontal limbic area, especially the anterior cingulate gyrus. This attenuation allows internally generated stimuli, together with the small amount of external stimuli that still gets through, to arouse the goal-seeking, appetitive, and volitional areas of the limbic system that are the middle forebrain dopaminergic areas mentioned above. Simultaneously, other limbic areas contribute affective input. When there is nonspecific forebrain activation, the result is the generation of abstract (symbolic) thoughts derived from past experiences that are prevented from awakening the sleeper by sleep activated inhibitory influences from the frontal cortex. These thoughts act in a reverse direction from that occurring during waking on perceptual and memory mechanisms, resulting in symbolic and primarily movie-like visual-spatial hallucinations. Meanwhile, the "reflective mechanisms" of the frontal limbic area, located in the dorsal lateral prefrontal cortex, are not operative during sleep and thus do not distinguish these resulting hallucinations from reality. In this way, dreams are the result of "abstract thinking ... converted into concrete perception" (p. 241).

Based on his results, Solms tentatively expresses some support for Freud's ideas about the source of dreams. Freud maintained that dreaming was the guardian of sleep, because the impulses of the appetites were deflected by censorship into the disguised hallucinations of dreams rather than awakening the sleeper. Similarly, Solms's model shows arousing stimuli being channeled away from the mechanisms of waking into the hallucinations of dreaming. Indeed, neurological patients reporting the cessation of dreaming also describe their sleep as disturbed (which Solms admits needs to be objectively verified in a sleep lab). Furthermore, patients who exhibit loss of inhibition and regulation following damage to, or disconnection of, deep prefrontal regions report an absence of dreaming which is consistent with the loss of functioning of Freud's censor. Finally, Freud said that wishes, meaning motives, instigate dreams. Solms agrees with this assertion, because the only thing that eliminates dreaming is damage to the area of the brain involved with motivation.

Solms's theories have been criticized from a number of fronts on a number of grounds. Yet his data and some of their implications have had a major effect on how dreaming is viewed by theorists from a number of perspectives. In particular, Hobson's group has recognized much of Solms's data as being important and informative but disagree on the interpretation of some of the data. For example, the damage Solms describes to the motivational system that eliminates dreaming, according to Hobson's group, is really damage to much more than the motivational system. Others criticize Solms for being too neurological and not psychological enough in his theory.

Cognitive Dream Theories

Cognitive dream theory approaches dreams not as brain processing of perceptual experiences but as a type of cognition (information processing) (Carskadon, 1993). These theories assume that dreams reprocess memories and knowledge using the same basic methods that the waking mind does. The focus is more on the process of dreaming than on the particulars of dreams' contents, sources, or significances. Unlike neuroscience approaches, they are not reductionistic. Unlike clinical approaches, they do not see unconscious motivation for dreaming nor hidden meanings in dreams. The interest is on how dreaming is similar to and how it differs from waking cognition. Within this framework, there are different cognitive dream theories. We will examine two of the more prominent ones.

Foulkes[30]

David Foulkes (1999), as a cognitive dream theorist, maintains that dreams are not simple perceptual phenomena but are a way of thinking. Dreams result from the somewhat random activation and reorganization of various semantic and episodic memory components in the mind. The main difference between waking cognition and dreaming is the dreaming mind is not regulated by sensory stimulation or even self-control. It processes information that is broader in scope and less associated than when awake. Yet, like during waking, the brain attempts to provide a coherent synthesis in a narrative format of the information currently available resulting in dream content that seems unusual to the waking mind. The result is recombinations of waking experiences, knowledge, and memory that simulate waking reality.

Dreaming thus depends on the ability to access and cognitively process recent experiences, knowledge, and other memories. It is also related to language production and high-level cognitive constructive processes of the human mind. For this reason, Foulkes maintains, animals do not dream, because they are not capable of such cognitive processes.

Foulkes comes to his understanding from rigorous series of studies of sleep laboratory dream recall from children of various ages (see Chapter 6). The ability to dream gradually develops during childhood beginning at about 5 years of age as language abilities and cognitive processes continue to develop. Although a few recalls could be obtained from children beginning at age 3, they were so short and undream-like that Foulkes dismisses them as evidence of real dreaming (see Chapter 6). The ability to dream becomes well formed by age 9 but continues developing through age 12–13.

Although dreams are the result of the "natural powers of the mind" that are the same as when awake and the content of dreams is systematic, coherent, and has a specific structure, there is no intention behind dream content. However, dreams do extend the dreamer's range of experiences and contribute to self-consciousness. They constitute a model of the waking world that is not a simple replay of the past but as something that could have happened.

Hunt[31]

Harry Hunt, a psychologist at Brock University in Canada, takes a broader approach than Foulkes. He says the study of dreaming needs to take information from a variety of sources, not just from subjects in the sleep laboratory or patients in the therapist's office. For Hunt, dream data also come from anthropological studies, dream journals, and those special dreams that people tend to notice and remember. In fact, he maintains, home dreams, not the ones from the lab, really tell what dreaming is all about. Such data show that there are a variety of types of dreams:

- Personal-mnemic dreams: containing everyday matters from the dreamer's waking life;
- Medical-somatic dreams: reflecting the physiology of the dreamer's body, especially illness;
- Prophetic dreams: Omens or other images of the future;

- Archetypal-spiritual dreams: encounters with ethereal or supernatural forces that are especially vivid and powerful often accompanied by very strong sensations;
- Nightmares: terrifying and upsetting;
- Lucid dreams: being conscious that one is dreaming while dreaming.

Some of these frequently occur such as the personal-mnemic dreams, while others such as the archetypal-spiritual dreams are rare but mostly intense and not likely to occur in the sleep lab. Each type has its own combination of cognitive processes and perhaps different functions.

Hunt also maintains that dreams are not limited to either being stories or imagery. They are both. One or the other can instigate the dream. Personal-mnemic dreams come from more grammar oriented processes while the rarer, intense dreams are more image oriented.

Hunt believes that Foulkes and Freud focus only on the personal-mnemic dreams, thus their theories are incomplete. Furthermore, some dreams are verbal propositions that are transformed into images (the theories of Freud, Foulkes, and Hobson focus on these), while other dreams start as visual-spatial images that are transformed into linguistic forms (the theory of Jung focuses on these types of dreams). This disparity leads to disagreements and disputes between the various theorists. But in reality, most of the various theorists have an accurate view of some dreaming, but none is comprehensive enough to account for all kinds of dreaming. In the end, a true theory of dreams and dreaming has to encompass all types of dreaming.

Hartmann[32]

The theory of dreaming by Ernest Hartmann, a Boston psychiatrist and long-time dream researcher, has three major aspects: the functional structure of the brain when dreaming, the emotional focus of dreams, and an aspect of personality related to dreaming. This theory is based in part on recent brain research and theories of others, his clinical impressions working with people and their dreams, and his and others' empirical research on dreams and dreamers.

For Hartmann, what is most important for understanding dreams and dreaming is what happens in the cortex, for it is there that conscious experience occurs. The functional structure of the brain is made up of neural nets. These structures are the synaptic connections between several or several hundreds of neurons active at any given time. Actually, it is a network of nets. That is, there are nets scattered about the cortex, sometimes widely scattered, that are networked together at specific times for specific functions. A mental event, be it a thought, memory, or an image, is the activation of a certain configuration of the net. There are different activation patterns for different contents of the mind.

Parts of the net are more tightly woven than other parts. A tight weave serves specific functions such as grammar, image recognition, or detailed memory recall.

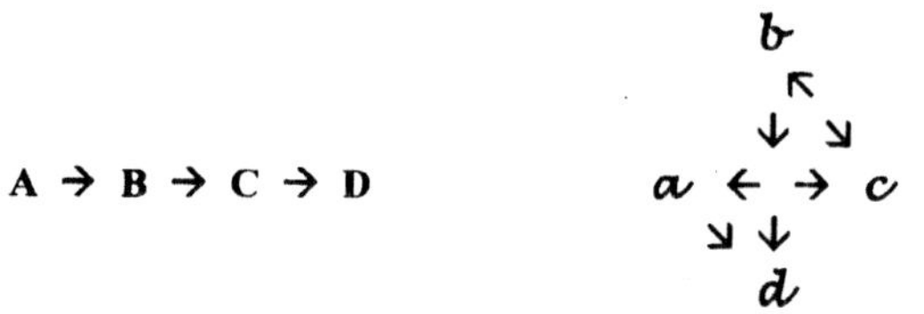

A → B → C → D

$$b$$
$$\nwarrow \;\; \downarrow \;\; \searrow$$
$$a \leftarrow \; \rightarrow \; c$$
$$\searrow \;\; \downarrow$$
$$d$$

Figure 32. On the left side is a representation of the organization of the functional neural networks during waking and on the right side a representation during dreaming. Additionally the nets represented by the letters are tighter during waking than during dreaming. (Modified from Hartmann (1998)).

They may have networked connections that are rather tightly defined with specified pathways. However, when dreaming, the network is more loosely and more broadly connected. When dreaming, neural activation tends to wander around networks and explore different connections more (see Figure 32). As a result, dreaming cognition is less linguistic, logical, and goal directed than is waking cognition. Additionally, there are fewer direct input to output paths. Deduction and making lists are not as possible. When dreaming, cognition is more metaphoric, bizarre, and novel.

There are always disturbances in the network of nets. These disturbances can be caused by things like behavioral stress, trauma, and conflicts, all with the common dominator of emotion. The greater the emotion, the greater the disturbance. The disturbance (emotion) focuses the content of the dream, and the nature of the network causes the disturbance to be metaphorically pictured rather than literally pictured. This process is most clearly seen in the dreams of adults following a trauma. They may dream of being overwhelmed by a tornado, caught in an earthquake, or some similar catastrophe. As the emotion changes with the passing of weeks and months, the metaphor also changes. For example, guilt may be represented as a hurt small animal or not supervising children who then get run over by a car. This same process also occurs, albeit not as obviously, in all dreams.

Hartmann also has found that some people apparently have looser, broader networks as their typical mode of functional brain organization. Behaviorally, he describes their personalities as having "thin boundaries." They have a rich fantasy life and have trouble telling reality from fantasy. They are daydreamers and are more open to experience. They have difficulty focusing on one thing. Their thoughts and feelings merge. Artists of various types tend to fall into this category.

In contrast, there are people who usually have apparently tightly woven, closely networked nets. They focus on one thing at a time. They clearly differentiate thoughts from feelings, reality from fantasy, self from others. They have a clear and well-compartmentalized sense of self that is well defended. They think of themselves as thought people. Many businessmen fall into this category.

These are the extremes. Most people are somewhere between these extremes, with thicker boundaries for some things and thinner boundaries for others.

The nature of individuals' boundaries relates to their dreams. People with thin boundaries have more dream recall, and their dreams have more vividness, more interaction between characters, and are more emotional than those of people with thick boundaries. People with thin boundaries are more likely to have nightmares.

One friendly critic (Domhoff, 1999) of Hartmann's theory says that parts of the theory are not well grounded in objective research. The idea that emotions direct the focus of dreaming needs to be tested rather than form the starting place for the theory. Further, Domhoff maintains that Hartmann does not have a reliable methodology to use in studying the place of emotions in dreams. Finally, Domhoff says that Hartmann presents no data that systematically show that dreams change over time in adults. In fact, much data (see Chapter 6) suggest otherwise.

Domhoff

Psychologist G. William Domhoff (2001) of the University of California, Santa Cruz has developed what he calls "A New Neurocognitive Theory of Dreaming." It is based on the data of Solms, brain imaging during sleep, Foulkes data and theory, and the Hall and Van de Castle method of studying dream content.

Domhoff sees dreaming as a developmental, cognitive entity resulting from the maturation and maintenance of a network of certain forebrain structures. Dreams are produced in accordance with a "continuity principle" using the present concerns of relevance to the dreamer and a "repetition principle" based on emotional concerns from the dreamer's past. The brain structures involved are those described by Solms and studies of the functional images of the brain during sleep. The cognitive development aspect is from Foulkes's research showing that dreaming develops gradually during the first decade of life. Domhoff points out that this cognitive development may be the result of the maturation of the brain structures necessary for dreaming. The continuity and repetition aspects come from his findings and others using the Hall and Van de Castle scales, showing that most recalled dream content is continuous with the dreamer's waking life yet with considerable repetition of characters, social interactions, misfortunes, negative emotions, and themes unique to the individual dreamer. The repetitive content may emanate from the activity in the portions of the brain responsible for emotionality.

Studies (see Chapter 6) using the Hall and Van de Castle system also show (1) dreams of college men and women in the United States have stayed unchanged during the major cultural changes of the latter half of the 20th century; (2) dream content changes little as adults age except for less physical aggression and negative emotion; (3) cross-cultural comparisons show many similarities in what people report they dream about with a few differences based on cultural differences; (4) the deviations of frequency of recalled dream aspects from the Hall and Van de Castle norms by individuals are consistent with their waking conceptions and emotional preoccupations past and present showing a continuity of dreams and current or past waking psychological issues. Additionally, the parallels between waking cognition and recalled dream content suggest that figurative thinking, using symbols and metaphors, may also be an important element of dreaming. The emphasis on dreams are concerns about self and others (see Chapter 6). Yet, recalled dreams having psychological meaning does not imply that dreaming is purposeful. Rather, he agrees with Flanagan (see Chapter 12) and Foulkes that dreams are the spin-off of the evolutionary development of sleep and consciousness.

SUMMARY

In this chapter, we have reviewed several important and representative theories of dreams. Some of these theories are basically psychological in their nature, while other theories are more based in the physiology of the brain. Some see dreams as "improvisationist" in that the dreamer combines whatever elements of mental activity happen to occur. Others see dreams as a "stage play" in that the dreamer starts with a story and brings in the elements necessary to portray that story. Hobson and colleagues would be an example of improvisationists, while Freud and Jung are examples of stage play. Other views are that dreams are either a compromise between primitive and disruptive tendencies and more advanced mental processes, or as non-linguistic, emotional expressions on the same level as waking mental processes. Examples of the first type are Freud and Hobson and colleagues, while an example of the second is Jung. There are those who insist that we reject subjectivity and study dreams only in the lab, believing that method is of prime importance. In contrast are those who place the dream itself first, saying the methods should follow.

Not everyone agrees that dreams are meaningful or even that a chapter such as this one should be included in this book. Many of my colleagues in the Sleep Research Society conclude that since the activation-synthesis theory has shown that dreams are a result of random activation of the cortex by the pons, dreams are a meaningless epiphenomenon. Others reach the same conclusion from a psychological perspective— dreams are the result of the lawful integration of more or less, randomly activated, recent and long-term memories. Although this process results in a structured story-line, there is no communicative intent. Hence, dreams do not mean anything, and interpretation of them is meaningless. Flanagan (1995, 2000) arrives at much the same conclusion from a philosophical approach.

Each of these dream theories has been criticized. The proponents of one theory have easily found and often vocally proclaimed the weaknesses of the others. It is not necessary to detail the individual criticisms of these theories since, in the end, we would be left with a welter of confusion or with nothing. We included the theories in this chapter—however imperfect—for two reasons. First, they are all we have at the moment. While not perfect, some, if not all, may contain aspects of the truth about what dreams really are. In the future, more accurate theories will probably adapt the best parts of them, or at least use them as a springboard to even better theories. Second, current approaches to dreams in the scientific laboratory, in the therapists' offices, in the popular press, and in the minds of modern humans are heavily influenced by these theories. Until something better comes along, they cannot be ignored.

Meanwhile, we recognize that such theories can even be useful. Such theories help organize the available knowledge and suggest further research. They also offer opponents of one or another of the theories, a clear and focused target for criticism. Both the research and criticisms generated help further our knowledge and perhaps will be the basis from which a future "Sleep-Einstein" will develop an equation that more truly shows the nature of dreams.

Part IV

Problems with Sleeping and Dreaming

To this point, we have concentrated on the normal processes of sleeping and dreaming, but things do not always go as intended. In this section, we will explore problems and difficulties of sleeping and dreaming. In Chapters 10 and 11, we will take a look at problems that typically come to the attention of one of the many sleep disorders treatment centers in the United States and, increasingly, in the rest of the world. Before that, Chapter 9 discusses things that are somewhat less severe in that they do not usually present themselves at a sleep disorders treatment center but are nevertheless problems of inconvenience, discomfort, and sometimes problems of great concern.

In the 1970s, a new aspect of medicine evolved—sleep disorders. Previously, physicians, as well as lay people, knew that sleep could be problematic; however, knowledge of both the kinds of problems people could have with sleep and the extent to which people suffered from them was limited, as was the knowledge of effective treatment for these problems. Insomnia, for example, has been well known for centuries, but knowledge of the number of different contributing factors to insomnia was minimal, and treatment consisted primarily of prescribing sleeping potions and pills.

As researchers in sleep laboratories around the world began to learn more and more about normal sleep, interest in abnormal sleep grew. Thus, during the decade of the 1970s, sleep disorder centers were developed in many medical centers for the purposes of learning more about the disorders of sleep and to providing clinics for accurate diagnosis and effective treatment.

CLASSIFICATION OF SLEEP DISORDERS[33]

People show up at sleep disorders centers with one, or a combination of, three kinds of complaints: not being able to sleep, being sleepy during the day, or abnormal

Table 5. The International Classification of Sleep Disorders

1. Dyssomnias
   A. Intrinsic Sleep Disorders
   B. Extrinsic Sleep Disorders
   C. Circadian Rhythm Sleep Disorders
2. Parasomnias
   A. Arousal Disorders
   B. Sleep-Wake Transition Disorders
   C. Parasomnias usually associated with REMS Sleep
   D. Other Parasomnias
3. Medical/Psychiatric Sleep Disorders
   A. Associated with Mental Disorders
   B. Associated with Neurological Disorders
   C. Associated with Other Medical Disorders

From American Sleep Disorders Association (1997).

events that occur during their sleep. However, any one of these problems may have very different underlying causes. For these reasons, sleep disorders are usually classi-fied and discussed by causes. There are three main categories of causes called dyssomnias, parasomnias, and sleep disorders associated with medical or psychiatic disorders (see Table 5).

Dyssomnias are problems with sleep that result in difficulties in initiating or maintaining sleep or in being excessively sleepy during the day. There are three sub-categories of dyssomnias. *Intrinsic sleep disorders* have their primary source from within the body—either physiological or psychological. Several of the most common sleep disorders that are found here are discussed in Chapter 10, including insomnia, nar-colepsy, sleep apnea, idiopathic hypersomnia, and periodic limb movement disorder. The *extrinsic sleep disorders* result primarily from causes outside the body. The prob-lems range from sleep disturbing environments and ascent to high altitudes to acute stress and food allergies. Also, sleep disorders resulting from being dependent on alcohol, stimulants, or sleeping pills fall under this classification. Some of these prob-lems will be discussed in the context of insomnia. Beyond that, there will be no fur-ther discussion, because they are all fairly obvious and are similarly treated by removal of the extrinsic factor. *Circadian rhythm sleep disorders* are primarily related to a problem with the timing of sleep in the nychthemeron (see Chapter 2). Jet lag and shift work can be found in Chapter 9. Delayed sleep phase disorder can be found in Chapter 11 along with brief mention of advanced sleep phase disorder and non-24-hour sleep-wake disorder.

Generally speaking, parasomnias are occurrences during sleep that are unde-sirable. Either they do not normally occur during sleep, such as bedwetting, or sleep makes an existing problem worse, such as abnormal heart rhythms. Hence, the term parasomnia is a kind of grab bag rather than a well-defined category. The key to understanding the parasomnias is to realize that sleep and wake are not always mutually exclusive states. Rather, they result from a recruitment of various components (see Chapter 13 and epilogue).

Parasomnias have four subcategories. *Arousal disorders* are a result of partial (incomplete) arousal during sleep. It is as if parts of the brain mechanisms for sleep and wake (see Chapter 4) are activated simultaneously or out of sequence. Included from this group in Chapter 9 are sleepwalking and sleep terrors. *Sleep-wake transition disorders* occur primarily during sleep stage transitions or transitions to or from wakefulness. Sleep talking is the example discussed in Chapter 9. *Disorders associated with REMS* are parasomnias that occur in or start in REMS. Nightmares is presented in Chapter 9 and REM behavior disorder in Chapter 10. *Other parasomnias* are those that do not fit in the first three categories. Chapter 9 focuses on bed-wetting and nocturnal teeth grinding from this category.

The sleep disorders associated with medical or psychiatric disorders occur in cases where sleep is a major component of the problem but is not the primary problem. Included in this category are people with major mental disorders (such as schizophrenia, depression, anxiety, and alcoholism), neurological disorders (such as Parkinsonism, Alzheimer's, and Huntington's disease), or other medical problems (such as sleeping sickness, peptic ulcers, and emphysema). We will not review these disorders, since the sleep problem is secondary to the medical or psychiatric disorder, which goes beyond the scope of this book.

A word of caution is in order here. As we examine these disorders, you may recognize some of these problems as occurring in yourself or someone you know. Indeed, your observations may reflect a genuine sleep disorder that should be evaluated by professionals at a sleep disorder clinic. However, more often than not, you may be suffering from the medical student syndrome. Medical students sometimes begin to see in themselves, and others, many of the diseases and disorders they are studying, although in reality there is no problem. This experience happens, because often there is no clear distinction between health and disease, but rather the difference is a matter of degree. So, too, with sleep disorders; everybody has had trouble sleeping sometime or has had occasional sleepiness during the day without having a dyssomnia. Likewise, jet lag is a frequent occurrence, but usually it is not severe enough to require a visit to a sleep disorder center. Only when the problems become excessive and debilitating, do they become sleep disorders.

Chapter 9

Some Difficulties That People May Have With Sleep[34]

Sleep is like food for the brain, yet getting enough quality sleep is a problem for many people. Some of these problems are the fault of circumstances that the sleeper is in, others are due to choices made by the sleeper, while others are things that happen to the sleeper. Sometimes the problem is not sleep itself but what happens during sleep. First, we will explore problems people have with getting enough quality sleep. Then we will turn our attention to some of the things that happen during sleep that are a problem for some people.

PROBLEMS WITH GETTING ENOUGH QUALITY SLEEP

Sleep Need and Sleep Debt

Many people in the Western world do not get sufficient sleep through their own choice or demands imposed upon them. Although most people often minimize the effects of sleep deprivation, they have been shown to be quite substantial. For many people, the only experience they have is being continually sleep deprived, which they take as normal. Robert J. Thomas said in a presentation at the Association of Professional Sleep Societies Meeting in Las Vegas, June 20, 2000, "We have insufficient RAM when sleep deprived." The effects, generally negative, of total sleep deprivation from one to several continuous days have been well researched. But most people do not often experience continuous, total sleep deprivation. More common is the accumulation of insufficient sleep night after night or irregular sleep patterns from night to night. Recent research has been showing that accumulated sleep debt from nights of insufficient sleep also has detrimental effects on both the body and the mind.

The National Sleep Foundation (2001, 2002) annually conducts a survey of sleep and sleep related habits of people in the United States. Results from 1998 through 2002 consistently showed that the average adult reports sleeping almost seven hours during the weekday, which is one hour less than the average recommended by sleep experts. Only about one-third of adults report getting 8 hours or more of sleep per night during the week, while two of five say they get less than 7 hours. Almost one-half of the respondents say they are likely to increase their sleep time on the weekend as compared to weekdays by about 45–50 minutes. The amount of sleep obtained during the workweek is strongly related to the number of hours worked each week; the greater the number of hours worked, the less sleep obtained. Additionally, caregivers, those caring for one or more individuals who could not live alone, and people with children report averaging slightly less sleep than do noncaregivers. Nearly two-thirds of people report having or having had at some time difficulty sleeping. As a counterpoint to these statistics, almost 90 percent of those surveyed said they believe that obtaining good sleep is important to enhance their lives.

But things may be even worse than the self-report surveys show. In a series of experiments (reported on by Adler, 1993), Tom Roth and colleagues at the Henry Ford Hospital in Detroit tested 300 healthy young adult normal sleepers. All slept about 7 hours per night outside the lab, and none said they felt particularly sleepy during the day. However, when tested in the sleep lab, one quarter of them regularly fell asleep within 6 minutes. When the others were allowed one hour less of sleep than they normally get for five nights, they too then fell asleep within 6 minutes. The subjects who normally fell asleep within 6 minutes also did worse on performance tasks, had slower reaction times, and were more affected by alcohol. All subjects did better when they had slept for 10 hours per night for 6 days, but the improvement was greater for the people who earlier had fallen asleep more quickly. These same people also got 7 more hours of sleep than the others when asked to sleep as much as they could in 32 hours. From these data, it appears that this group biologically requires more sleep than average and are sleep deprived when they try to get along on an average amount of sleep, although they apparently were not aware of this fact.

Box 25

The Effect of Music on Sleep

Some people like to fall asleep to music. This fact prompted Ramiro Sanchez, while an undergraduate at Northwestern University in Evanston, Illinois, to study the effect that different kinds of music have on sleep with sleep researcher Richard R. Bootzin (Sanchez & Bootzin, 1985). Forty-eight students took a two-hour evening nap while listening to white noise (like static when a radio is tuned between stations), classical music, soft rock, or hard rock. The results of the experiment revealed that static "white noise" is more conducive to good sleep than is any kind of music. Those who slept with white noise averaged 15 minutes to get to sleep and slept for 103 minutes. Those who slept to classical music slept for 66 to 73 minutes. Soft rock listeners averaged a total sleep time of 38 minutes. The hard rock listeners did not get much sleep, only 5.4 minutes. Comparison data for those listening to nothing were not provided.

The researchers posited that music disrupted sleep to the extent that the sound was unpredictable. Those who choose to fall asleep to music with screaming guitars and drum solos or similar sounds are cheating themselves out of a good night of sleep.

Effects of Sleep Deprivation

Chapter 2 reviewed the general effects of sleep deprivation. Here we explore how these effects can make a difference in people's lives.

The 2002 National Sleep Foundation poll (2001) found that nearly 25% of people in the United States are not getting the minimum amount of sleep they said they need. For people 18–29 years old, the percentage was higher at 29% but lower for people 65 and older at 12%. The report further showed that people who sleep less and have more daytime sleepiness were less likely to have positive feelings such as a sense of peace, satisfaction with life, and feeling full of energy and, have more negative moods such as anger, stress, pessimism, and fatigue. Almost two people out of every five said that their sleepiness also interferes with their activities at least a few times a month, and one in six said the interference occurs a few days every week. Respondents who said they got less than 6 hours of sleep on weekdays felt sleepier during the day than those who got more than 8 hours. They said they were more likely to get impatient or irked by common irritations on days when they were sleepy. They also said they were more likely to make mistakes and had problems getting along with others. Especially prevalent was the number of respondents who said that sleepiness impaired their performance at work, increased their chances of injury, and made it more difficult to make decisions and listen carefully to others.

As mentioned in Chapter 2, sleep debt can result in lapses in attention due to microsleeps plus general mental inefficiency. Whatever persons may be doing stops during a microsleep. They appear to stare off into space, and they cease whatever they were doing. Lapses due to microsleeps are especially prevalent during the absence of external stimulation. But sleep deprivation also results in more general decrements in performance. There is evidence for a general decrease in perceptual, cognitive, and psychomotor CAPACITY (Dinges, 1989; Harrison & Horne, 1999; Hauri, 1979; Horne, 1988, & MacLean et al., 1990) plus a decrease of alertness short of microsleeps (Thomas et al., 1990). The effects of lack of sleep on performance are more akin to an overworked automobile engine rather than a battery running down (Dinges & Powell, 1989; Horne, 1988). The overworked engine loses some peak horsepower as well as the occasional misfiring of a spark plug, causing the engine sometimes to sputter. Giving the engine more gas can compensate for these engine deficits early on, just as a person can reduce the effects of sleep deprivation by extra effort and motivation, but eventually even this attempt does not help much. Likewise, revving the engine occasionally may help at first, just like stretching or splashing cold water on your face helps, yet the engine becomes less and less effective as time goes on just as stretching or cold water cease to be very effective over time.

Recent studies using functional imaging of the brain show that people who have lost one night of sleep have noticeable differences in brain activity (Drummond et al., 2000). It was especially noticeable in the prefrontal cortex. These studies also show that in a fully rested person, the prefrontal areas and left temporal area of the brain become active when processing language. In the sleep-deprived person, the prefrontal areas become more active, but the left temporal area becomes much *less* active. To compensate, the parietal areas, typically not used by the rested person for this task, take over, resulting in only some deficit in performance.

Earlier this group (Drummond et al., 1999) had shown that the prefrontal brain regions activated in rested persons when doing arithmetic problems were not active when sleep deprived, but no other area appeared to take over this task resulting in considerable errors and omitted responses.

In a third experiment (Drummond, Gillin, & Brown, 2001), subjects had to do both the verbal and the arithmetic tasks at the same time. They again found various levels of deficits in performance when sleep deprived, less activation of the left temporal lobe, and increased activation in the prefrontal and parietal areas. Additionally, there was greater activation in the areas involved with maintaining attention and monitoring errors when sleep deprived.

Collectively, these studies show that sleep deprivation causes a change in the distribution of activity in the brain when doing a given task. Depending on the task, some areas may become more active, others less active, and others newly recruited in an effort to accomplish the task. Yet even when there is greater brain effort, there are usually still deficits in performance.

Effects of Sleep Deprivation on Performance[35]

For many years, research has shown that sleep deprivation has a very negative effect on long, dull, repetitive, and monotonous psychomotor tasks as well as reaction time, short-term memory, and other aspects of visual and auditory memory. The greater the monotony of these tasks, the more quickly the negative effects of sleep deprivation are manifested. In contrast, there appears to be no effect on other kinds of tasks such as those that are complex but rule based, involve logical deduction, have high intrinsic interest, are relatively short (less than 10 minutes), are strongly externally motivated (such as by money rewards), involve critical reasoning, or are well practiced. Generally, people seem to overcome the effects of sleep deprivation by exerting

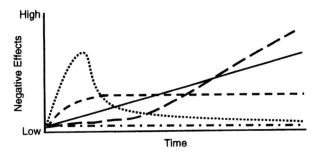

Figure 33. Hypothetical trends in how different people think sleep deprivation will effect them. See text for explanation.

compensatory effort. Yet, new research coupled with informed speculation suggests that these findings have helped perpetuate the myth that sleep is not really all that necessary. It is now known that the effects of sleep deprivation are much broader than previously understood.

Many people wrongly believe that they can adapt sleep deprivation and perform well. There are four general beliefs about the pattern of the ability to adjust to sleep deprivation (see Figure 33). Some people think that they will suffer effects for a while but then "get used to them." These persons are represented by the line of small dashes on Figure 33. Some think that they will suffer for awhile but then adapt and do as well as they would with more sleep. These people are represented by the dotted line. The big dashed line represents those who believe they can do okay for awhile, but eventually "it will catch up" with them. Finally, there are those represented by the dash–dot line who think there are no effects of sleep deprivation. The objective truth is shown as the solid line; a continually worsening linear trend.

There now appears to be a variety of tasks that are negatively affected by sleep deprivation. These tasks include those that are not routine and where higher-level cognitive skills are required. The list includes dealing with the unexpected, when innovation and flexibility is needed, where plans need revising, where great amounts of information need to be quickly assimilated, where information is ambiguous, where there are competing distractions that need to be sorted through to determine what needs attention and what can be ignored, where risks need to be realistically assessed, where it is important to keep track of when things happened, and when the big picture needs updating. Additionally, sleep deprivation may have negative effects on the ability to communicate with others because of flattening of voice, problems retrieving words, and shorter and less frequent utterances. Sleep deprivation also causes problems with controlling negative moods or excessive euphoria, inhibiting immature or inappropriate behaviors, keeping the lid on emotional outbursts, being empathetic, anticipating the range of possible consequences, having insight over one's own performance, and being more susceptible to argument and suggestion. Sleep deprivation can increase errors of omission, increase errors of commission, and decrease time spent on task. Many of these things depend on a fully functioning prefrontal cortex, which functional brain imaging studies show is greatly affected by sleep deprivation. While some effects of sleep deprivation, such as general arousal, are lessened by caffeine, the functions dependent on the prefrontal cortex are not.

Van Dongen and Dinges (2001) report that performance decline resulting from sleep deprivation is influenced by several individual characteristics. These characteristics include the phase of the individual's circadian rhythm at the time of the performance, the individual's sleep need per nychthemeron, and the individual's vulnerability to sleep loss.

Several studies have looked at the effects of accumulated sleep deprivation on the performance of medical interns (reviewed in Patton, Landers, & Agarwal, 2001). Medical interns have work schedules that require them to be available for 24 hours at a time, sometimes longer. It is not unusual for them to get little sleep during this time. Although they are apparently able to do things like grasp technical information from medical journals, studies have concluded that sleep deprived interns show greater hesitancy in decision making, are not as well focused in their planning, not as innovative, and have impaired verbal fluency.

Another line of research involves military personnel in simulated or real operations for 48 to 80 hours (see Harrison & Horne, 2000). Performance noticeably deteriorated at 36 hours when the individuals had problems keeping track of critical tasks, failed to use incoming information to update maps, and put off tasks that required immediate attention. They became less flexible when generating possible responses to unpredictable problems. They became more docile, more resigned to their situation, yet focused more on personal survival rather than the overall tasks at hand. Some lower level officers no longer acted as leaders. Planning ahead was reduced, and behavior sometimes became disinhibited. Communication became less accurate or misinterpreted.

Another approach has been to put people into game-like situations in the laboratory to see the effects of sleep debt. Harrison and Horne (1999) used their Masterplanner game for this purpose. This game simulates marketing strategy for managers and business students where greater innovation in the face of changing events increases potential sales. The game becomes more and more difficult as it progresses. After 36 hours without sleep, it was apparent that players were no longer able to do what was required for success in the game and their "sales" results deteriorated as they increasingly relied on previously successful solutions that were no longer successful. Non-sleep deprived participants were much more successful in comparison. The critical reasoning ability of the participants was concurrently tested showing both groups equally able to digest and comprehend large amounts of printed information. What the sleep deprived participants eventually lacked was the ability to use this information in new, useful ways.

Many of these findings are based on single bouts of sleep deprivation of 24, 36 or more hours. And the studies have typically used young adult males, mainly college students or young soldiers. More recent research is beginning to show that the effects are "dose dependent." That is, the greater the degree of sleep deprivation, the greater the degree of effects. Likewise, recent research is showing that accumulation of partial sleep deprivation over a number of days may have similar effects to a night or two of continuous sleep deprivation. Still more research is needed to show how age and gender influence these kinds of effects of sleep deprivation. For example, a couple of older studies that used simple types of performance tasks showed middle aged subjects believed they were less affected by sleep deprivation than did younger subjects but actually did worse on tasks involving persistence and attention, meticulousness, and mental processing. Finally, more attention is beginning to be paid to individual differences in susceptibility to sleep deprivation.

Effects of Sleepiness on Driving[36]

Driving a car and sleeping are incompatible. Although this statement is obvious, at least 100,000 crashes, 71,000 injuries, and 1,500 fatalities reported by police each year involve drowsiness as a major cause according to conservative estimates by the (U.S.) National Highway Traffic Safety Administration (no date). In the National Sleep Foundation annual polls from 1998 to 2002, over 50–60% of respondents said they had driven while drowsy in the last year, and 17–27% said they had actually fallen asleep while driving. These percentages are much higher in young adults. Twenty to 30% of shift workers reported a fatigue related driving misfortune in the last year and one-fourth admit actually to falling asleep while driving (National Sleep Foundation, 2001, 2002). Almost one-half of medical interns say they have fallen asleep while driving, most often after getting off work. More traffic accidents occur during times of greater circadian sleepiness, with the major peak in the early morning hours and a smaller peak in the late afternoon. When differences in the number of people driving at different times of the day is taken into account, at 6:00 a.m. the risk of a sleep related accident is 20 times greater and at 4:00 p.m. is 3 times greater than at 10:00 a.m. Drivers who work long hours, night shifts, or multiple jobs are the most likely to be involved in a sleepiness related car accident, especially if their commute lasts longer than 20 minutes. Other factors include getting less than 6 hours of sleep per night, being awake 20 or more hours, taking medicine for colds and flu that cause sleepiness, and lack of sleep and long drives during holiday seasons. The cost of incidents due to falling asleep at the wheel has been estimated to be $12.5 billion per year (National Sleep Foundation, 2000).

Self-awareness of drowsiness is sufficiently obvious that virtually no one should fall asleep at the wheel. However, what most people do not realize, or at least do not act upon, is that drowsiness can very easily and very suddenly become sleep. At 55 miles per hour, a vehicle will travel more then 100 yards during a 4 second microsleep—enough for a vehicle to become involved in a dangerous, sometimes fatal, situation. After 17 hours without sleep, performance on a cognitive psychomotor task such as driving is equivalent to someone with a blood alcohol level of 0.05 (Dawson & Reid, 1997). After 24 hours without sleep, this figure rises to be equivalent to 0.10.

Powell and associates (2001) directly compared reaction times to several hazards in 16 healthy, adult volunteers following sleep deprivation or intake of alcohol while driving on a 1.4-mile performance course at GM's proving grounds in Arizona. After an initial round of testing, when fully rested, the subjects were split into three groups (1) after one night without sleep, (2) sleeping for no more than two hours for seven consecutive nights, and (3) after consuming alcohol to a mean blood alcohol level of the 0.089 percent. Changes in driving performances of all groups were similar in the second round. The average reaction time of the alcohol-impaired group was 294 milliseconds, while the average for the sleep-deprived groups 300 milliseconds, both about 20% longer than baseline. Conclusion: driving sleep deprived can be as bad as driving drunk.

Belenky and colleagues (Johnson et al., 1998; Thorne et al., 1998, 1999; Welsh et al., 1998) have shown that accumulated sleep debt can impact negatively on driving ability. They use commercial truck drivers as their subjects. One study lasting two weeks centered around 7 consecutive days of either 3, 5, 7, or 9 hours in bed. All subjects spent 8 hours in bed for 3 days before and after this regimen. Sleep and wake were measured continuously, and the subjects were repeatedly tested on a psychomotor vigilance task that required no learning and in a driving simulator. On the vigilance task, the greater the accumulated sleep deprivation, the greater the decrement of performance. This decline in functioning carried over into the recovery period in spite of large sleep recovery. Additionally, the greater the accumulated sleep deprivation, the greater decrease in performance as the task went on. In the driving simulator, problems with staying in the lane increased as sleep deprivation accumulated and did not totally diminish during the recovery days. Speeding increased progressively in the 3-hour deprived group. There were a large number of accidents in the 3-hour deprived group, but this number diminished with recovery sleep. Microsleeps were not the sole cause of the accidents, because over one-half of them were not preceded by falling asleep. Peripheral attention also showed decrements in the 3-hour deprived group. Large individual differences were apparent throughout these data. The authors concluded that even modest accumulated sleep deprivation leads to distinct decreases in performance that can fail to recover completely even with 3 days of recovery sleep.

The Better Sleep Council and the American Automobile Association's Foundation for Traffic Safety list the following as some of the danger signals for impending sleep onset while driving: feeling drowsy, eyelids feeling heavy, eyes burning or feeling strained, problem keeping eyes focused, incessant yawning, no memory of driving the last few miles, and lane drifting or missing traffic signals. At this point you must stop driving immediately and take appropriate counter measures (see below).

Few drivers admit to having fallen asleep after an accident. For some, it may be the fear of reprisal or liability lawsuit that causes conscious denial. For most, however, it is likely that they did not even realize that they had fallen asleep for a few seconds. Laboratory studies have shown that most people do not report falling asleep until they have been asleep for a couple of minutes. The result is that far too many people continue driving when feeling drowsy. They will attempt to use countermeasures such as opening the window to let cold air blow on their faces, turn the radio or CD player up loud, or frequently change position in the car. Some will stop briefly and do a bit of exercise. However, laboratory research with driving simulators has shown that such measures are effective for 15 minutes at best. This brief period may buy the driver enough time to find a safe place to stop but not to continue driving for long periods of time. Also, if someone is seriously sleep deprived, the loud radio or CD player may divert attention enough that response to a dangerous situation may be too slow or even missed.

The most effective counter measures to sleepiness when driving are consuming caffeine or napping. About 150 mg of caffeine, about two cups of coffee, is needed to be beneficial, but more than this amount can cause unpleasant and potentially disrupting side effects. Also a 15-minute, but not more than 20-minute, nap helps greatly. The ideal solution is to use both the caffeine and the nap during a 30-minute break. Drink the coffee. Then take the nap. It takes about 30 minutes for the caffeine to become effective, about the time the nap should end. This combination has been shown to provide enduring effects that significantly reduce the likelihood of having a sleep related accident.

Awareness of Sleepiness

Many people are not aware of just how sleepy they are. They may say they do not feel sleepy most of the time, especially if they are active and busy. What is really happening though is that arousing activities and situations mask their sleepiness (see Chapter 2). A better indicator of whether you are sleepy or not is what happens when these masking stimuli are not present (see Chapter 3).

Box 26

Sleeping with Pets

John Shepard, medical director of the Mayo Clinic Sleep Disorders Center, had a patient tell him that she often had to get up in the middle of the night to let her dog out. She had to wait up to 15 minutes before getting back to bed with her pet. Curious about how common this experience was, he asked the next 300 patients at the Mayo Clinic Sleep Disorders Center about how often and to what extent their sleep was affected by their pet. Of the 157 who said they had pets, mainly cats and dogs, almost 60% said their pet slept in their bedroom. Fifty percent of the pet dogs slept in the bed. An even greater percent of cats were allowed to sleep in the bed. Over one-half of the pet owners said their pet disrupted their sleep in some way every night, but only 1% said the disruption averaged more than 20 minutes. Twenty-one percent of the pet dogs snored, as did 7% of the pet cats.

Managing Sleepiness

Not getting enough sleep is nothing to be proud of. According to the 1999 National Sleep Foundation poll (2001), 58% of the respondents mistakenly said they believed that people can learn to sleep less while still being able to function normally. Charles Czeisler of Harvard University (personal communication) has compared sleep need to a semitrailer with a circadian driver that accumulates its load as the wakefulness goes on. The load is unloaded twice as fast during sleep. But without enough sleep, the trailer is only partially unloaded. When this deprivation happens night after night, the load accumulates, and the speed and efficiency of the semitrailer suffers.

Most sleep debt can be alleviated by simple changes:

- Recognizing the importance of sleep and allowing enough time every nychthemeron for it is often helpful.
- Following good sleep hygiene (see Box 14 in Chapter 5).
- Taking steps to manage stress.
- Planned short naps.

Fulfilling our sleep quota leaves us more energetic, alert, happy, creative, productive, motivated, and healthy (Maas, 1998). Some people may have difficulty obtaining enough sleep or have a sleep disorder that requires seeking professional help from a sleep disorders treatment center (see Chapter 10).

PROBLEMS INVOLVING THE CIRCADIAN RHYTHM OF SLEEP

Jet Lag

Jet lag can occur when there is rapid travel east or west across time zones. Travel to the north or south may cause some fatigue, but not jet lag per se. Jet lag is caused by a mismatch between the phase of the body's internal circadian rhythm and the phase of the local nychthemeral time. For example, the body may think it is morning, but according to local time it is the middle of the night. When traveling east the circadian rhythm of the body is behind that of local time and needs to be advanced, and the opposite occurs when traveling west.

One-third of people do not seem to be affected by jet lag. For the rest, it can range in severity from mild to strong. Symptoms last for a few days and include sleep disturbance, daytime tiredness, reduced concentration, slower reaction times, irritability, and general disorientation. Other common symptoms are headaches, digestive problems, and intestinal problems. In the extreme, it can contribute to "travel paranoia." There are also problems with sleep at night—difficulty getting to sleep when having traveled eastward or awakening too early when traveling westward. These events occur because the body's internal clock is not yet preparing the body for sleep for the former and prepares the body to be awake earlier than local time for the latter. Additionally, the sleep that is obtained is disturbed and not entirely restful. The net result is that individuals suffering from jet lag may have performance problems due to both trying to perform during the low phase of the circadian rhythm and insufficient and poor sleep.

Generally, there is greater jet lag when traveling toward the east than when traveling toward the west. For example, professional baseball teams lose more games when they have just traveled from the west to the east than when traveling east to west. As a rule of thumb, it takes 1 recovery day for each time zone crossed when traveling to the west but $1\frac{1}{2}$ recovery days for each time zone when traveling toward the east for the effects of jet lag to completely remit. This difference occurs because the body's internal circadian rhythm is a bit longer than 24 hours and thus tends toward phase delaying. When traveling east, this natural tendency must be opposed. In a few individuals who have traveled to the east, recovery takes longer because the body's circadian rhythm insists on delaying instead of advancing. For example, it may delay by 16 hours rather than getting to the same phase by advancing 8 hours. In all cases, if several time zones have been crossed, adaptation is more rapid in the first few days before gradually tapering off. However, it is not unusual for some people at some times to find traveling east easier than traveling west.

Countermeasures may be applied to attempt to assuage the effects of jet lag or to speed recovery. Some aim at improving the quality and quantity of sleep while others aim at more quickly resynchronizing the circadian rhythms of the body to local time. Some do both simultaneously. One bit of advice: when possible, leave early in the day when traveling east but in the evening when traveling west.

Sleep deprivation resulting from jet lag can be improved in several ways. Using a short acting (3–5 hours) sleeping medication can improve sleep while traveling and upon arrival at the destination. En route, you should try to sleep when you would be sleeping at the destination and awaken when you would be awakening there. A short acting sleeping pill can facilitate this process, especially when trying to sleep on an airplane, but must be timed so that the effects are gone at or before the destination awakening time. It also helps to optimize the sleeping environment by reducing noise and light and improving body comfort as much as possible. Altering the environment can be done on the plane by using earplugs, eyeshades, and a c-shaped pillow at the back of the neck. Avoid alcohol and big meals while traveling and drink coffee only at the time you would do so at the destination, but drink a lot of water.

The key to getting circadian rhythms synchronized to local time is to adopt local time quickly for your schedule of eating, sleeping, and generally being active. Begin this routine as much as possible en route or even a few days before leaving. Timing of exposure to bright light and darkness is critical. Although more research is needed, the following tentative advice can be given at this time. Keep track of your subjective nighttime (= night according to the internal rhythm of your body; see Chapter 2) as the process of synchronizing to local time is occurring. While there is no easy way to be absolutely sure of this timing, you can use this rule of thumb: your circadian rhythm moves from where it was at departure toward synchronization with your destination at the rate of one hour per day. If for some reason your rhythm may not be synchronized with your departure location, such as if you have been traveling about with many different destinations through several time zones or rotating through different work shifts, it is not possible to estimate where your body's circadian rhythm is, and you will not be able to use this plan. If you need to phase advance, because of traveling east, seek several hours of bright light in your subjective morning, which on the first day at the destination would be afternoon if you crossed several time zones but in the morning after a few days at the destination, and avoid light during your subjective evening and night. If you need to phase delay, because of traveling west, seek several hours of bright light in your subjective evening but avoid light during your subjective night and early morning. Avoiding light at the wrong time is as important as seeking light at the right time. Computer programs that more precisely specify when to seek and when to avoid light have been developed and are undergoing tests and refinements but may soon be available.

Even more tentative are suggestions for taking melatonin to both reduce sleep deprivation and speed resynchronization of circadian rhythms. Not enough is known about optimal doses, individual differences in sensitivities, interactions with drugs, or long-term effects for this substance. Additionally, melatonin is not regulated in the United States, and the purity or amount may not be as indicated on the label. In some countries, it is illegal to possess it without a prescription. Also, be aware, since it can produce sleepiness, you should not drive or engage in other potentially dangerous activities that may require your full alertness. This being said, I can report that much research indicates positive results from taking melatonin to aid recovery from the effects of jet lag. It can both improve the quality of sleep and act as a zeitgeber (see Chapter 2) to speed synchronization of circadian rhythms to local time. However, just like exposure to light, timing is critical. It should be taken before or early in the subjective night to phase advance for eastward travel and late in the subjective night to phase delay for westward travel. Note that this practice is just the opposite of when to seek light, since melatonin and light move the circadian clock in opposite directions. As with exposure to light, there are computer algorithms that have been developed and are being tested and refined for when to take melatonin to combat jet lag.

Daylight Savings Time

Related to jet lag is a phenomenon experienced by many in the United States and other parts of the world who have Daylight Savings Time (Coren, 1996). Every spring on a given date, there is a 23-hour nychthemeron ("spring forward") requiring you to phase advance and every fall on a given date there is a 25-hour nychthemeron ("fall back") requiring you to phase delay. It is as if you and everyone else took a jet trip one time zone east in the spring and one time zone west in the fall. Many of people suffer for a day or so from mild jet lag symptoms. There are beneficial effects on mood at awakening and the perception of sleep quality for about a week after going off daylight savings time in the fall but opposite effects on mood in the spring when going on it (Monk & Alpin, 1980). Also, there is about a 7% increase in traffic accidents the day after the time change in the spring but about a 7% decrease in them in the fall. There are similar changes in hospital admissions for other kinds of accidents.

Sleepiness and the Workplace[37]

Sleepiness in the workplace is a serious problem. Some of the sleepiness is due to the job, and other aspects are due to the worker. The sleepiness that workers bring with them to work cause them to perform worse on a variety of tasks and have less healthy interpersonal relationships (Patton, Landers, & Agarwal, 2001) as well as affect other aspects of their lives including at home and when driving. But the workplace may also be a contributing factor in sleepiness. The cause and effects of accumulated sleep deficits because the demands of the job that often leave their workers inadequate time to sleep has been the focus of a lot of research attention in long haul truck drivers, airline personnel, military, and medical interns.

Some of the National Sleep Foundation annual polls have also looked at the effects of sleepiness in the workplace (National Sleep Foundation, 2001). In 1997, it was found that sleepiness cost employers in the U.S. about $18 billion per year due to lost productivity. When mistakes, damage, and health problems caused by sleepiness were included, the costs were even greater. One out of every 7 workers surveyed said they were sometimes late for work because of sleepiness. For young adults, it was over one in five. Close to one in five workers reported sometimes making mistakes at work due to sleepiness. Respondents said sleepiness made concentration harder (65%), stress was more difficult to handle (65%), solving problems and making decisions was more difficult (58%), and listening to others on the job was harder (57%).

A variety of factors in the workplace contributes to employee sleepiness. These factors include schedules of working (shift work, long hours, overtime), nature of the

---

Box 27

The Effect of Sleep Habits on Academic Performance

A random sampling of 200 on-campus students at a large private university showed that sleep habits, especially wake-up times, correlated with grade point averages (Trockel, Barnes, & Egget, 2000). Specifically, later awakening times were correlated with lower average grades. This correlation was greater than for any other factor studied, including exercise, eating habits, mood states, perceived stress, time management, social support, spiritual or religious habits, number of hours worked per week, gender, and age.

Other research has shown that university students who averaged less than 7 hours of sleep per night averaged twice as many visits to physicians and reported two times as many infections than those who averaged more than 7 hours (Coren, 1998).

In contrast, Gray and Watson (2002) found little evidence that sleep quality or quantity impact academic performance, but being a regular early riser does have a positive effect.

---

tasks (prolonged vigilance, high stress), and the physical nature of the workplace (lack of bright lights, poor temperature control).

Unfortunately, there are no perfect solutions to these problems (Rosekind et al., 1996). Yet, there are many things workers can do for themselves to improve their sleep and sleep time to minimize sleepiness (see Chapter 5). Likewise, there are things employers can do to help minimize the sleepiness of their workers including education and training, improving work schedules, and improving the workplace.

Shift Work

Shift work loosely means working anytime other than during the day. It also can refer to rotating between working during the day and at other times. Either way, shift work presents a challenge for workers (currently 20% of the workforce in the United States) in getting enough good quality sleep. Shift work is even more difficult for people over 50 years of age, morning types (see Chapter 2), long sleepers (see Chapter 3), those with chronic illnesses, or those who have a sleep disorder (see Chapter 11). It is estimated that 20% of workers cannot tolerate shift work (Coren, 1996). There are three interacting sources of problems for shift workers—poor quality and quantity of sleep, disrupted circadian rhythms, and domestic/social problems. These problems in turn cause significant problems with mood, health, mental skills, and performance (Harrington, 1994). Additionally, 12-hour shifts are becoming more popular especially in some chemical and plastics industries as well as with nurses (Coren, 1996). The buildup of sleepiness, accompanied by feelings of fatigue and decreased alertness, is greater during a 12-hour shift than an 8-hour shift. This buildup tends to accumulate as the workweek goes on. The result has been found to be errors in work and judgment.

Shift workers typically do not get enough sleep or good quality sleep. The average shift worker in the United States and Europe gets 5 to 7 hours less sleep per week than their non-shift working counterparts. This disparity occurs because of both social/domestic pressures to be doing other things during the day other than sleeping and because they are trying to sleep when their circadian rhythm is in its wake maintenance zone (see Chapter 2). The sleep that is obtained is of poorer quality, because it is fragmented (see Chapter 3) by arousals. Research studies have shown that SWS sleep is less affected than are stage 2 and REMS. The flip side is the struggle to remain awake when working. About 75% of shift workers experience sleepiness every shift, and at least 20% fall asleep at work (Coren, 1996).

Most shift workers have disrupted circadian rhythms. Rotating shift workers may, at best, successfully get their circadian rhythms synchronized to their current shift for a few days before they have to rotate to the next shift. Some never shift, and a few even shift the wrong way. Even those who permanently work a non-day shift without rotating may be frequently desynchronized, because on their days off they often assume a diurnal pattern of waking and sleep at night in order to take part in social/domestic activities. Since the many different body functions resynchronize at different rates, their bodies are operating like various instruments in a band playing the same song but at various notes ahead or behind the others.

Shift workers are forced to cope socially and domestically with a world that is diurnally oriented. For example, on their time off from work, they often must participate in activities during the day even if they are sleep deprived and synchronized to a different schedule. This pattern is especially true for women shift workers who are expected to continue to run the household on a "normal" schedule. But it can also affect men in their roles as a sex partner, social companion, father, and so forth. In addition, religious, recreational, and entertainment functions are mainly orientated toward a diurnal cycle. Many permanent night shift workers find that they need to be awake during the day on days off, requiring them to sleep at night. Just a weekend of night sleep can quickly cause resynchronization. They are like salmon trying to jump waterfalls to get up stream, finding that it is hard to advance but easy to fall back. It takes longer, up to a week, to resynchronize to working at night and sleeping during the day, because humans are biologically organized for night sleep, and daylight acts as a strong zeitgeber.

As a result of disruptions to their sleep, circadian rhythms, and social/domestic lives, shift workers often experience more problems than their day working counterparts. They complain of social isolation and have 57% higher divorce rates. They report more negative moods and have more emotional problems. They have higher incidences of sleep disorders, stomach and intestinal problems, and cardiovascular ill-nesses. They have a higher than average number of car accidents when driving home from work. An increasing amount of research shows there are more mistakes and acci-dents on the job among shiftworkers during the nightshift (Akerstedt, 1995).

A special problem that some shift workers experience is "night shift paralysis." It is the inability to move for a few minutes to more than 5 minutes (Coren, 1996). It has been observed in flight controllers, especially when working successive night shifts, and in those with the most sleep deprivation. It has also been observed in nurses on 12-hour shifts.

There are several things that can be done to ameliorate the problems of shift work, but none are completely successful. Both workers and employers benefit from education about the interrelationship of changes in the body's circadian rhythms, sleep problems, and social/domestic stresses that result from shift work. Teaching shiftworkers about good sleep hygiene (see Chapter 5) and about how to manipulate zeitgebers (see Chapter 2) can also be beneficial. Prescription sleeping pills, if prop-erly used, can improve sleep quality and quantity but seem to have no effect on reset-ting circadian rhythms or result in no improvement in waking, night alertness and performance. However, given the potential for overuse and misuse, sleeping pills are not generally recommended. Over-the-counter sleep aids may cause more problems than solutions, since they can leave a person drowsy for hours after awakening. Taking melatonin prior to attempting sleep during the day can help with getting more and better sleep as well as acting as a zeitgeber for resynchronizing the circa-dian rhythms, but there is nothing known about the effects of its long-term use as well as other potential problems (see section on Jet Lag). Maintaining a bright (more than 7000 lux) workplace and a very dark bedroom can also help. Avoiding light during your subjective night (see Chapter 2) is important because even short exposure to daylight at the wrong time can negatively affect the synchronization of the circadian rhythms. Very dark wraparound sunglasses or even dark welders glasses can help with this problem but pose a risk for driving and doing other potentially dangerous things. Finally, judicious use of caffeine or the new arousal drugs that are being developed may help mitigate the effects of sleepiness on the job.

Some shift rotation schedules are better than others for countering the problems. Schedules that rotate with the clock (days to afternoons to nights to days and so on) are the best. Working no more than five nights in a row followed by two nychthe-merons off, no more than four 12-hour shifts in a row, not starting the day shift before 7 a.m., and avoiding complicated schedules are also beneficial. There are two schools of thought on how rapidly to rotate shifts. Both agree that weekly rotations are not good, but in the United States less frequent rotations are preferred so that workers can be synchronized at least for some of the tail end of each rotation. In Europe, more rapid rotations are favored, such as every two nychthemerons, with the idea that the person will not even try to resynchronize. It is recognized that neither scheme is perfect, but each has some advantages over the other, and both are better than other alternatives.

There are also some unique aspects of what can be done to lessen the effects of shift work. Morning types are less flexible about their sleeping times but get more out of a 20-minute nap. Evening types are more flexible and can recoup faster after sleep deprivation. If the situation requires sustained wake, try for several short naps, especially when sleepiness is felt. Even better are several short naps and one 2–3 hour one. (c.f. Mason, 2000).

DIFFICULTIES WITH SLEEP WITH ADVANCED AGE[38]

Advanced age has several effects on sleep that can cause problems. In fact, more than half of those over age 65 report disturbed sleep. One cause is the natural change in circadian rhythms in adults. As adults age, they tend to phase advance their internal circadian rhythms. But there is evidence that the rhythms also begin to flatten, so there is less difference between the nadir and the acrophase, and the response to zeitgebers gets a bit weaker. Additionally, the amount of slow wave sleep diminishes with age in adults, as does the release of melatonin and growth hormone. The net result is that by retirement age, sleep is shorter, shallower, and more fragmented, making sleep seem like more of a problem than it was before. Also, getting to sleep and staying asleep is frequently more of a problem. Yet, it is easier to doze off more during the day when engaged in quiet activities. Many of these changes occur sooner in males than females. Additionally, as people age, they are more likely to develop chronic medical illnesses that can affect sleep. Also, sleep disorders are more common later in life.

Many of these things develop gradually during adult life. Some changes begin to manifest themselves earlier than others. For example, beginning as early as the 40s or 50s, some people may have more trouble adapting to jet lag or shift work, because it becomes harder and harder for them to sleep during their subjective day (Carrier, 2001).

PROBLEMS THAT OCCUR DURING SLEEP

Snoring[39]

Mark Twain called snoring "sleeping out loud." Other wags have called snoring "sound sleeping." Snoring, however, can indicate serious problems and may cause some of those problems. It occurs when there is less room for the air to travel through the upper airways during sleep. The air has to move faster through the space and causes vibrations of the soft tissue of the throat, like a flag flapping in a stiff breeze. Anything that constricts the upper airway passages or results in there being more flaccid tissue in the throat can contribute to snoring, including relaxation of the throat muscles that normally contract when inhaling, excess tissue, inflammation, inherited differences in the shape of the upper airways, and diminished elastic content of the tissues with age. Allergies, infection, respiratory irritants, and smoking can cause swelling of these tissues. Alcohol and some drugs can cause the muscles of the throat to relax. Lying on the back can cause the tongue and other throat tissue to be pulled back by gravity. Large tonsils and adenoids may constrict the size of the throat. Nasal congestion may force more mouth breathing. Even depression, stress, or anxiety can cause changes in blood flow to the nose, causing swelling.

There is general agreement that snoring is common, males snore more than females, and the incidence of snoring increases with age from about 20 to 60 years. One study shows a linear trend from 10 to 60% in males and 5 to 45% in females during this age span. Seventy percent of children snore occasionally, but 7 to 10% do so every night. There are thought to be over 40 million people who snore in the United States.

There are degrees of differences in snoring, ranging from mild and only occasional to what has been called heroic. The latter group snores virtually every night and can be heard by others in distant rooms or even by neighbors! Loud and frequent snoring can be a sign of obstructive sleep apnea (see Chapter 10), but not all people who snore have apnea. It is thought that some snoring progresses to apnea over time. Snoring can occur in all sleep stages but can be more common in stages 2, 3, and 4. It may be more common in some families and some forms may have a genetic basis. Not that there is a specific gene for snoring, but predisposing characteristics of the upper airway may be inherited.

Snoring has long been recognized as being a problem for sleeping partners and others nearby. However, more recently, snoring, even without apnea, has been linked to a number of medical and behavioral problems in many people. Persistent daytime sleepiness, tiredness, problems with concentration, subtle cognitive deficits, and declines in performance have all been found in some people who snore. To a lesser extent, so, too, have headaches, increases in blood pressure, increased sympathetic nervous system activation, cardiac disease, cerebrovascular disease, and hormone problems. Some of the behavioral problems seem to occur because snoring causes fragmented sleep resulting from the increased effort needed to breathe. The heart and vascular effects are thought to be related to the increase in chest pressure caused by the constriction of the upper airways.

There is a long and continuing history of various treatments for snoring, many of which did not work or were even dangerous. Even today there are claims made for various treatments that are questionable and could be dangerous if they keep people from seeking medical treatment for sleep apnea (see Chapter 10). Acceptable approaches to treatment start with lifestyle changes, move on to oral appliances, then CPAP, and, finally, to surgery if necessary. Lifestyle changes may include weight loss to reduce the excess soft tissue in the throat, reduction of the use of alcohol or medications that cause the muscles of the throat muscle to relax, cessation of smoking, efforts to avoid irritants to the upper airways, and not sleeping on the back. Oral appliances are mouthpieces that keep the tongue forward or advance the lower jaw. CPAP will be explained in chapter 10 under apnea. Surgeries to the throat or nose may enlarge the upper airways and/or remove soft tissue. The treatments beyond lifestyle changes need to be made by qualified medical personal.

There are products available without consulting a physician or dentist that claim to cure snoring, but such claims are usually dubious and typically unsubstantiated. Among these treatments are devices that hold the mouth closed as a treatment for snoring under the mistaken idea that the sole cause for snoring is breathing through the mouth. Such devices can be dangerous and should not be used.

Nightmares[40]

Nightmares

The term **nightmare** comes from night + mara, where mara means to crush. It originally referred to a specific kind of night experience when persons would awaken with the experience of a demon, also called an incubus, sitting on their chest causing suffocation. In the last century, nightmares came to include other negative, upsetting sleep experiences including all sorts of bad dreams. While there are similarities between the experiences we commonly group together as nightmares, there are important differences between true nightmares and bad dreams, night terrors, and post-traumatic stress disorder nightmares.

The official definition (American Sleep Disorders Association, 1997) for a nightmare is a frightening dream that awakens the sleeper. The frightening aspect most commonly is intense fear but may also be anxiety, sadness, anger, guilt, disgust, helplessness, or grief. There is full alertness upon awakening, often with a moderate increase in heart rate and breathing rate and immediate recall of the content of the nightmare. Nightmares usually occur after at least 10 minutes into a REMS episode during the last half of the sleep period.

Bad Dreams (a.k.a. Anxiety Dreams)

Bad dreams (a.k.a. **anxiety dreams**) are sometimes distinguished from nightmares by the fact that the person does not awaken during the dream but recalls the disturbing content upon awakening later. Another approach says this difference does not matter. More important is how distressing either is to the person when awake. Some people are greatly distressed by them, but an equal number very little, if at all. Some people look upon their nightmares and bad dreams as creative, interesting, and fascinating and even enjoy them as much as they would enjoy a horror film. Others simply dismiss and ignore them. Some experts believe that the important factor is whether the nightmare or bad dream has a negative effect on waking life, not whether the person is awakened during the experience.

Almost everyone can recall at least one nightmare or bad dream during their lifetime. Nightmares or bad dreams are most frequent between 3 and 8 years of age. Women also report having more nightmares and bad dreams than do men. As many as one out of every four college students report having one nightmare or bad dream per month with 5% reporting them once per week. This number declines to 1 to 2% in adults and the elderly. From another perspective, 4 to 8% of all people report that nightmares and bad dreams are a "current problem," and another 6% say they were a past problem. Yet, retrospective self-reports underestimate nightmare and bad dream frequency by a factor of $2\frac{1}{2}$ when compared to daily logs in young adults and by a factor of 10 in the elderly.

Nightmares and bad dreams are more frequently reported during times of crisis, loss, and trauma. They are a natural response to such things and can help us psychologically recover from them. In such cases, the nightmare or bad dream changes over time, then seems to gradually fade away. In some cases, the content of the nightmare is directly tied to the precipitating event, but the terror and vulnerability triggered by the event can also be metaphorically represented by nightmares and bad dreams of tidal waves, big whirlwinds, and so forth. The nightmares and bad dreams occurring soon after the trauma may result in a lot of terror and fear, sometimes accompanied by feelings of great vulnerability. Survivor guilt, and sometimes grief and anger, may follow directly or indirectly. After a period of weeks or months, dreams return to their normal patterns, but nightmares or bad dreams may return in the future when some new experience revives memory of the trauma that originally precipitated the nightmare or bad dream. Nightmares and bad dreams can also be caused by general stress, normal childhood fears and problems, illness and fever, and be a side effect of some medications.

Contrary to widespread belief, nightmares and bad dreams are not a sign of mental disorder. If anything, it is the concern about them that contributes to anxiety, depression, and other psychological problems. Those who suffer from nightmares and bad dreams often share the psychological trait of what psychiatrist Ernest Hartmann calls "thin boundaries." People with thin boundaries are more open, sensitive, and vulnerable and, as a result, view more events as personally traumatic than do most people. Nightmare and bad dream distress has also been found to be more likely in those more susceptible to hypnosis, as well as those who are creative and absorbed in fantasy and esthetic experiences. Nightmares are also more frequent in people who have suffered trauma or abuse. But there are also people who have nightmares who fit none of these categories. Being distressed about nightmares and bad dreams is only weakly related to psychopathology, if at all, and is only weakly related to nightmare and bad dream frequency. Nightmare and bad dream sufferers report more sleep problems, such as taking longer to get to sleep, more awakenings, and less sleep quality, all of which improve as the nightmares and bad dreams abate.

While traditional psychotherapy has not been shown to be effective for treating nightmares and bad dreams, there has been much support for cognitive-behavioral interventions. These treatments include relaxation techniques, systematic desensitization, and the counterconditioning of a relaxing response to the nightmares and bad dreams. Even more effective has been the recent use of imagery rehearsal that has sufferers write, talk, paint, or draw about their nightmares and bad dreams, then go on to change the recalled nightmare and bad dreams by rehearsing new scenarios, changing the negatives into positives. In the context of a safe and supportive relationship with a therapist, sufferers may also be encouraged to adopt a more playful attitude toward such dreams and to be aware that the content of the dream cannot really hurt them. Sometimes persons are encouraged, when awake, to converse with the characters in their nightmares and bad dreams. Other approaches encourage sufferers to become lucid during the nightmare or bad dream and change it then. For some people, hypnosis has proved to be effective.

Night Terrors

Night terrors are different from nightmares and bad dreams in several significant ways. Typically, the child partially arouses suddenly from SWS and emits a piercing scream that awakens parents who rush into the room to see the child sitting up with a terrified facial expression and maybe thrashing about. The child's eyes may be wide. The child may be sweating, have a racing heart, and be breathing rapidly. Although not apparent, the child may also have an elevation in blood pressure and a decrease in skin resistance. The attempts of the parents to soothe the fear of the child are unsuccessful, for the child is in a dazed state and not readily responsive to them. After about 1 to 5 minutes, the child does calm a bit and returns to sleep. The next morning, the child has no recall of the incident and little or no dream recall. If there is recall, it is only of an image of something like a monster or a wall closing in.

Night terrors are generally considered to be benign and are usually outgrown, much to the relief of the parents. They occur in about 3% of children, peaking at 3–5 years of age with two-thirds ceasing by adolescence. Their occurrence in adults is less than 1%. They tend to be found in others in the family and may overlap with sleepwalking. Sleep deprivation and emotional stress may increase their frequency, but there is no relationship with psychopathology. Severe cases that do not remit over time may be successfully treated with prescribed medications.

Post-traumatic Stress Disorder (PTSD) Nightmares

Post-traumatic stress disorder (PTSD) nightmares are a key component of what some people live with following a very intense traumatic experience. The nightmares are a repetitive reexperiencing of the traumatic event, although some details may be changed or missing. Up to 90% of people with PTSD report experiencing them. They can occur during any stage of sleep, although they are more likely to occur early in the night, and are more emotionally intrusive and anxiety causing than most nightmares. They also are a cause of sleep disruption including more awakenings, fear of sleep, and various changes in REMS. Gross body movements and activation of the autonomic nervous system accompany the nightmare and subsequent awakening. When aroused from the nightmare, the person will be confused and anxious but not always remember the entire nightmare.

Treatment for PTSD nightmares is complex and difficult, but recent new approaches are showing much promise. The treatment has to be individualized because of related psychological and medical conditions. The cognitive-behavioral techniques used with other nightmares and bad dreams can also be helpful with PTSD nightmares, but additional psychotherapy, psychosocial therapy, and medications are often helpful, too.

Box 28

Sleep-Related Violence[41]

Mr. Parks was a young married man who had fallen asleep on the couch, then in the early morning hours got up from the couch, put on his shoes and jacket, and drove his car 23 Km along a well traveled road, with turns and traffic lights, for about 20 minutes. At the home of his in-laws, he carried the tire iron in from the car and retrieved a knife from the kitchen, killed his mother-in-law, and attempted to kill his father-in-law. After testimony by sleep disorder specialists based on their examination of Mr. Parks and the circumstances of the incident, the court acquitted him of responsibility for the murder and attempted murder on the basis that he was sleepwalking.

There are other well-documented cases of sleep-related violence including other homicides, attempted suicides, self-injury, damage to objects, and indecent exposure. These reports have been found to be due to sleepwalking, sleep inertia, REMS behavior disorder (see Chapter 10), nocturnal seizures, or excessive sleepiness due to sleep deprivation (but often accompanied by alcohol intake), jet lag, or sleep disorders such as narcolepsy and sleep apnea (see Chapter 10). Such incidences are more common than might be expected, generally thought to involve 2% of adults. However, individuals rarely repeat these behaviors.

Such cases are examples of automatisms—complex behaviors that occur without conscious awareness or voluntary intention—and, therefore, the person is not held responsible and punished because in the United States and the United Kingdom a person must "knowingly intend to commit the crime." Instead, they may be required to get treatment for their sleep problem (see Chapter 10).

Table 6. Some common repetitive metaphorical elements reported in dreams

---

Being chased
Appearing naked in public
Falling
Ghosts returning from the dead
Being kidnapped
Rejection, humiliation
Loosing teeth
Being trapped
Large scale disasters such as floods and tornadoes
Being paralyzed and unable to move
Being endangered
A violent attack
An out-of-control vehicle

Recurrent Dreams and Repetitive Nightmares

Recurrent dreams and repetitive nightmares range from virtual duplication of the entire dream or nightmare to the recurrence of themes or components in different dreams. Typical are recurrences of metaphorical depictions of conflicts or stress such as tidal waves, tornados, and hurricanes (see also Table 6). Their occurrence correlates with increases of waking anxiety, depression, stress, or personal adjustments. Resolution of waking situation usually is accompanied by less frequent repetitive elements in dreams or their complete disappearance.

Sleepwalking

Sleepwalking is not what most people think it is. It is not acting out a dream (however, REM Behavior Disorder is; see Chapter 10). Sleepwalking begins during SWS, not REMS, typically occurs in the first half of the night, results in little if any dream recall, and can be induced in the predisposed by forced arousal. It occurs when the brain does not fully awaken from a deep sleep. Sleepwalking begins with the person moving about in bed, then suddenly sitting up with a glazed look on their face and in their eyes. Next, they may repeatedly engage in stereotyped behaviors such as picking at their covers, undressing and dressing, and so forth. Simultaneously, they may mumble or make other sounds. The event may end at this point as they lay down and resume normal sleeping. Or the next step may be for them to get out of bed and walk around the room. Sometimes, they may walk to nearby rooms, the yard, the neighborhood, or even further. The frequency of these components diminishes the further they get from the bed.

Movements during sleepwalking appear purposeless and tend to be clumsy. The person may trip, bump into things, or knock things over. Injuries can occur, but violent acts are rare. Yet, at other times, they may do something very complex like prepare a meal, play a musical instrument, or even drive a car. They may vocalize or even have conversations, yet screaming is highly unusual. Responsiveness to the environment, including to their own name, may be greatly reduced. Most instances last from less than a minute up to 15 minutes but have been reported to sometimes last an hour or more.

Several things contribute to the occurrence of sleepwalking. Eighty percent of sleepwalkers have an immediate family member who also sleepwalks or has night terrors. Studies of twins show a pattern of genetic inheritance. People who sleepwalk are more likely to talk in their sleep, wet their beds, and have confusional arousals or sleep terrors. It is most common in children, with 15–30% having done it at lease once and 3–4% frequently. The peak of onset of sleep walking is 5 years of age, with the peak occurrence at 12 years of age. It most often abates by 15 years of age. Sleepwalking is not associated with any psychological pathology in children but tends to occur more in children who sleep very deeply. Sleepwalking in adults is a different matter. About 1 of every 100 adults sleepwalks chronically. It usually continues from adolescence but is rare in the elderly. Sleepwalking in adults may be associated with Personality Disorders, Mood Disorders, or Anxiety Disorders (DSM-IV, 1994) but a large majority have no underlying psychiatric or psychological conditions.

There are several things that can be done for people who sleepwalk. Awakening a person who is sleepwalking is difficult and may be met with resistance or even violence. It is sometimes possible and more successful to lead them back to bed gently. By all means, the sleepwalker should be kept out of harm's way. Since most children outgrow sleepwalking, the best thing for parents to do is simply to wait for the child to grow out of it. While waiting, they can try to reduce the things that trigger sleepwalking events, such as stress and sleep deprivation. Making the bedroom and the rest of the house safer is also advisable. However, if the sleepwalking is intense, frequent, potentially dangerous, or if it occurs in adulthood, then one of the following might also be tried: psychological treatment, relaxation therapy, stress management skills, hypnosis, or medications.

Sleep Talking[42]

Sleep talking is often related to sleepwalking and is most common in children, but also occurs in adults. Estimates of people who have sleep-talked one time or another range from 20% to nearly 100%. Most often, sleep talking consists of a few mumbles to, occasionally, a few understandable words to, more rarely, to a hundred or so intelligible words. People have been known to sing, laugh, and make other kinds or utterances. Most often, sleep talking lasts for only a few seconds. Although you may have heard accounts of two-way conversations with a sleep-talker, verification of this occurrence in the sleep lab has only been partially successful. Although occasionally used in literature, such as Othello being convinced by Iago's relaying the supposed sleep talking of Cassio, secrets are seldom spoken.

While sleep talking can occur during any stage of sleep at any time during the night, most of it occurs during stage 2 sleep and only 10–20% during REMS. Partial awakening may occur during sleep talking. Although sleep talking during REMS tends to be more grammatically correct and more emotional, it usually is without reference to the person's surroundings. Rarely has it been shown to be related to the content of the ongoing dream, and attempts to use it as a play-by-play narration of the dream have failed, because the speech is too frequently garbled or nonsensical.

Sleep talking tends to occur more frequently among related family members but is considered benign and therefore not treated. There is only one reported case of serious consequences resulting from sleep talking; a firefighter who frequently talked in his sleep in the fire station dormitory was in danger of losing his job because he was keeping other firefighters awake!

Bedwetting

Bedwetting (enuresis) is considered an annoying but otherwise typically benign problem. It is much more common than generally realized but is usually outgrown. It is better not to make a big issue out of bedwetting that occurs in children under 6 or 7 years of age if they have never been dry for more than a few successive nights. For some children, neurological control of the bladder sphincter can even come as late as 12–15 years of age. Parents of older children may want to try any one of several training methods involving gentle alarms that have been shown to work quite well. The reemergence of wetting the bed after a number of dry months or years can indicate genito-urinary problems, psychological problems, or even neurological problems such as epileptic seizures and should be brought to the attention of a medical doctor.

Teeth Grinding (Sleep Bruxism)

Ten to twenty percent of people may grind or click their teeth frequently during sleep, but it is most prevalent in adolescents. For the vast majority of these people, bruxism is not serious, but it can cause damage to the teeth or sore jaw muscles for some. While bruxism has not been shown to be associated with any psychological problems, it may be more prevalent during times of stress. Bruxism occurs most frequently during stage 2 sleep and REMS but has also been observed during other stages of sleep. It may be accompanied by a partial arousal, yet the sleeper has no awareness of it and seldom awakens. Other body movements and an increase in heart rate frequently accompany it. Dentists can treat bruxism by fitting the sleeper with a guard worn over the teeth during sleep.

Chapter 10

Disorders of Sleep, Part I[43,44]

The typical sleep disorders clinic in many ways resembles the sleep lab described in the prologue, since it contains the facilities to measure the nighttime and daytime sleep of patients. The standard EEG, EOG, and EMG measurements are used to assess the states of sleep, but, as we shall see, other bodily functions during sleep are also measured to aid in effective diagnosis of sleep disorders.

The typical sleep disorders clinic has technicians, just as the research lab does, and clinicians/researchers who are typically Ph.D.s and M.D.s. The Ph.D.s are most often psychologists or psychobiologists and the M.D.s are usually pulmonary physicians, neurologists, psychiatrists, internists, and other related specialists. They meet regularly as a team to review and discuss patient histories and to confer on newly admitted patients about possible diagnosis and potential treatments. In addition, they usually meet once a week for about an hour with other interested professionals to discuss specific topics or patients in depth. These case studies, or "grand rounds" as they are sometimes called, provide a forum for sharing knowledge and ideas among the participants. In this chapter, several of the major sleep disorders will be presented as grand rounds case studies followed by discussion of the disorder in general.

NARCOLEPSY

L.I.[45] is a 35-year old-female who said her symptoms first appeared as a teenager when she noticed a weakness in the knees when shooting free-throws during basketball games or on other occasions when she laughed at something funny. Eventually, she began to drop things she was holding, and her eyelids would often droop. Gradually, the symptoms became more frequent and more intense. She stated that she was always somewhat sleepy as a teenager, but she began to feel sleepier during the daytime at approximately the time she started college. Even after a long night of sleep, she would fall asleep in class, at movies, after dinner, and at other quiet times. These behaviors

Much of this chapter is adapted from Moorcroft (1993) with permission of the publisher.

began to affect her functioning, especially in social situations. Her symptoms became worse if she became emotionally aroused; the example she gave was that a number of times she had "passed out" while kissing her date.

Frequent visits to physicians provided no relief. She was diagnosed in the past as having a variety of physical problems, such as hypothyroidism, and psychological problems. However, neither medication—she was at various times placed on thyroid hormone, tranquilizers, and other medications—nor psychotherapy provided any relief, and her symptoms gradually became worse.

She was obliged to take frequent naps, after which she felt refreshed. If she tried to "fight off" the need to nap, she would subsequently fall asleep in inappropriate places, such as the dinner table. She had tried "sleeping-in" in the morning but was unable to do so.

About once a week, usually when going to sleep, she experiences hallucinations, called hypnogogic hallucinations, that are strong and frightening, such as someone in the room holding a knife about to stab her. Usually at these times she is unable to move for 1–2 minutes, even after awakening. The same thing also sometimes happens when awakening from sleep, called hypnopompic hallucinations.

In the past, she experienced blackouts. She reported having periods of time for which she had no memory of what she was doing. For example, she noted several instances of driving home, then suddenly becoming aware of having driven many miles past her home.

L.I. is an unemployed nurse, recently divorced with two pre-teenage children who live at home with her. She maintains that child support and alimony do not provide enough money and she needs to find a job, but her symptoms of narcolepsy have prevented her from finding and keeping one.

At times, although totally awake, she complains that she has experienced muscle weakness and even collapse, especially during times of emotional arousal such as dealing with her two pre-teenage children. This has forced her to avoid confrontations with them and try to "control" her emotions. As a result she is usually "emotionally flat." Both her father and grandfather were "nappers" and were very calm, "unemotional" men. She appears slightly depressed and desperate.

L.I.'s sleep was assessed in the lab for one night followed by a MSLT (see Chapter 3) the next day. Figure 34 shows the results of her night in the sleep lab. Comparisons with the typical night of sleep of the young adult (Figure 8 and Table 1 in Chapter 1) revealed several characteristic things. First, she experienced a hypnogogic hallucination with some sleep paralysis within the first few minutes after the lights were turned out and just when the polysomnogram showed she had fallen asleep. She reported a vague awareness of someone "lurking in the shadows" of the room and feeling very frightened but being unable to call out.

Second, she fell asleep quickly after the second time the lights were turned out and went into REMS almost immediately, followed by a relatively normal cycle of REMS periods.

Third, her sleep was fragmented with more stage 1 and less stage 2 and SWS than is typical, as well as a high number of awakenings. This entire pattern reflects a low sleep efficiency for her age.

The MSLT (Figure 35) likewise showed some unusual characteristics. During each nap period, she fell asleep very quickly, in contrast to the normal pattern of taking over

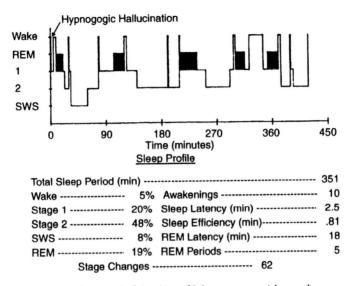

Figure 34. The record of the sleep of L.I.—a person with narcolepsy.

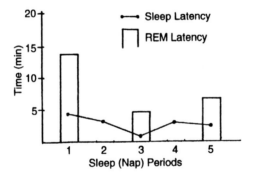

Figure 35. The results of L.I.'s Multiple Sleep Latency Test.

15 minutes to initiate sleep. In addition, during three of her five naps, she quickly went into REMS. A normal young adult might, on a rare occasion, go into REMS during one of the naps, especially an earlier one, but not during several of the naps.

Treatment consisted of keeping her on a stimulant drug during the day. In addition, a second drug was prescribed to control her cataplexy- muscle weakness, collapse, and sleep paralysis.

Overall, this case is fairly typical of narcolepsy. The most common complaints are those of excessive, seemingly perpetual, sleepiness and sleep attacks that are irresistible, even in arousing situations. The resulting sleep may last up to an hour and be refreshing. The next most common complaint is that of cataplexy, ranging anywhere from weakness in the limbs, face, or speech muscles to total, wilting collapse. Cataplexy is often triggered by emotions. During brief cataplectic attacks, a person is conscious, but longer attacks, those over one minute long, may quickly progress into sleep.

Hypnogogic and hypnopomnic hallucinations (or imagery) and sleep paralysis occur together, or singly, in almost one-half of people with narcolepsy. These hallucinations are vivid, brief, dream-like occurrences at entry to and from sleep that sometimes leave the person with a sense of fear or dread but may also be reenactments of a part of the past few hours. Sleep paralysis is the inability to move that occurs on awakening or when attempting to fall asleep. Both hypnogogic and hypnopomnic hallucinations and paralysis occur in individuals without narcolepsy, especially children and sleep deprived adults without narcolepsy.

About one half of all people suffering from narcolepsy report experiencing automatic behavior or blackouts (see Chapter 2). During these episodes, persons may continue behavior associated with wakeful consciousness but later have no memory of what they did. These episodes can last minutes or even hours. Naps, although inconvenient, are often refreshing to people with narcolepsy.

Narcolepsy appears to be a problem of REMS. Cateplexy and sleep paralysis are the muscle paralysis of REMS, while hypnogogic hallucinations are the dreams. REMS occurring soon after sleep onset is not typical of normal adult sleep. The excessive sleepiness may result from overactive REMS-on mechanisms in the brain or from the poor nocturnal sleep, including frequent awakenings, less SWS, and fragmented REMS, that have been shown frequently, but not always, to accompany narcolepsy. Blackouts are probably similar to sleepwalking.

Typically, narcolepsy begins to appear in the teens, with sleep attacks as the first symptom, although onsets in younger and older people do occur. Over several years, the sleep attacks worsen when cataplexy and other symptoms begin to appear and then become more frequent. Patients often report, however, that their problem has been unrecognized as narcolepsy for many years, and that they were treated for many other problems or even called lazy.

Overall, narcolepsy impairs a person's life. Divorce is frequent, reflecting interpersonal complications caused by the symptoms. Likewise, the social life of people with narcolepsy is impaired, for they cannot go to movies, concerts, dinner parties, play cards, or participate in other "quiet" activities. The sleepiness of persons with narcolepsy even affects their participation in more active social events such as sports. Since cataplectic attacks are likely to be triggered by strong emotions, people with narcolepsy tend to guard their emotions, thus appearing dull and emotionally flat. Many have a history of being fired for falling asleep on the job, and people with narcolepsy frequently have had a number of accidents, both while driving automobiles and on the job. They also complain of problems with their memories, which may really be a problem of paying attention. As a result of these problems, they often are somewhat depressed, anxious, and frustrated. Others describe them as being unmotivated, withdrawn, and aggressive or believe they are lazy, bored, slothful, or depressed.

Narcolepsy occurs in over 5 out of every 10,000 persons. There are thought to be over 250,000 people with narcolepsy in the U.S. today. There appears to be good evidence that it is at least partially inherited, but narcolepsy may also be caused by damage to the brain. Recent findings have shown people with narcolepsy are less responsive to their own orexin/hypocretin (see Chapter 4). At this time, control of symptoms with drugs—a stimulant for the sleepiness and other drugs for the cateplexy—is the only effective treatment. In some countries, an additional drug is used to improve nighttime sleep, which in turn lessens daytime symptoms. Several short naps of 15–20 minutes also help reduce sleepiness. Psychological support and family therapy are also important.

SLEEP APNEA

R.P. is a 43-year-old high school math teacher who came to the lab—or rather was pushed here by his wife, his third—because of excessive snoring. During the interview, he indicated that he had "always been a snorer." While in the military, his buddies kept threatening to throw him out of the barracks because of his snoring. His snoring got worse in his late 20s, coinciding with a 40-pound weight gain. He says that he is never aware of snoring, because he is a very, very deep sleeper who awakens slowly and in a "fog." Even in a cool room, he will wake up with sweaty pajamas.

His wife reported that he sometimes snores so loudly that, even when she goes to another part of the house in a desperate attempt to get her own sleep, she can still hear him "through closed doors and with a pillow over my head." She said his snoring has a gagging, choking quality separated by a minute or so of silence. She mentioned that he "flails around a bit" in his sleep sometimes hitting or kicking her. He blamed his snoring as part of the cause for his first two divorces, and said he would like to get it under control before a third divorce happens.

During his teaching, he always had to be moving or standing at the blackboard. Even during tests, he paced around. During teacher's meetings, he often had to fight off the urge to sleep by sitting in uncomfortable positions. When grading papers, he drank a lot of coffee, got up frequently, and sometimes splashed cold water on his face. Naps had never been refreshing for him.

He says that he doesn't attend movies, watch TV, or play cards, claiming to be bored by them. ("They must be boring because I always fall asleep!") He and his wife do bowl in a league once a week. He avoids long drives because of accidents he has had sleeping behind the wheel. He used to coach basketball but had to give it up. "The practices were O.K.—I could keep moving around, but during the bus trips, in the locker room, and even during the games, I would drift off to sleep!"

R.P. is overweight by about 50 pounds. He appears to have no neck; rather his head continues straight down to his shoulders. He has a history of high blood pressure and heart problems. Otherwise, he appears to be in good health.

R.P. recalls that his father, who died of a heart attack at age 51, also snored heavily. In addition, his father appeared to be overweight and frequently napped.

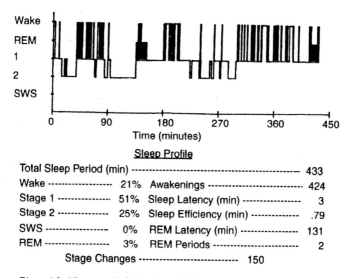

Figure 36. The record of the sleep of R.P.—a person with sleep apnea.

R.P. reported trying several methods to stop snoring, including a special collar he purchased through the mail. Nothing helped. He also related that he had tried hypnosis. When asked if that had helped, he hesitated, showing a wry smile and replied, "Well, yes." When asked to elaborate, he continued, "The hypnotist gave me a post hypnotic suggestion—every time I would start snoring, I would turn over."

"And did it work?"

"Well, I spent the next three nights spinning!"

Subsequent to his first visit, we had his wife send a tape recording of his snoring. The tape revealed that he did indeed snore loudly, but that the snoring was intermittent, not continuous. Five or six snores were followed by a minute or so of silence. This pattern continued over and over again with the first snore of each series having a gagging, gasping quality.

In the lab, R.P. fell asleep within 3 minutes of lights out (see Figure 36) but awakened 62 seconds later with a gasping, snoring sound. This cycle continued throughout much of the rest of the night; as soon as he was in stage 1 or 2 sleep, his breathing ceased, then he would awaken a minute or so later, gasping and snoring loudly. He woke 424 times in 433 minutes of the sleep period.

The profile of his sleep was very abnormal. In addition to the frequent arousals, he never reached SWS and had very little REMS. Most of his sleep was stage 1 with the rest stage 2. Time awake totaled about 1/5 of the sleep period. Sleep efficiency was low. Violent body movements accompanied most of his arousals.

Additional data were included on the polysomnogram about his breathing by electronically measuring the air going into or out of his mouth and breathing movements of the chest. The amount of oxygen in the blood was continuously indirectly measured by a device called an oximeter from a lead placed on his finger. His sleep position was automatically recorded by placing a matchbox size monitor on his chest.

These measurements confirmed that, although the chest was making breathing movements, no air was entering or leaving his body between the bouts of snoring. This condition is called obstructive sleep apnea (= absence of breathing), due to his upper air passages collapsing shut while he is asleep.

At other times, the air passages were only partially blocked, allowing some air to move in and out of his body but at well below normal levels. This condition is called sleep hypopnea (= partial breathing). The average number of apneas plus hypopneas per hour was 57. His blood was desaturated (= blood oxygen 4% or more below what it was at the time of lights out) a total duration of 108 of the 433 minutes of the sleep period. The average low value of oxygen saturation of the blood was 81% of its capacity with the lowest saturation reaching 58%. Normal percentages of saturation during sleep are in the high 90s, and physiological consequences may occur at saturations of less than 88%.

R.P. stated the next morning that he had a typical night of sleep for him and thought he had awakened maybe 8 to 10 times. He did not feel refreshed, and he had a headache. He asked if we could help him.

Treatment consisted of placing Mr. P. on a CPAP (= continuous positive air pressure) machine. Each night, he placed a small, soft plastic breathing mask over his nose. This mask was connected to a specially designed air pump placed close to the bed that was carefully adjusted so that air pressure would keep the throat open to allow normal breathing. A check with Mr. P. a few days later revealed a dramatic change. He said he felt alert and rested during the day. Although sleeping with the mask on was a bit uncomfortable, he loved it because of the rest he was now getting. And his wife said he was no longer keeping her awake with his snoring.

A few months later, R.P. spent another night in the sleep lab while using the CPAP machine. This time his sleep was essentially normal for his age. He showed only few apneas and almost no oxygen desaturations. He stated his sleepiness during the day had almost disappeared. His blood pressure was also much improved.

Because of his obstructive sleep apnea, R.P. woke up regularly throughout the night in order to take several breaths accompanied by loud snoring, as the air was forced through the narrow air passage. Obviously, under such conditions, the result is very poor sleep. Little, if any, SWS occurred and REMS was reduced, which results in excessive daytime sleepiness. Some people with sleep apnea complain of snoring, but only a few are aware of the frequent awakenings during the night. Those who do complain of the awakenings tell of the choking or suffocating sensations at such times that are accompanied by anxiety. Some patients show sleep apnea for only a part of the night or only in some sleep positions, such as on the back.

At least 4% of adult females and 8% of adult males and 2–3% of children suffer from obstructive sleep apnea. Obstructive sleep apnea is at least three times more frequent in males than in premenopausal females, but the ratio for females is 1:1 after menopause. It tends to run in families. Many sufferers are overweight and have thick necks.

Sleep apnea is frequently accompanied in middle age patients by high blood pressure and various heart problems, especially arrhythmias. Sleep apnea gets progressively worse with time. The hypertension and heart problems may be caused, at least in part, by the fall in blood oxygen associated with the apnea, for the blood pressure increases dramatically during periods of apnea. Some people with long-term obstructive sleep apnea are in danger of dying in their sleep from heart failure during one of their apnic episodes. On the other hand, following successful treatment, some people with obstructive sleep apnea show dramatic reductions of high blood pressure and heart problems.

People with sleep apnea may complain of other problems such as blackouts, automatic behaviors, night sweats, and morning headaches. They frequently maintain that they sleep deeply and are hard to arouse, yet they often awaken disoriented and "foggy headed." They may complain that they gag easily and that naps are not refreshing. Alcohol, antihistamines, tranquilizers, and sleeping pills make their symptoms worse. Some individuals may show symptoms only after having several alcoholic drinks prior to going to sleep.

Since sleep apnea has only been recognized since the mid 1970s, many people with apnea have a history of misdiagnosis and failed treatment attempts. Often, they were simply called lazy or crazy. Because of the excessive sleepiness, they frequently have a history of divorce, multiple car accidents, and employment problems. It is not unusual for them to become depressed and irritable because of the symptoms and also because of diminished sexual desires. Many also complain of concentration, judgment, and memory problems, as well as changes in personality marked by irritability and hostility.

CPAP has become the most commonly prescribed treatment of obstructive sleep apnea. In some cases, other treatments are often tried first. Weight loss may be prescribed, especially in those patients who showed a dramatic gain in weight prior to the onset of the apnea. People who only have obstructive apnea when sleeping on their backs may be advised that sewing a tennis ball into the upper back of their pajamas prevents them from sleeping in that position. Use of alcohol and other sleeping pills should be significantly reduced or eliminated. The use of one of a large variety of dental appliances, that hold the lower jaw or tongue forward, for the treatment of obstructive sleep apnea is increasing. Some of these dental appliances mouth guards worn by some athletes, others are more metallic and mechanical looking. A qualified dentist must fit them.

Abnormalities of the upper airways, especially involving the throat, are sometimes found and surgically corrected in adults with obstructive sleep apnea. This type of surgical treatment is becoming more common for the treatment of obstructive apnea when other treatments fail, even if there is no outstanding abnormality. Abnormal constrictions of the respiratory passages are frequently found in children complaining of excessive daytime sleepiness. Surgery correcting the airway abnormality most often corrects the sleepiness.

IDIOPATHIC HYPERSOMNIA

Some people are sleepier than others for no known reason. A few feel tired almost all of the time, and others sleep a great deal longer than the average. Some of these very sleepy people are classified as having idiopathic, meaning not caused by something else, hypersomnia. It is not common, but it is striking when it occurs. It is not a result of insomnia, poor sleep, or other known sleep pathologies. It just happens. Beginning sometime between ages 15 and 25, they feel almost constantly tired, but can resist naps. Short naps, when taken, are not refreshing, yet, without sufficient sleep, sufferers may begin to display automatic behavior, blackouts, and microsleeps (see Chapters 2 and 3). Most commonly, family members show a similar condition, although many report that they are unlike any relatives. They sleep deeply at night, but only slightly longer than average. They awaken easily and spontaneously in the morning. Their sleep pattern is normal, but prolonged. However, they frequently are subject to fainting and migraine headaches. There is no known treatment.

Idiopathic hypersomnia needs to be distinguished from the long sleeper syndrome. Long sleepers may arrive at the sleep disorders clinic complaining about many of the same things as people with idiopathic hypersomnia, but careful history taking and polysomnographic testing reveal differences. Long sleepers need 10 or more hours of sleep per night. If they try to get along on less, they show the effects of continuous partial sleep deprivation (see Chapter 3), including excessive daytime sleepiness, shown both by their own subjective reports of a constant struggle to stay awake, multiple napping, and blackouts and automatic behavior, and by a low average MSLT sleep latency. They usually report having difficulty arousing and often experience "sleep inertia" (foggy-headedness for a long time with confusions and commission of often impulsive and irrational, socially embarrassing or criminal acts; see Chapter 2). They are hard to awaken and can be abusive and aggressive if awakened, even when they themselves have requested it. If they do get the 10 or more hours of sleep per night they require, the daytime sleepiness remits to normal levels.

Prescribed treatment is usually simple for both idiopathic hypersomnia and long sleeper syndrome—more sleep every night.

PERIODIC LIMB MOVEMENT DISORDER

E.C. is a 51-year-old woman, who came to the clinic complaining of insomnia and serious sleepiness during the day. She was without problems as a child but has had trouble sleeping as an adult, apparently getting worse in recent years. She has been a housewife much of her adult life.

She reports having to get up during the night to "stretch her legs" because of an uncomfortable feeling in them. When she does get to sleep, however, she says she sleeps very deeply, but awakens not feeling refreshed or rejuvenated. Her husband reports that she often shakes the bed during sleep and kicks off the bedcovers.

E.C. reported trying many things for her "insomnia" including many drugs, both prescribed and over-the-counter, but to no avail. Likewise, six weeks off caffeine was of no help. She exercises on an Exercycle or plays tennis daily. She occasionally takes voluntary naps, which help. When trying to nap, she falls asleep quickly, but the creepy sensation in her legs awakens her every 10 minutes or so. Her naps are not refreshing. Even when she is just sitting still, she feels the discomfort inside her calves and must get up every 15 minutes to walk it off. These sensations are getting worse as she gets older. They are also worse when she is tired. Her sleepiness has caused her to have a car accident and many near misses.

She was not sure if her parents suffered from similar problems, but did remember that her father couldn't stand deskwork and would rather have a job that kept him moving around.

The polysomnogram showed that Mrs. E.C., after walking around the bedroom for about 20 minutes, got into bed and fell asleep quickly, but her sleep was punctuated with many, usually brief, awakenings. Most of these awakenings were caused by a series of leg kicks measured by placing a pair of electrodes on the front of each leg half way between the knee and ankle. These movements were very stereotyped (that is, identical to one another), abrupt contractions of certain lower leg muscles occurring about every half minute. The typical pattern was for early kicks in a series to disturb and lighten sleep, with only the later jerks causing actual awakening. Upon returning to sleep, the legs were occasionally quiet for several minutes allowing sleep to proceed normally, but then the kicks would begin again, thus disturbing her sleep.

The kicks each lasting a few seconds, tended to come in bursts of 30 or more with 20 to 40 seconds between individual kicks. The quality and characteristics of the overall sleep pattern were not good, as can be seen in Figure 37. Both the amounts of time to get to sleep and the REMS latency were very long. Note the high percentage of wake time and stage 1 accompanied by lowered amounts of stages 2 and SWS. The number of awakenings is very high as are the number of movements and stage shifts. Sleep efficiency was a very poor 0.70. During the 425 minutes of the sleep period, she had 353 kicks with slightly more of them during REMS. The next morning, she reported that her sleep was typical and that she felt tired and unrefreshed as usual. She had no awareness of the many awakenings or leg kicks during the night.

Periodic limb movement disorders (PLMD) patients may complain of insomnia or excessive daytime sleepiness. There is usually no awareness of the movements during sleep however, and awareness of only a few of the multiple awakenings caused by them.

Typically, both legs are involved, although it is not unusual for movement of other body parts to accompany the leg kicks. Kicks occur in clusters ranging from several minutes to hours, with individual movements of 1/2 to 5 seconds each, occurring every 20 to 40 seconds. In some cases, only one leg kicks. Estimates have been made that PLMD accounts for up to 15% of insomnia and 7% of excessive sleepiness. PLMD tends to be more frequent early in the night, but it rarely occurs in REMS. Yet, there are many people with PLMD who have no sleep problems.

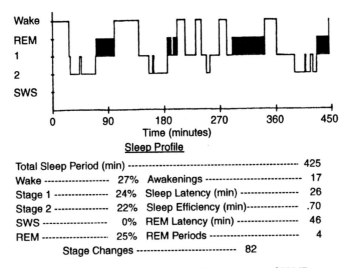

Figure 37. The record of the sleep of E.C.—a case of PLMD.

PLMD tends to run in families, where it is frequently associated with leg cramps. It is mainly seen in middle-aged and older persons, and tends to get worse with age, lack of sleep, stress, or emotional upheaval. Over 40% of retirees have PLMD. A person may have PLMD every night or only occasionally. Although often occurring spontaneously, PLMD may be precipitated or caused by other medical conditions or drugs.

People with PLMD may also have restless legs. It is the deep ache or creeping sensation inside the calves that occurs if the legs are stationary, such as when sitting or lying, that necessitates the individual to keep moving and, thereby, may interfere with sleep onset. It is very disagreeable and relentless.

Restless legs are reported by 15 to 40% of people with kidney failure requiring dialysis. It also is reported by up to 20% of pregnant women. Iron deficiency is reported in many persons with restless legs, and dietary iron supplement may improve the disorder. Patients with Parkinson's disease may develop restless legs when treated with drugs that enhance dopamine in the brain. Caffeine, warm rooms, and exposure to cold can intensify restless legs symptoms. Strangely, restless legs has been reported to disappear with fever.

Exercise, stretching, and certain anti-convulsants have helped in some cases of restless legs. More recently, drugs that deepen sleep, but that have no effect on the kicks, have helped some sufferers of PLMD obtain more satisfying sleep. Avoiding elements that intensify either of these disorders, such as stress or tiredness, is recommended.

REM BEHAVIOR DISORDER

The following is a dramatic case presented at the start of one of the grand rounds sessions:

> Mr. R.D. is a 73-year-old male, retired librarian. He is a very pleasant, mild, and considerate person who came to us because of hitting, slapping, and even choking his wife "a couple of times a week" during his sleep. He has also bolted from the bed, breaking objects on dressers and damaging furniture. He had injured himself. These incidents are often accompanied by sleep talking or more precisely, sleep yelling. The most recent event, which resulted in his hospitalization and referral to our sleep/wake disorders clinic, occurred when he dived from the bed into a dresser, breaking his nose. He said that he was diving out of the boat to escape ugly enemy thugs who were making threats and pursuing him.
>
> When questioned, he said that some of his dreams had become very vivid and violent in the last decade or so. His wife of 47 years reported that he always jerked a lot during his sleep, but this kind of behavior only began around the time he was forced to retire due to age. She said she could awaken him during these incidents, but only after screaming his name many times for what seemed like several minutes. When awakened, he reported vividly dreaming of protecting himself and/or her from a variety of threatening criminals, terrorists, and monsters.
>
> They both agreed that there were not marital problems or personality changes—only these sleep outbursts. His psychological tests showed no depression or pathology.
>
> Mr. R.D. was only able to spend one night in the lab during which there were no incidents or vivid dream reports. His polysomnogram was normal except for (a) somewhat more SWS, (b) high rem density, (c) random, irregular limb movements and twitches in all sleep stages, and (d) brief loss of muscle paralysis during REMS.
>
> Mr. R.D. was diagnosed on the basis of these facts and findings as having REM Behavior Disorder (RBD) and was put on a daily dose of a drug that eliminated his symptoms.

RBD is a parasomnia characterized by unusual dreaming and nightmares whose content is vividly filled with a great deal of activity and violent confrontations. The sleeping person actually engages in complex, vigorous behavior including punching, kicking, grabbing, and leaping from bed, which are often accompanied by vocalizations. Usually the dreamer is experiencing fear, and the behaviors are defensive against what was reported to have been happening in the dream. Injury to the dreamer and sleeping partner is common.

Sleep laboratory studies confirm that these events occur during REMS. The typical rems and characteristic EEG of REMS are present, and the events tend to occur in the latter half of the night. Muscle tone, as shown in the EMG, may be absent during non-eventful REMS, but is sometimes present when these events occur. There is no arousal from sleep during the event.

Other changes in sleep have been noted in people who suffer from RBD. They have more SWS than typical and more rems during REMS. Limb movements in all stages of sleep are also common. Other aspects of sleep are within normal limits.

Most of the patients with RBD observed thus far are elderly males, with the average age of onset in the early 60s. However, it has been observed at other ages, including in children. Forty percent of patients were found to have brain disease or damage of some kind, including Alzheimer's Disease. In other cases, no psychopathology is associated with RBD. In fact, most sufferers are very pleasant when awake and tend to be happily married. RBD sometimes runs in families.

The striking similarity in behavior between RBD and cats with damage to specific parts of the brainstem (see Chapter 4) has been noted. In these animals, just as in RBD humans, animated and violent behaviors occur during REMS. In RBD, it appears as if something goes awry with the pontine REM-ON system (see Chapter 4), such that the motor inhibition that is normally a part of REMS, sometimes malfunctions. At the same time, cells that produce complex sequences of movement are activated, resulting in the behaviors. The cortex responds to these movements by synthesizing the dream content (see the Hobson-McCarley Activation-Synthesis model of dreaming in Chapter 8). A temporary version of RBD may also occur in alcoholics going through delirium tremors ("DTs") and in other people following psychoactive drug withdrawal. Effective treatment of both the vivid dreams and the behaviors has been achieved with low doses of drugs.

Chapter 11

Disorders of Sleep, Part II[46,47]

INSOMNIA

Instead of individual case conferences for our study of insomnias, we will focus our attention upon a special symposium at the annual meeting of the Associated Professional Sleep Societies (APSS). A panel of experts on insomnia from five different sleep clinics review and discuss insomnia. Rather than relating what each said verbatim, the following is a summary of the symposium. A moderator is asking the questions.

What is Insomnia?

Essentially, insomnia is not being able to get enough quality sleep efficiently. It has many different causes. Many have likened it to a fever. Just as a fever may be caused by many different things, insomnia is a symptom resulting from any number of causes. Since insomnia may have various causes, it may be classified either as a type of dyssomnia or as a type of sleep disorder secondary to medical/psychiatric disorders.

How Prevalent is Insomnia?

Studies of insomnia in the Western industrialized world show 30 to 35% of all people report that they have at least mild or occasional insomnia, with about 15% saying they have serious problems. Thus, about 35 million Americans label themselves as people with serious insomnia. But this varies with age and gender, with almost no complaints of insomnia in 8–10-year-olds, but serious complaints in 25 to 35% of retirees and a 1.5 times greater prevalence in females than in males. Insomnia occurs more often in people with depression, anxiety, substance abuse, and recurrent problems with their health.

Much of this chapter is adapted from Moorcroft (1993) with permission of the publisher.

What are the Characteristics of Different Kinds of Insomnia?

Figure 38(a) shows the typical sleep profile of insomniacs who have difficulty falling asleep. They lie in bed wanting to get to sleep, but remaining awake. Typically, we say that if a person takes longer than 30 minutes to fall asleep, **sleep onset insomnia** has occurred.

Some people have no problem falling asleep, but are unable to maintain sleep throughout the night. Such a night of sleep is shown in Figure 38(b), with several relatively long awakenings punctuating the sleep period. Specifically, we say a person

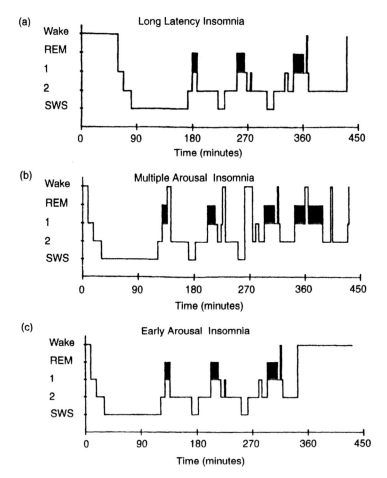

Figure 38. Sleep patterns of insomnia.

has **sleep maintenance insomnia** if the person is awake for more than a total of 30 minutes during the sleep period and/or has five or more awakenings.

Others awaken earlier than desired from sleep, as shown in Figure 38. In these people, sleep onset is reasonably rapid and sleep continuity is good, but the length is inadequate. We say **early arousal insomnia** occurs when there is less than 6.5 hours of total sleep.

On occasion, a fourth type is seen. The problem here is not how much sleep is obtained, but how good it is. **Light sleep insomnia** is said to occur if the person has more than 12% of stage 1 sleep and less than 5% of SWS if 20 to 30 years of age, or less than 3% of SWS if 30 to 40 years old.

So, Insomnia is a Problem with Sleeping?

Yes, but it is also a 24-hour problem because, by definition, the person's waking life must also be affected by the troubled sleep. Usually this means complaints of depression, fatigue, or of being washed-out, as well as a lack of concentration and alertness.

Is Anyone who Meets these Criteria an Insomniac?

Yes, but duration of these problems also needs to be considered. Almost everybody has experienced a night or two of poor sleep, followed by a day or two of fatigue. This experience may be caused by stress or excitement, hospitalization, sleeping in a different bed, or a host of other causes. It is called **transient insomnia**, because adequate sleep and alert days soon return. It is seldom a cause for treatment.

Short-term insomnia has a duration of several days to a few weeks. It often results from ongoing stress, such as school, work, or family problems, or a personal loss that takes some time to resolve. Usually once the person adjusts to the stress or the loss, normal sleep returns, but sometimes treatment intervention is beneficial.

When the symptoms of poor sleep with waking consequences persist for more than three weeks, it is labeled **persistent insomnia**. In practice, many people with persistent insomnia have slept poorly and suffered the waking consequences for months or even years. It is these people with persistent insomnia that require, and benefit from, treatment.

Is Persistent Insomnia Life Threatening?

As compelling as sleep is for us, lack of it is seldom directly life threatening (see Chapter 3), but it can greatly affect the quality of life. It can cause physiological problems, is frequently reported to be mentally and emotionally distressing, and can secondarily lead to grave consequences, such as automobile accidents and interpersonal problems in the family, on the job, and elsewhere.

Can You be More Specific about the Causes of Insomnia?

In some cases, the way insomnia manifests itself may give a clue to the cause. Sleep onset insomnia is associated with anxiety and/or over arousal of some kind. Depression, on the other hand, often results in early arousal insomnia or maintenance insomnia. However, insomnia can be caused by many other, more complicated, factors. There are four major groupings of persistent insomnias—insomnia caused by medical problems, insomnia associated with psychological problems, insomnia associated with lifestyle, and primary insomnia.

Insomnia caused by medical problems.   Some long-term illnesses cause persistent insomnia because of pain and discomfort. But other relationships between illness and persistent insomnia are not so obvious. For example, sleep apnea and PLMD sometimes result in complaints of insomnia, because the people lack awareness that they stop breathing or kick their legs during sleep.

Psychological problems insomnia.   One-third to one-half of people seeking medical help for persistent insomnia have a psychological problem as the primary cause. Both mild and severe psychological problems may affect sleep. Persons with schizophrenia, for example, often complain of sleep onset problems and generally poor sleep. People with phobic disorders, anxiety problems, or those who are obsessive-compulsive, have sleep onset difficulties, as well as some sleep maintenance problems. People with adjustment problems like continuing marital or job stress may also experience sleep difficulties. However, depression is the most common psychological problem causing persistent insomnia.

While about one out of five depressed people report hypersomnia, most complain of insomnia. Depressed individuals may have trouble falling asleep. However, they more commonly show sleep maintenance disturbances with multiple awakenings and premature final awakenings. As a result, they feel achy and washed-out, although not really tired. Frequently depressed people have much shorter REMS latencies than normal and longer REMS periods earlier in the night. They also show reduced SWS. The reduced REMS latency is so dramatic in endogenously depressed individuals that it is considered a biological indicator that a person is depressed and may even be used as a very early sign of depression. Some of these disturbances of sleep tend to persist even when the behavioral indicators of depression are in remission.

Insomnia associated with lifestyle.   For about one-fourth of people with persistent insomnia, behaviors are the root cause. These behaviors are divided into two subgroups: **persistent psychophysiological**, about 15% of all people with insomnia, and insomnia as a result of substance consumption, about 12%.

Psychophysiological insomnia is often termed "learned" or "behavioral" insomnia because of the presence of maladaptive learning or behaviors incompatible with sleeping. There appear to be several subtypes.

Some people are chronically tense. When awake, they tend to be restless, overactive, nervous, and apprehensive. It should not be surprising that such people also sleep poorly. Their general bodily tension carries over into sleep. In the laboratory, their sleep recordings may reveal higher than normal activity in the neck muscles, as well as other muscles, and their pulse rate tends to be high. They report and demonstrate numerous, sometimes prolonged, awakenings later in the night that are often associated with worried thoughts and anxious dreams. Often this sleep disturbance results in reduced REMS and SWS. Sometimes, they also show sleep onset difficulties. They describe themselves as light sleepers.

These people are more fatigued than truly sleepy. They seldom nap, and when they do make attempts, they often fail to fall asleep. On the other hand, they tend to sleep better at the start of vacations. It is as if they feel they have permission to relax since they are on vacation.

Another subgroup of people with psychophysiological insomnia has learned not to sleep! They have unconsciously learned to associate bedroom cues such as the bed, nightclothes, etc., with not being able to sleep. Typically, these people will sleep better in a new and strange environment, such as a motel room, whereas most of us find we sleep a bit worse in a new situation. An extreme example of this problem was a student who, while mountain climbing, was forced to sleep on a narrow ledge tied to the rocks, yet had his best night of sleep in a year! He did so, because the sleeping situation was so different from his bedroom that he did not have enough learned associations to it to keep him awake. People with conditioned insomnia often report frequently falling asleep when not trying, such as when reading, driving, or watching television.

How does Learned Insomnia Come about?

For most of us, the bedroom stimuli become cues to sleep. They are always present just before we successfully fall asleep, so we learn that when these cues are present, we will soon fall asleep. For people with insomnia, however, something goes wrong. Perhaps, for a short period in their life something made sleep onset more difficult, such as excessive noise, poor weather, or emotional problems. For most people, this phenomenon is temporary, and normal sleep quickly returns. But some susceptible individuals begin to unconsciously associate the bedroom cues with not sleeping. Even after the original cause is long gone, the learned insomnia remains, because it is self-perpetuating. The bedroom cues lead to poor sleep onset, and poor sleep onset occurs in the presence of these bedroom cues. So, on and on it goes. Left untreated, learned insomnia seldom disappears but usually gets worse.

How are Substances Involved with Insomnia?

Many drugs, legal and illegal, taken to affect behavior also affect sleep. While some drugs make people extra sleepy, the side effects of others reduce the amount or disrupt the normal pattern of sleep.

Alcohol is a common substance that can produce insomnia. While many people self-medicate with alcohol because it makes them sleepy, once asleep alcohol eventually disrupts sleep (see Chapter 5). Persons with alcohol in their blood will toss and turn more frequently during sleep. Additionally, alcohol reduces the amount of REMS during sleep, with REMS rebound following cessation of intake. Alcohol, however, does increase total sleep time.

Sleep will progressively disintegrate with continued, excessive alcohol use, resulting in a reduction of total sleep time, breaking up of REMS periods, and less REMS overall. Severe alcoholism can lead to a permanent, irreversible reduction of both REMS and SWS. Sudden abstinence in alcoholics usually results in severe sleep onset problems, sharply reduced SWS, and a dramatic increase in REMS. This withdrawal pattern typically lasts 10–14 days after the last bout of drinking.

People also use substances to keep themselves awake and alert—drugs such as **amphetamines** and substances such as **caffeine**. Some weight reduction agents have the side effect of increased arousal. Depending on the amount used, length of use, and individual susceptibility, the user may suffer various degrees of sleep disturbance. These disturbances include sleep onset delays, less total sleep time, reduced SWS and REMS, and, with continued use, sudden daytime sleepiness. Some coffee drinkers are so sensitive to caffeine that even one cup in the morning may disturb their subsequent night of sleep.

What about the Fourth Major Subgrouping, Primary Insomnia?

Primary insomnia comes in several varieties. In one variety, we find those people with insomnia who are their own worst enemies; they **try too hard** to fall asleep. When an individual consciously tries hard to do something, and works at it mentally, the brain is aroused. This arousal tends to oppose the brain mechanisms that bring on sleep. So, the person is trying to use the activated, awake brain to force the sleep control parts of the brain to induce sleep. Since the two oppose one another (see Chapter 4), insomnia results. Frequent glances at the clock to see how long it is taking to fall asleep, calculations of how much sleep can be obtained before the alarm goes off, and concern about poor functioning the next waking day if "enough" sleep is not obtained are all often a part of this type of insomnia.

In about 5% of persistent insomnia cases, the cause is not easily attributed to medical or psychological problems or to life style. In such cases, the insomnia is considered **idiopathic**. One example is childhood onset insomnia. The name is an adequate description: the person has had insomnia all of his or her life and for no apparent reason. However, it is presumed that there is a malfunction of the sleep/wake mechanisms of the brain. Sometimes hospital staff or parents note the remarkable lack of sleep in these people even as babies. Their memories of childhood are of long, lonely, sleepless nights followed by days of struggle, constantly fighting off fatigue. In many of these people, neither sleeping pills nor stimulants are of much help. Extensive medical examination and testing during the person's life do not uncover any physical or psychological problems causing the sleeplessness. Often these people show both onset and maintenance sleep problems, and the sleep they do get is light. That is, they are easily aroused with reduced SWS and reduced REMS.

Sleep state misperception accounts for about 7.5% of people who complain of persistent insomnia. While subjectively they think they have insomnia, they fail to meet criteria. Some are simply short sleepers who are worried, because they have heard that healthy individuals need 7 to 8 hours of sleep per night, but they get much less. The key is that they do not suffer the waking symptoms typical of others with insomnia. Their short sleep is simply adequate for them.

Others with primary insomnia have complaints of tiredness and fatigue when awake and all of the disruptions to life that result from insomnia. However, their sleep length and sleep profile are entirely within normal limits. Although it is typical for most people with insomnia to underestimate their sleep time and sleep efficiency while overestimating their sleep latency, they, nevertheless, do not have normal sleep. With this group, however, there are no objective indications of poor sleep. Some sleep disorders experts have speculated that their insomnia is real but that we have not discovered what to look for or how to measure it in them. Another believes that "they think all night long," and that such mental effort is fatiguing rather than restful. In any event, many of these patients report benefit while awake from the same treatments as other people with insomnia, even though such treatments make no change in their sleep as measured in the laboratory.

Just what are the Treatments for Insomnia?

While a good physician would not treat a patient with a fever simply by prescribing aspirin, insomnia should not be simply, reflexively treated with sleeping pills. The most effective and long lasting treatment for insomnia is directed at changing the behaviors and cognitions that contribute to the insomnia. This approach is called cognitive-behavioral treatment for insomnia, or CBT-I. It has been shown to be as effective as sleeping pills in the short run of a few weeks and superior to them for subsequent months and years (Backhaus, Hohagen, Voderholzer, & Riemann, 2001). It also is effective with most people with any type of insomnia and even helps when other medical or psychological conditions are present.

CBT-I begins with taking a thorough history of the sleep, medical, and psychological status of the person. What is the nature of the sleep problem, and how long has it existed? A week of two of the person keeping a sleep log can be very useful for discerning this. Most sleep logs include space to record daily such things as time of going to bed, amount of time to get to sleep, number and duration of awakenings, quality of sleep, level of daytime wakefulness, naps, etc. What was sleep like previously? What are the differences between good and bad nights of sleep including differences in the wake period that proceeded such nights? It is also important to ask questions that screen for other sleep disorders that may be causing or contributing to the insomnia. A complete medical history and exam may reveal causal or parallel conditions that need to be treated if not being done so already. What medications is the person taking? Some medications used to treat various illnesses may have side effects that contribute to insomnia. Since depression is a leading cause of insomnia and other psychological conditions may also influence sleep, the psychological status of the person should also be assessed and any problems treated. However, simply treating a causal or co-morbid medical or psychological condition may not necessarily help the insomnia, so concurrent CBT-I should also be considered.

There are several components to CBT-I. Which components are used, in what order, and when to use them depends on the nature of the insomnia as determined from the history of the person. The goal is to improve the person's sleep compatible with desired outcomes by changing those behaviors that are incompatible with sleep. The major components include education, cognitive changes, stimulus control, arousal reduction, sleep restriction, and circadian rhythm maintenance. Specific activities may encompass more than one of these categories.

Education about the basics of sleep can help dispel the misconceptions that many people have. Some of the type of information in Chapters 1 and 2 about sleep, especially its changes with normal aging and our propensity to sleep during certain parts of the nychthemeron, may be new to them. Information about good sleep hygiene such as in Box 14 in Chapter 5 is also important. This information can help lead to a change in attitude about sleep and a change in beliefs and thoughts that can interfere with sleep. However, studies have shown that such information alone is not enough to help most people with persistent insomnia.

Cognitive changes continue and extend what was begun with education about sleep. Many people engage in thoughts and behaviors that are counterproductive even when attempting to achieve better sleep. For example, they may "try harder" to make themselves fall asleep and stay in bed longer in order to get enough sleep. While lying there, they focus on how they need to get to sleep so that they will feel rested and able to function the next day. But these thoughts and behaviors only cause frustration, tension, and anxiety that are incompatible with sleep and perpetuate the insomnia in a vicious cycle.

Many people may also have negative thoughts that exacerbate their insomnia. They may believe that their sleep is much worse than it actually is. They may blame poor waking performance solely on their poor sleep. They may be unrealistic about how much sleep they require. They may tell themselves they are terrible sleepers. When trying to fall asleep, they may think to themselves over and over things like:

- Everybody needs exactly 8 hours of sleep per night.
- The best sleep occurs before midnight.
- I know I'll be a wreck the next day if I don't get enough sleep.

Changing these, and any other, negative ruminations will frequently contribute to better sleep by reducing the overall level of anxiety and encourage a positive outlook the next day, regardless of the length of the previous night of sleep.

This objective may be accomplished by encouraging the person to write down comments about sleep and then redefine the negative statements such as:

- I'll never sleep well.
- I cannot get to sleep the night before an important meeting.
- Sleep is a waste of time, but I cannot do without it.

to positive comments:

- Everybody, including me, can sleep well.
- Maybe it will take a little longer, but I can get to sleep and sleep well before an important meeting.
- Sleep takes time and is necessary, so I'll just enjoy it.

The person must practice these positive comments aloud several times during the day for a while until they become ingrained.

The cognitive component also involves creating a set of realistic expectations in the person. People with insomnia often want and expect immediate improvement. However, they need to realize that insomnia took time to develop and will take time to dissipate. Often, sleep will get worse for a week or so during CBT-I, before it gets better. It is not unlike having surgery; there is a period of increased inconvenience and suffering one must go through in order to return to health. Continuing to keep a sleep log during the course of treatment can help persons see eventual progress and encourage them to adhere to the CBT-I treatments.

Stimulus control involves making the bedroom conducive to sleep. Some of these habits are incorporated into sleep hygiene but may have to be more intensely targeted in some insomniacs. The process begins with providing a comfortable sleeping environment conducive to sleeping, but more intensive focus may have to be made on reversing the learned associations that many people with insomnia have that inhibit getting to sleep. For example, if the person has spent hours in bed trying unsuccessfully to get to sleep or doing things like studying, doing taxes, or watching exciting movies on TV, then the bed becomes a conditioned stimulus for the conditioned response arousal and anxiety, rather than relaxation and sleep. This needs to be changed by implementing a rigid adherence to avoiding bed unless sleepy, getting up if sleep does not come in a reasonable time and going to another room and returning only when sleepy, sleeping only in the bedroom, and using the bed only for sleep (and sex). The goal is to classically condition the bed as a stimulus for the response of sleep.

Arousal reduction may be necessary, because many people with insomnia have elevated levels of arousal and tension in their mind and body. These levels may be true for the entire nychthemeron or only when sleep in attempted. Arousal reduction can be accomplished in several ways but must be learned and practiced first while awake for about two weeks before applying them at bedtime. **Progressive muscle relaxation** involves learning to relax groups of muscles in the body by first tensing them and then letting them relax. Eventually, the person learns what relaxed muscles feel like and can more easily cause them to relax when desired, such as at bedtime. Biofeedback can achieve a similar result by providing auditory or visual information from a piece of equipment monitoring some aspect of the body that tells persons to what degree they are able to achieve a relaxed state. Eventually, they learn how to achieve this state and no longer need the external feedback. **Guided imagery** training enables people to imagine vividly a pleasant experience or situation. The image itself is not only calming, but diverts attention from arousal-provoking thoughts. **Abdominal breathing** involves concentrating on breathing using the diaphragm rather than the chest. It is easy to learn and promotes a slower and more relaxing breathing rate while also diverting attention from arousing thoughts.

Another technique that may be helpful to some people is to schedule "worry time." For some people, problems and concerns seem to pop into their minds when they want to go to sleep. This practice keeps them awake. It is better to schedule a half-hour or so in the evening, but not just before bedtime, to worry. If when attempting to go to sleep, a worry comes up, they can then say, "I have worried about that. It's taken care of." or "I forgot to worry about this, but I can do it during my next worry time. Goodnight." The idea is to think of and deal with problems when the mind is fresh and can do something. This practice clears the deck for sleep.

Sleep restriction is counter-intuitive to many people with insomnia and may be initially resisted as a treatment modality. It is intended to increase the person's sleep efficiency by limiting the time in bed to the time actually spent sleeping. Many insomniacs have done the opposite. They have increased their time in bed attempting to get an "adequate" amount of sleep. The result is they spend a great deal of time in bed awake, not asleep. Sleep restriction therapy is designed to reverse this pattern.

Based on sleep log data, the average amount of time person actually sleeps is determined. Their time in bed is then restricted to that amount of time, but never less than 4.5 hours. Bedtime is established counting backwards from a desired regular time of awakening by the number of hours allowed in bed. Typically, the result is even less sleep for a few days, but as fatigue builds, more of the time in bed is spent sleeping. When sleep efficiency reaches .85 to .90 as determined by the sleep log, then 15 minutes is added to the time allowed in bed. An additional 15 minutes is added every time sleep efficiency reaches .85 to .90. However, each increment should be maintained for at least 5 days before adding another. Eventually, a desirable amount of efficient sleep is achieved and maintained.

Circadian rhythm maintenance is also a component of CBT-I. Establishing and maintaining efficient sleep in a person with insomnia requires sleeping and waking at about the same time every nychthemeron. Irregular times for sleep can result in poor quality sleep (see Chapter 2). Getting out of bed at the same time each morning regardless of the amount of sleep obtained is critically important in maintaining stable circadian rhythm sleep/wake phases.

CBT-I generally takes several weeks, although there are shorter variations that have shown some success. It has proved successful when done on an individual basis or in groups. The components need to be gradually introduced over the course of the treatment, compliance and progress monitored, and adjustments made. It needs to terminate with instruction on how to maintain gains and prevent relapse.

There is a need for people well trained in the principles of psychology to provide CBT-I for people with insomnia. Although it sounds like many of the CBT-I components can be done by individuals without needing someone to guide them, in reality a trained professional working with people with insomnia individually or in groups has proved to be much more effective. The professional can tailor and pace the treatment better, as well as provide support and encouragement. Also, the professional can trouble-shoot problems, answer questions, and make appropriate adjustments.

What About the Use of Sleeping Pills?

We are now into the second generation of prescription sleeping pills that are much safer and have fewer side effects than the first generation. The second generation pills far outsell the first generation ones. They are shorter acting, so there is less carry over of sleepiness into the waking period. They have less disruptive effect on the components of sleep, especially less or no reduction of REMS. Some are much better for helping with sleep onset, while others are also effective for sleep maintenance. Like the first generation, they have been shown to be effective for 2 to 3 weeks. Beyond this period of time, their effectiveness may begin to diminish in some, but not all, people with insomnia. They can be very effective for transient or short-term insomnia but should not be used on a regular basis except in certain cases as determined by a specialist in sleep disorders. Prescription sleeping pills should not be used by people with various medical or psychological conditions or who are employed in jobs that might require immediate response during sleeping hours. Whether or not an individual should be taking sleeping pills is best determined by the physician before prescribing this kind of medication.

Over-the-counter (non-prescription) sleep aids are, at best, poor in producing sleep. In spite of the many different brand names and expensive advertising campaigns to convince us that each is unique and most effective, they are all very similar and relatively ineffective. These sleeping pills usually contain some kind of antihistamine, which is often also one of the main ingredients in cough medicines and decongestants. In some, the main ingredient is combined with other things such as aspirin. At best, they produce some drowsiness in some people, but at worst, they may produce troublesome side effects, including arousal that can interfere with sleeping. None is very powerful in producing sleep in any natural and consistent way. Most sleep professionals do not recommend them.

Most sleep professionals also give the same negative recommendation for other kinds of things used to obtain sleep. Many people drink alcohol to facilitate their sleep. However, in the long run this practice is counterproductive (see Chapter 5). Alternative therapies, such as the use of herbs or magnets, have been poorly studied but are of doubtful value. There is little or no objective evidence that they really work. Also, as discussed in Chapter 5, you cannot be sure of their purity or of the actual amount in commercial preparations of them. For a person who has enduring insomnia, such treatments are not likely to be of much help.

Can Sleeping Pills and CBT-I be Combined?

It would seem to make sense to combine prescription sleeping pills and CBT-I. The sleeping pills could provide immediate relief, while the person is gradually acquiring the long-term benefits of the CBT-I. While this idea seems reasonable, experience has tended to show otherwise. The combined use of CBT-I and sleeping pills seems to reduce the eventual effectiveness of the CBT-I. It may be that the person is less motivated to do the CBT-I, since the sleeping pills are providing them good sleep. Or, it may be that the person learns to, or continues to, rely upon external means to obtain good sleep rather than develop and rely upon internal resources. For whatever reason, the combination does not appear to be as effective as CBT-I in the long run. Also, many people with insomnia who have been using sleeping pills for a long time find that they are no longer effective, or they may turn to CBT-I to kick the sleeping pill habit.

We now conclude the symposium on insomnia. Thanks to all our participants. Your comments have been very useful.

Box 29

Sleep Related Nocturnal Eating Disorder[48]

A relatively recent discovery has been the Sleep Related Nocturnal Eating disorder. This disorder occurs when a person almost nightly gets up and eats after falling asleep. It usually occurs about an hour after sleep onset but can occur up to eight times per night in some people. The preference is for eating high-calorie foods, and the result can be weight gain. Yet, over 80% are unaware, or only somewhat aware, that they do it. The missing food, open refrigerator, or partially eaten food may be the most obvious clue. The onset is typically in the late teens to early 20s and two-thirds of those with the disorder are female. It is unrelated to waking eating disorders or any kind of hunger. Eating prior to bed has little effect on its occurrence. Although a number of possible precipitating causes have been noted, including medications, other sleep disorders, stress, and giving up smoking or alcohol, the most common finding is that over one-half of the suffers have a history of multiple abuse of some kind during childhood. There is no consensus for effective treatment as of this writing.

CIRCADIAN RHYTHM SLEEP DISORDERS

W.N. is a 20-year-old student living in the dorm at a nearby college. During the intake interview, he was reasonably alert and energetic, yet looked tired. He was 20 minutes late for his 11 a.m. appointment.

He described his problem as insomnia. "I just can't get to sleep." The problem started this semester, midway through the first semester of his junior year, when he had to take a required course only offered at 8 a.m. He said he was lucky when he started college to have no early-morning classes. He could "take advantage of college dorm life" at night without having to worry about getting up early. As a result, he typically went to sleep between 3 and 4 a.m.—even later on weekends. After that, he carefully selected his courses in order to avoid those that met early in the morning—until he had no choice this semester.

Because he could not get to sleep early enough at night, he had missed many of his 8 a.m. classes this semester, since he "just could not wake up." He had repeatedly tried going to bed at midnight, but just lay awake for several hours. He had tried "everything," including: warm milk and graham crackers, sleeping pills, herbal teas, exhaustive exercise, alcohol, a dull textbook, and, on the advice of a friend, facing his bed due north to get the "proper magnetic pull" on his brain. Nothing worked. He was desperate, because when he did get up after only a few hours of sleep, he was so "wiped out" that he got little out of the 8 a.m. lecture. He actually fell asleep in the class several times. He missed so many classes that his professor threatened to drop him from the course.

Upon questioning, he related how weekends and breaks were his salvation, because he slept in until mid-afternoon. When asked when he felt most alert, he immediately and emphatically stated "in the evening—once I make it past supper, I'm O.K." He scored 15 on the Smith, Reilly, and Midkiff (1989) questionnaire (see Chapter 2), which classified him as a strong evening type. His psychological tests were within normal limits.

His polysomnogram showed a sleep latency of 233 minutes after lights out at 23:30 hours, but otherwise normal sleep for his age, other than a high normal amount of SWS, indicating a possible sleep deprivation. He awoke without much difficulty at 10:30 a.m. when called over the intercom by a polysomnographic technician who needed to analyze his sleep record before an 11:30 appointment. He said the night was a typical night of sleep for him.

It is apparent that W.N.'s problem was not insomnia, but a sleep phase delay disorder (see Figure 39). He can fall asleep only when his body is in its circadian primary sleepiness zone (see Chapter 2), which, for him, occurs after 3 a.m. His body stubbornly refused to advance that zone when he tries going to bed earlier, thus he was unable to get to sleep until much later. He is not a sleep onset insomniac for two reasons. He falls asleep easily if he goes to bed around 3 a.m. and he has much difficulty arising before 10 a.m. but otherwise seems to get good sleep.

He was treated with **chronotherapy.** Chronotherapy consists of having the person go to bed 3 hours later each day or two, and getting out of bed after exactly 8 hours, no matter what time of day or amount of sleep has been obtained. No napping is allowed until the next bedtime. This delay of sleep each "day" is greater than the person's typical phase delay, and thus, sleep onset is rapid and sleep is sound. This regimen seems to allow the person to recapture control of sleep onset after about 8 days. At this point, the person is usually able to establish and maintain a normal, stable bedtime in the late evening and arise regularly mid-morning. The treatment was successful for W.N., and he passed his course.

People with delayed sleep phase syndrome resemble people with insomnia in that they seem to have trouble getting to sleep. But unlike people with sleep onset insomnia, they fall asleep about the same time every night. Thus, if they go to bed at this time, they have no problem falling asleep, but if they go to bed earlier, their sleep onset problems occur. Furthermore, they tend to have problems awakening before a certain, relatively fixed clock time. Thus, they are on a stable 24-hour rhythm, and their primary sleepiness zone (see Chapter 2) is during the same clock hours every nychthemeron. It is just that these clock hours are delayed from those desired or those demanded by the environment.

These people can be considered extreme night owls. No amount of willpower or sleeping pills are able to help. These people show peak alertness and efficiency only late in the day. The problem often starts in childhood perhaps with late-night study habits or illness. It does seem to run in families, suggesting that some people may be more prone to develop it. Chronotherapy and/or bright light therapy are used to treat these sufferers.

Light therapy takes advantage of the fact that bright light is a major zeitgeber for human circadian rhythms (see Chapter 2). Light in the early morning (before dawn) tends to phase advance circadian rhythms (i.e., make them earlier), while light in the evening (after dusk) tends to phase delay them (i.e., make them later). Thus, for phase delay syndrome, several days of 1 to 2 hours of bright (2500 or more lux) morning light is often sufficient to move the phase of the person's sleep cycle to the more desired and adaptive time. Continued exposure to light in the morning may be necessary to maintain the change.

Delayed sleep phase syndrome, such as in this case, is not the only kind of rhythm disruption that can occur. Other types are the result of the effects of shift work and jet lag (discussed in Chapter 10), and the apparently rare advanced sleep phase syndrome, non-24-hour sleep/wake rhythm, and irregular sleep/wake rhythm.

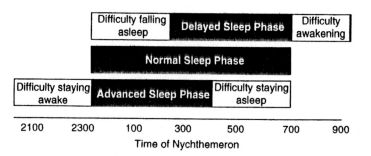

Figure 39. The differences between normal sleep, delayed sleep phase, and advanced sleep phase.

There are relatively few reports of people with advanced sleep phase syndrome. People with the inability to remain awake and alert in the evening and who typically go to sleep between 8 and 9 p.m. awaken at about 4 to 5 a.m. and are unable to return to sleep. Like phase delay persons, they are on a 24-hour schedule, but they are unable to modify the placement of their sleep period during the 24 hours. These people are true day larks. The reason so few cases of sleep advance syndrome have been reported is unclear. Perhaps it is not as troublesome to job and school schedules, and no sleep loss occurs, so these people have no need to seek help. Or perhaps there truly are few of them, since the propensity for people is to phase delay (see Chapter 3).

Non-24-hour sleep/wake rhythm is characterized by progressively later sleep onset and arousal times, that is, a person's body is on a 25 or 26-hour sleep/wake schedule. For part of each month, things are relatively fine for these persons. They go to sleep and arise more or less as the world expects. But eventually, they drift out-of-phase with the world—desiring sleep when the world is awake and wake when the world is asleep. Chronotherapy or light therapy is used to treat these cases unless the person is blind. (Many blind people have a non-24-hour sleep/wake cycle showing how important light is in entraining the circadian clock—see Chapter 2).

The final type of rhythm disruption is the lack of any well-defined rhythm at all. The persons' nychthemeron consists of many daytime naps and shortened nocturnal sleep. Meal patterns also often become disrupted, and they simply eat whenever they feel like it. Weakness, languor, and many bodily complaints typically also occur. These people usually complain of insomnia, not realizing that the inability to sleep well at night is caused by their disordered schedules. Treatment is difficult when the absence of circadian sleep/wake schedule occurs, and any success may not last. It consists of enforcing a more typical 24-hour cycle of rest/activity as well as regularizing other aspects of daily living, such as meals. Often, this treatment requires someone living with the person to be responsible for establishing routines until the person becomes synchronized.

CONCLUSION

Sleep/wake disorders medicine has a relatively brief history. However, since the first sleep/wake disorders center opened in the early 1970s, many people have been assessed and treated. Many of these people were found to have serious sleep/wake disorders that were not even known to exist prior to research conducted at sleep/wake centers. Today, the majority of people with any kind of sleep complaint have a condition which is potentially diagnosable and, more importantly, treatable. Many people can now live better quality lives as a result. The likelihood is for even more improvement of life for countless numbers of people as they too are diagnosed and treated and as research finds out more about these disorders, how they affect our lives, and how they can be treated.

Part V

Why We Sleep and Dream

Sleep has persisted in evolution even though it is apparently maladaptive with respect to other functions. While we sleep, we do not procreate, protect or nurture the young, gather food, earn money, write papers, etc. It is against the logic of natural selection to sacrifice such important activities unless sleep serves equally or more important functions.

(Rechtschaffen, 1998, p. 360)

Some animals sleep when it would be much simpler not to do so. For example, the blind Indus dolphin lives in very murky water, so it does not need to see, it uses sonar to navigate, and it eventually became blind. Yet, in spite of the difficulties of sleeping in an aquatic environment—difficulties equal to those of trying to see in murky water—the Indus dolphin has retained sleep. Among mammals and birds, at least, there is some compelling reason to sleep. Yet, there is no complete understanding of, much less complete agreement about, the functions of sleep. It seems as if we are just on the threshold of understanding why we sleep. It is like being in a room with several doors that are just a bit open allowing us a peak of what is inside. With a bit of effort, we may be able, in the future, to open one or more of those doors and get a clearer view. Meanwhile, in the next two chapters we will peek into many doors in order to review many of the current theories of sleep, especially those that remain active and viable or that are new and exciting.

First, let us be clear on what is meant by function (Carskadon, 1993). Function means purpose. Function equals instrumental value, that is, it makes a difference. Function means the effect or effects accomplished. But there are different levels of purposes, instrumental values, and effects, ranging from essential to enhancing to convenient to trivial to detrimental. Consider the functions of your nose. It is a vital component of the respiratory system, a convenient place upon which to rest glasses, an enhancer or detractor of facial beauty, and a most annoying place of irritation when you have a cold.

A function may be but a component of a larger system or sequence. Again, your nose is a part of the respiratory system and a component of your face. Some of its functions are in relation to the greater whole.

Some functions of things are absolutely necessary; the system would fail without them. Other functions may not be necessary, but the system works better or faster with them. You can breathe through your mouth, but it is generally better to do so through your nose. Still other functions may be convenient but could be easily replaced or done

---

Box 30

Historical Review of Theories of Sleep[49]

Throughout recorded history, speculations on the causes and functions of sleep usually reflected the prevailing understanding of physiology of the time subsequently to become modified to be consistent with new discoveries in physiology. Along the way, prevailing psychological and religious ideas also have had an influence.

The ancient Greeks often viewed sleep as caused by and causing distributions of heat in the body. A slight cooling of the temperature of the blood was thought by Aristotle to cause sleep because of a resulting redistribution of warm blood into the center of the body. He also stated that heat causes fumes from eaten food to leave the veins and go to the head. There the fumes cool and sink to lower parts of the body, which draws heat away from the body thereby rendering one sleepy.

A rather curious explanation came out of the 12th century by Hildegard von Bingen (who often wrote about medicine and nature in a mystical way). She made a connection between sleep and food and the Fall of Adam. She described how food and rest nourished the body. Prior to the Fall, the sleep of Adam was a kind of deep contemplation, and food was partaken visually—simply delighting and edifying the soul and spirit. The Fall weakened and enfeebled the body though, and thus made necessary eating and sleep to rejuvenate it once again.

The sixteenth century physician Paracelsus endeavored to relate medicine and nature. His advice was to rise with the sun and retire at sunset. This habit would eliminate tiredness caused by working and thus refresh the body.

During the 17th and 18th centuries, physiology and metaphysics were combined to explain sleep. Sleep resulted when the "animal spirits" were drained off from the body by work and activity, resulting in exhaustion. Or, sleep occurs when the brain separates nervous spirits out of the blood during wakefulness. Or, sleep happens when the liquor in the brain gets used up or thickens while being awake and thus cannot fill the small vessels and nerves that serve the sense organs and muscles. Interestingly, these notions led to opposing views on how to improve sleep: some espousing no pillows so that blood flows to the head while others suggesting many pillows to encourage blood to flow from the head.

The discovery of oxygen led to a new theory of sleep around the turn of the 19th century. Oxygen in the air we breathe yields an "ether of life" which the blood transports to the brain for storage. From here, it is distributed into nerves and muscles to produce motion, but it is apparently used up during wakefulness, only to be replenished by sleep. Later in the 19th, century, other oxygen-based theories were enunciated. Sleep was seen as a result of a lack of oxygen, especially in the brain. This phenomenon occurred, according to one theory, because certain substances, such as lactic acid and creatine, were higher in the tired body and these substances absorb oxygen.

Passive theories of sleep were also common during the 19th century—especially the notion that sleep is due to a lack of stimulation. Dr. Edward Elapariede of France developed one such popular theory of the time. He saw sleep as an active instinct—like a process that serves to avoid fatigue. In short, we cease sleeping when we have had enough sleep.

Early in the 20th century, many "bottle" theories were produced. These theories see the body as a bottle that gradually fill up with one or another substance ("humors") that induce sleep. Sleep rids the bottle (body) of this poison. These theories see sleep being due to the accumulation of one or another substance ("humors") that induce sleep, gradually eliminated during sleep. The putative humors included known substances such as lactic acid, carbon dioxide, and cholesterol, as well as poorly defined things given names like leucomaines and urotoxins. There was a flurry of research on these substances early in the 20th century, especially with the "hypnotoxin" of Legendre and Pieron. Later, in the 1960s, research again flourished, this time with success, leading to a current knowledge of several sleep substances including DSIP, muramyl pedtides, and adenocine (see Chapter 5).

During the 20th century, as the understanding of brain functioning advanced, there have been many neurophysiological theories of sleep. Early theories posited inhibition as a key factor. Prominent among these theories was Pavlov's notion of "cortical inhibition." He saw sleep resulting from inhibitory influences located in the cerebral cortex. Subsequent theories and research have shifted the location of such inhibitory areas to lower parts of the brain and have included active excitatory areas as also being important.

Today, most people, when asked, would probably say the function of sleep is for some kind of rest and restoration. Intuitively, this idea seems to be so. We go to bed tired, "worn-out," exhausted, and so forth, but usually awaken refreshed and revived following a night of sleep. Yet, simple rest and restoration ideas of the function of sleep are too simple to be the only answer. Left unanswered are questions such as what is restored and why is sleep the only, or best or utilized, means of doing so? Restoration may be a part of the explanation, but only a part.

without. There are ways that glasses could be kept on your face rather than to rest them on your nose. Finally, other functions may be superfluous or even detrimental. A stuffy nose is a good example.

Often the search for function has concentrated on that which is essential or primary (Kreuger & Obal, 2002; Nicolau et al., 2000). The organism has no other way to initiate this function and would suffer from its loss. It is why the function developed during evolution. Yet, the next two levels of functions, enhancing and convenient are also important and are worthy of search and research efforts and should not be quickly discounted. We may find that the functions of sleep are of these latter types more than of the former type and are just as important as practical answers to the version of the question, "What is the function of sleep?" that means "What is sleep for?" We also must realize that it is more difficult to discover a non-essential function than an essential function. Yet, it is possible to determine such functions by careful research and reasoning. Then, too, the essential function of sleep may not be readily apparent from the characteristics of sleep or its mechanisms of generation (Kavanau, 2001).

Often the question is put too simply: "What is the function of sleep?" Turn the question around and ask, "What is the function of wakefulness?" There is no one, simple answer to either question. Thus, we must ask, "What *are* the functions of sleep?" and seek answers on many levels, from molecular to behavioral (Hauri, 1979). Furthermore, we need to remember that "sleep and wake are mutually interacting and cyclic phenomena" (Hauri, 1979, p. 252), and thus a theory of sleep necessarily involves implications for wakefulness, also. Then too, a theory or explanation of the functions of sleep must be consistent with the other myriads of details that are known about it—many of which have been presented earlier in this book. Most importantly to Kreuger and Obal (2002), the loss of consciousness that occurs during sleep must be explained in an adequate theory of sleep.

There are essentially four scientific strategies used in the search for the functions of sleep: description, correlation, stimulation, and deprivation (Rechtschaffen, 1998). Each has its strengths and weaknesses.

- Description: points to possible functions, but there may easily be other explanations for the observations. For example, it is easily observed that sleeping animals typically close their eyes, but that does not mean that the function of sleep is to protect the eyes. It is more likely that closing the eyes facilitates sleep.
- Correlation: sleep correlated with something suggests possible function, but other explanations are possible. For example, if sleep is correlated with some aspect of personality, we do not know if sleep causes that aspect, or that aspect causes sleep, or a third factor causes both.
- Stimulation (experimentation): suggests internal changes to which sleep responds, but stimulation can increase or decrease sleep independent of need. For example, a sleeping pill is shown to stimulate sleep. Research can show the brain mechanisms by which the pill stimulates sleep, but it may have nothing to do with natural mechanisms, hence function.
- Deprivation: reveals what happens without sleep, but the results could be responses to sleep-preventing stimuli themselves rather than affecting sleep directly. For example, rats kept awake by forced running show consequences, but it is not clear if the consequences are from the lack of sleep or the continuous running.

The best clues to the functions of sleep come when there is research using several different methodologies from more than one type of strategy that consistently leads to the same conclusion.

You may ask, "Why is it important to seek out and understand the functions of sleep and dreaming?" The answer is, we can never really know what sleep is until we understand its functions. This in turn influences our (Meddis, 1979):

- attitudes toward our own sleep;
- research endeavors (a good example is the dramatic change in sleep research that occurred when it was realized that sleep is active and not passive);
- treatments for sleep/wake disorders;
- and contributions to our basic understanding of human beings and the world in which we live.

In an interesting new paper, Nicolau and colleagues (2000) posit that it is not so much that sleep has evolved, but that it is waking that has evolved. With the development of the forebrain during evolution, homeotherms developed a new wake that is different from their reptilian forbearers. The old wake of reptiles became SWS.

We will begin our review by examining the overall functions of sleep and NREMS in Chapter 12, then look at the functions of REMS and dreaming in Chapter 13.

Chapter 12

Functions of Sleep and NREMS[50]

As a to our exploration of the possible functions of sleep, let us briefly review the many unique characteristics of sleep (after Rechtschaffen, 1998). Sleep:

- is found in all mammals, birds, and apparently reptiles; it may also occur in some or all amphibians, fish, and invertebrates
- cannot be replaced by waking rest
- is homeostatic—deprivation leads to rebound
- is rhythmic—it tends to occur at regular times each nychthemeron
- results in physiological and psychological changes that do not easily occur otherwise
- is a time of unconsciousness with reduced interaction with the external environment
- is actively produced by the brain
- has two distinct components that alternate in mammals
- has similar development in all mammals

Generally sleep is somewhat responsive to what happens in the daytime. Some waking activities have been found to affect sleep, such as increasing body temperature by exercise or sitting in a hot tub of water, weight gain or weight loss. Equally important are things during waking that do not affect sleep or do so to a very limited extent. Among them are exercise, increased metabolic rate, prolonged bed rest, intense sensory stimulation, sensory deprivation, and mentally stimulating activities (Rechtschaffen, 1998). Certainly what waking influence there is cannot be said to be the determining factor of why we sleep. Instead, sleep appears to be a need in its own right. In fact, the most consistent thing that sleep deprivation

Parts of this chapter are adapted from Moorcroft, 1993 with permission of the publisher.

does is increase the need for sleep and the need for the things that happen during sleep (Rechtschaffen, 1998).

FUNCTIONS FOR ALL SLEEP

Rest and Restoration

One of the oldest and most intuitive notions is that sleep is for rest and restoration of the body and mind. It seems to be a time of quiescence when the body appears to be able to generally reverse the wear and tear accumulated when awake. We feel bad when we do not get sleep or enough of it. In fact, sleep may have evolved out of rest that alternates with activity in most animals. It is possible that this pattern occurred to enable even greater rest and even restoration of tissues and organs worn down by waking activity.

Sleep researchers are confident that there is some kind of recuperation that occurs during sleep because of the presence of a drive to sleep in all higher animals, the deficits that occur with lost sleep, and the rebound after lost sleep (Bennington, 2001). The greater the sleep lost, the greater the rate of recuperation with subsequent sleep. Yet, there needs to be a minimum amount of continuity during sleep for it to be recuperative, and both REMS and SWS appear necessary for complete recuperation. Additionally, sleep researchers are fairly sure that recuperation needed and obtained is proportional to basic waking activity, and that the recuperation occurs at a cellular or brain circuit level. What is less certain is the precise nature of the recuperation, the relationship between NREMS and REMS, and why there is cycling between them.

In addition to being an intuitive notion, the notion that sleep is for rest and restoration is supported by the fact that some hormones are primarily released during early SWS. Growth hormone is released in its highest levels in young, growing humans during sleep and only during the first SWS period of the night in adults. The levels of other anabolic hormones (prolactin, leutenizing hormone, testosterone) are also highest during sleep. In contrast, catabolic hormones such as the corticosteroids are low during normally phased sleep periods (see Chapter 5).

More recently, research out of Van Cauter's laboratory at the University of Chicago has shown that sleep is necessary for certain body functions to stay within normal limits (see Chapter 5). Additionally, NREMS is hypothesized to replenish cerebral glycogen stores depleted during waking (Bennington and Heller, 1994, 1995).

However, there is evidence contrary to the hypothesis of a rest and restoration function for sleep (Rechtschaffen, 1998). There is a mean decrease in protein synthesis during sleep due mainly to fasting and the fact that level of muscle activity, hence wear and tear, during waking has a very low correlation with sleep length. While there is an increase in growth hormone during sleep, there is not an increase of overall protein synthesis. Also, there is not convincing evidence that energy is replenished during sleep. Glycogen restoration is increased only during early sleep with little change during the rest of sleep. Furthermore, sleep deprivation does not result in obvious dramatic and permanent breakdowns of the body or the mind. The physiological effects of acute sleep deprivation are generally small.

Also, logically, it is not clear why unconsciousness, a key component of sleep, is necessary for rest and restoration, when simple inactivity while awake would seem to accomplish the same ends. There is, too, a great variation in sleep in various species of mammals and other animals for it to be necessary for rest and restoration. And, the fact that some mammals sleep half a brain at a time because they need to keep their bodies moving (see Box 1 in Chapter 1) suggests that the benefit of sleep is not primarily for the body. We will look at these concepts more fully later in this chapter and the next.

Conservation of Energy

Sleep is a time of reduced levels of activity, body temperature, and energy consumption. This notion leads to the hypothesis that sleep serves the function of conservation of energy, especially when little is to be gained from being awake and active (Obál, 1984; Webb, 1979). The conservation of energy that occurs during sleep comes from more than a lack of activity, since a period of simple rest would accomplish that goal. Rather, it is the decrease of body temperature during sleep that conserves considerable energy (Berger & Phillips, 1995). The cost of maintaining temperature in warm-blooded animals is high—metabolic rate is 7 to 10 times higher in endotherms than in ectotherms at the same body temperature—and a reduction of only a few degrees is cost-effective (Walker & Berger, 1980). A decrease of $1°-2°$ in endotherms causes a 10% decrease in metabolic rate at neutral ambient temperatures and even greater savings at ambient temperatures that are cooler than neutral.

There is the apparent concurrent evolution of NREMS during evolution as homeothermy evolved with a similar concurrent development during ontogeny. Parallel development of sleep in mammals and birds occurred with the advent of endothermy. NREMS, with its turning down the thermostat of the bodies, matures concurrently with endothermy during maturation. Additionally, there is a greater requirement for sleep in animals that have less energy reserve. Finally, it is noted that there may be a continuation from sleep into hibernation with its even greater reduction in body temperature and energy usage. In contrast, others have pointed out that sleep may simply permit hibernation and, since there is a rebound of SWS following hibernation (see Box 1 in Chapter 1), sleep and hibernation may not be continuous.

A second version of this purported function for sleep focuses on energy expenditure. Sleep is a time of enforced rest that sets limits on activity and energy expenditure in order to help balance an animal's species-specific energy budget to keep it at a level that is affordable. There is a correlation of 0.63 between sleep length per nychthemeron and metabolic rate in mammals. Metabolic cost of activity varies inversely with body size, and food requirements are proportionally higher in smaller animals. Longer sleeping species tend to be small with higher metabolic rates. There is greater sleep in immature animals when more energy must be directed toward growth. The effects of terminal sleep deprivation studies in rats (see Box 31) are also consistent with this version of the hypothesis.

Box 31

Rechtschaffen's Sleep Deprivation Experiments in Rats

Starting in the mid-1980s Al Rechtschaffen and colleagues have done a series of experiments involving depriving rats of sleep in an attempt to learn more about the functions of sleep (c.f. Rechtschaffen et al., 1989; Rechtschaffen & Begrmann, 2002). In their basic procedure, an experimental rat and a control rat share a horizontal disk that is mounted over a shallow pool of water. The rats are separated from each other by a wall and have constant access to their own food and water. When a computer that continuously monitors the experimental rat for electrophysiological signs of sleep detects sleep-onset, it causes the disk to rotate slowly, preventing the animals from continuing sleeping. As a result, it gets only 10% of its normal total sleep, but the control rat gets almost 75% of its normal amount, because it can sleep whenever the experimental rat is awake and the disk is not moving. Michael Bonnet, (personal communication) maintains that it is really sleep fragmentation that is occurring in the experimental animal, not sleep deprivation, since it does get brief snatches of sleep before being quickly awakened. Whatever the interpretation, when deprived of sleep in this way, the experimental rats died after 2 to 3 weeks.

For some of the experiments, the rats were selectively deprived of either REMS or SWS, rather than all sleep. Unless otherwise noted, the results were the same except that they survived about twice as long with the selective deprivation. In some of the experiments, the rats were allowed uninterrupted sleep when they approached death (12 to 20 days of sleep deprivation); they recovered completely within a couple of weeks.

During individual experiments in this series, the rats were variously monitored for numerous physiological parameters and examined postmortemly for many more. Surprisingly few abnormalities were found. The rats did become disheveled looking, lost weight, and preferred a much warmer room temperature. Most notably, they showed double their food intake, followed by deficits of temperature regulation and excessive heat loss, followed by a breakdown of their defenses against common bacteria. However, extensive investigation (1) was not able to pinpoint the causes of many of these effects, and (2) ruled out all of these effects as the direct cause of death.

Notably, the researchers could find no major changes in the anatomy, microanatomy, synaptic activity, chemistry, or functioning of the brains of these animals. While narrowing the number of possible functions of sleep, they nevertheless were forced to conclude that these studies failed to specify the essential function of sleep. Yet, sleep appears to be of some biological necessity, at least in the rat.

A major criticism of these conclusions is that the effects may have been caused by stress (c.f. Horne, 2000). These experiments caused stress for both the experimental and control rats by confining them in a small space with little opportunity for normal activity. Also, the experimental rat occasionally would get wet from falling into the water while asleep as the disk rotated. In the experimental rat, the stress was coupled with sleep deprivation and, since REMS may be an anodyne for stress, it may have shown more symptoms compared to the controls. However, Rechtschaffen counters that (1) many of the effects are the opposite of what others have shown that stress alone causes, (2) stress causes effects not seen in these rats, and (3) these rats show effects not seen in stressed rats. Horne also cautions not to generalize these results to humans, since rats do not spend much time in relaxed wakefulness, but humans do.

Rechtschaffen (1998) comments on these hypotheses by saying that some support can also be found in the negative correlation (-0.53) between total sleep time per nychthemeron and body weight. Animals with greater body weight have more stored energy and lower cost of locomotion. They also have lower heat loss due to their greater bulk and generally better insulation. Lacking these qualities, there is greater savings in sleeping in smaller animals. Yet, the reductions in energy expenditure during sleep are only modest.

Behavioral Adaptation

One of the behavioral theories of sleep can be summed up by the phrase, "It's safer to be asleep." There are times in the twenty-four-hour day when an animal may be less safe. The danger might be from other animals attacking it when it is more vulnerable. The immobility of sleep attracts less predator attention and reduced responsiveness to the environment. Webb (1983) has termed this "**adaptive non-responding**" during times of potential danger. Adaptive non-responding is under circadian control and resembles an evolutionarily developed instinct. It may be more important in more advanced animals (Horne, 1983c).

Another threat might be from an accident when the animal is less able to perceive danger in its environment. For many animals, including human beings, nighttime is more dangerous. Our main sensory receptor—our eyes—is built to respond best during daylight. We can see at night, but not well. This fact makes us, and other animals like us, more susceptible to stumbling over a cliff or other natural dangers. For other animals, daytime is the dangerous time. During such dangerous times, it is safer to be asleep (Meddis, 1983).

Paralleling the safety function of sleep may be a function related to food availability (see Box 1 in Chapter 1). It is not effective for an animal to be active during those parts of the day when its food is not as available—maybe because its food in the form of other animals is sleeping!. From a cost/benefit basis, it is better to be asleep if it takes too much energy and poses too great a risk to be awake and active with little likelihood of securing much food (Meddis, 1975).

This adaptive non-responding hypothesis, intuitive as it is, is almost impossible to test scientifically, because it is difficult to determine degree of predatory susceptibility. Also, it has been argued that sleeping animals may be less aware of potential predators, thus at greater, not less, risk of danger by sleeping. Support for this idea comes from data that show less NREMS and REMS in some animals in the presence of predators, and some species that are more likely to be preyed upon have less REMS. Some researchers counter that the nature of the typical sleeping habitat also needs to be considered. Animals who have a safe sleeping habitat tend to sleep more than those animals that do not have a safe place to sleep. Being immobile in a safe place is clearly an advantage. Also, for all versions of this hypothesis, it is not clear why sleep with unconsciousness is necessary when waking behavioral inactivity (or dozing—see Box 1 in Chapter 1) would do the same thing.

Benefits for the Brain

Horne (1983a; 1988; 1989) contends that human sleep does much more good for the brain than the rest of the body. At the time he published this conclusion, most of the positive findings on sleep deprivation studies were limited to effects on the brain and to psychological effects. These dysfunctions have been shown to be due to more than simply "lapses" caused by "microsleeps;" rather, they are also the direct result of cognitive deficits caused by the lack of sleep (see Chapters 3 and 9). It is the brain, more than the body, that becomes dysfunctional without sleep.

However, such dysfunctions may be due as much to the disruption of the circadian rhythms that accompany sleep deprivation. Whenever a person is awake, the brain is at maximal activity levels or very near to it. Even during quiet restfulness, when alpha waves are dominating the EEG, the brain cells are still considerably active, rather like a computer whenever it is turned on—it consumes about the same amount of power whether it is running a program or simply waiting for instructions. In order for maintenance to be done, brain activity needs to be reduced. Only during SWS is this condition met. This reduction in activity applies to the forebrain but not to the brainstem. The functions of the brainstem are rigidly determined, with little possibility for adaptability or change. In contrast, the forebrain is very plastic, allowing greater flexibility in behavior and learning. Such a system requires more upkeep and maintenance.

Rechtschaffen (1998) counters that while sleep deprivation worsens performance and higher order cognitive and creative mental processes in humans (see Chapters 3 and 9), these results would seem to have little parallel in animals, leaving no reason for animal sleep.

Hobson (1988) has some notions compatible with the conclusions of Horne. He focuses on small, neurons that use norepinephrine as their neurotransmitter and have large fields of influence on other neurons. He speculates that such neurons may deplete their levels of norepinephrine during wakefulness and need to regenerate during REMS when they are relatively inactive. At the same time, other neurons that are not as highly utilized during waking are being stimulated during sleep in a stereotyped, redundant, and highly organized manner, thus insuring their daily activation. They might otherwise deteriorate from disuse given the vicissitudes of external, waking stimulation. For these neurons, REMS may function as a reliable, patterned circuit check that, additionally, may improve the functioning of the nervous system rather than just maintain it. During growth in the young organism, this same mechanism helps insure proper construction of the brain (see Chapter 13).

Krueger (c.f. Krueger & Obal, 1993; Krueger et al., 1995; Krueger et al., 1999), as a part of a larger theory that sleep is for local cellular benefit (see below), also views sleep for the maintenance of synapses that have not been recently stimulated during wakefulness. This need arises because such synapses are components of important circuits for memories.

Kavanau (c.f. 1997), based on an extensive and wide ranging review of the literature, maintains that the primary reason for sleep is to reactivate periodically brain circuits containing memories, both inherited and acquired, in order to be maintained. Without periodic stimulation the synapses that are part of these circuits chemically degrade, resulting in weakened memories. Stimulation causes growth and maintenance of the synapses, hence the memories they subsume. In the higher animals, all of which have unambiguous sleep, such reactivation of brain circuits can only be done during sleep because, while awake, the same brain cells are too preoccupied with sensory input, especially visual, and body movements are too disruptive.

In contrast, it has been pointed out that there is no known way that the unstimulated synapses can signal that they need maintenance stimulation (Bennington, 2000). Likewise, it is not known how such a process might cause an increase in sleep pressure during sleep deprivation.

(We will explore this issue more in the sections in Chapter 13 on the role of NREMS and REMS in memory consolidation.)

Box 32

Can We Learn While We Sleep?

The idea of sleep-learning has been a topic of science fiction, as well as of scientific investigation. Numerous studies have been done to determine whether or not we can learn while we are asleep (Badia, 1990; Eich, 1990; Kleitman, 1972). In one experiment, sleeping subjects were presented 10 Chinese words and their English equivalents. Later, when awake, they were tested for their memory of these word equivalents. The data showed that learning had not occurred. In another study, 21 subjects were presented with 96 sets of subjects and answers at 5-minute intervals throughout the night of sleep. The EEGs of all the subjects were monitored, and it was discovered that the percentage of items recalled during wakefulness decreased as alpha wave frequency, a sign of wakefulness (see Chapter 1) decreased. It was concluded that sleep-learning is a very weak phenomenon at best and, therefore, an impractical way to acquire any new learning.

On the other hand, sleep-learning may possibly be state dependent learning. That is, what is learned when asleep may be capable of being recalled only when again asleep. Thus, you would have to be tested during sleep to demonstrate what you have learned during previous sleep. For example, sleeping subjects were instructed to make a specific response, such as, "your nose will itch and you will scratch it," to a word (such as ITCH). Later, these words, mixed in with other new words, were spoken to the still sleeping subjects. Sometimes the suggested response occurred, but only if the suggestion was given during REMS, and only if the cue word was spoken during REMS. Appropriate responses to the cue words were still seen 5 months later in some of the subjects. None of the subjects were able to recall any of the words or the suggested responses when awake.

There has also been some evidence that more elementary kinds of learning, such as classical (Pavlovian) conditioning and habituation involving things like heart rate and eye blinks, may occur during sleep (Carskadon, 1993). Suggestions that implicit learning, that is, learning without awareness, may take place during sleep have not been verified.

The data from studies on sleep-learning have been disappointing to those who expected useful, easy, and efficient learning during sleep. (Sorry about that.) Most authorities in the Western world do not believe new learning of any significance occurs while sleeping that transfers to the waking state. Neither explicit nor implicit learning have been shown to occur during sleep and be manifested during wakefulness when adequate measures have been taken not to present the to-be-learned material when alpha waves are present. In contrast, Russian researchers conclude that sleep-learning is a hardy, viable, and useful phenomenon. However, their conclusions are based on highly trained subjects but include no direct measurement of sleep. In fact, the information-to-be-learned was presented early and late in the sleep period when a lot of wake was likely to be occurring.

In addition to being almost effortless, the reason sleep-learning seems so appealing to so many students is the implicit assumption that nothing of value or use occurs during sleep, thus the unoccupied brain is available for learning. As apparent throughout this book, this assumption is unfounded.

Local Cell Benefits[51]

Another hypothesis holds that the primary reason for sleep is to benefit local groups of cells rather than benefit the entire organism or even individual organs. Moruzzi (1966) suggested that sleep is for the slow recovery and stabilization of synapses involved in plastic activities of learning, memory, and consciousness.

A related notion is that sleep strengthens and preserves synapses underused during waking so that they do not weaken so much as to be unavailable when needed in the future (Kreuger et al., 1995). Either way, sleep begins when groups of cells that have been active release chemicals, such as cytokines and nerve growth factors (see Chapter 4), that initiate several parallel, cascading biochemical processes that help strengthen the active synapses. The result is maintenance of individual synapses, but also the integration of new synaptic patterns initiated by new experiences. These integrated patterns result in greater flexibility in behavior but within a contextual framework.

Kavanau (c.f. 1997) has speculated that use-dependent synapses are stabilized during sleep, free of sensory input interference. The substances released from active synapses also cause the circuits to alter their firing patterns. When enough local circuits are in this altered state, sleepiness occurs. As more local circuits enter this state, sleep ensues. Thus, sleep is neuron use dependent, not wake dependent.

According to Kreuger, whole brain sleep onset and duration is coordinated and organized by specific brain areas, such as the basal forebrain area, thalamus, and pons (see Chapter 4). These special areas are influenced by local circuits that have entered the functional mode of sleep as well as by the suprachiasmatic nucleus for circadian rhythm control, thermoregulatory centers of the brain, and sensory input from the body (see Chapter 5). Numerous experiments have shown that destruction of these areas results in the absence of sleep that is only temporary, although the subsequent sleep may not be as well organized. These studies show that it is not these areas that actually initiate sleep but only play a role in organizing it. The difference between NREMS and REMS is the level of the coordinating brain areas. For REMS, these areas are in the brainstem, while for NREMS, these areas are in the forebrain.

Evidence that sleep occurs at a local level includes:

- Sleep patterns of electrical activity can be shown to occur in local groups of cells;
- Local cellular events combining to produce a coordinated output have been shown to occur elsewhere in the brain. For example, in the SCN, individual cells have their individual circadian firing patterns that coordinate to result in the circadian rhythms of the entire animal;
- Adenosine may build up in local areas because of activity in that area. The adenosine, in turn, causes a local slowing of EEG potentials;
- There is no area of the brain that when destroyed permanently eliminates NREMS
- Unihemispheric sleep in some aquatic mammals and in many birds (see Chapter 1) shows sleep is not a whole brain phenomenon;
- There are anterior–posterior and right–left differences in EEG power during sleep;
- As sleep progresses through the night, there are different changes in the EEG in different regions of the cortex;

- Extensive use of an area of the brain during waking due to sensory or cognitive activity results in greater intensity of activity in that area during sleep;
- There are regional differences in brain electrical activity during sleep following sleep deprivation. Such differences are not seen during waking;
- There is evidence that the transition from wake to sleep may not occur in all parts of the brain simultaneously;
- Research by Pigarev (c.f. Pigarev et al., 1996) shows that parts of the cortex may be asleep, while other parts are awake and vice-versa for 20 to 30 minutes;
- The symptoms of several sleep disorders, such as narcolopsy and RBD, are consistent with the idea that parts of the brain can be asleep, while other parts are awake. Also, lucid dreaming and the effects of sleep deprivation suggest the same thing.

Thus sleep, for Kreuger, is for synaptic efficacy and organization, which is dynamic and use dependent. The result is important changes in input–output dynamics that benefit the entire organism. This putative function requires loss of consciousness that many other posited functions of sleep cannot explain. The loss of consciousness is both a necessary condition for and a consequence of these local processes.

On the other hand, Rechtschaffen (1998) asks what processes in the brain identify such synapses, how such efforts are directed toward them, and why this has to be done during sleep rather than waking. Further, he points out that there is no direct evidence that sleep or lack of it has an effect on synapses, especially the weak ones.

Emotional Benefits

Sleep deprivation increases negative mood and decreases positive mood (see Chapter 9), strongly suggesting that a function of sleep is mood regulation. Sleep generally elevates mood. (We will explore this concept further in Chapter 13.)

A number of studies show that morning mood following nighttime sleep in non-depressed people is affected by the amount and quality of the prior sleep (Cartwright et al., 1998). Sleep of sufficient length and quality improves morning mood. When deprived of sleep for one night, morning mood scores are significantly lower.

It has also been shown that circadian phase interacts with amount of prior wake to influence mood, but the interaction is not simple (Boivin et al., 1997). Depending on circadian phase, mood elevates, deteriorates, or remains the same with increasing duration of waking. This interaction is complex and non-additive such that a slight change in timing of the sleep–wake cycle can have notable effects on mood.

THE FUNCTIONS OF INDIVIDUAL SLEEP STAGES

Some of the functions of sleep are best explored by considering each stage of sleep rather than sleep as a whole. Some of the putative functions are derived from the nature of each of the stages, and other functions are suggested by selective sleep deprivation studies. Although rarely occurring in the real world, stages of sleep have been selectively deprived in the sleep laboratory and the resulting changes in physiology or behavior used to infer functions of the deprived stage.

NREMS[52]

We will start examining the functions of NREMS. The functions of REMS are in Chapter 13. First, let us review some of the characteristics of NREMS that have implications for its functions:

- General slowing of the body and brain activity and functions;
- Decreased body temperature;
- Changes in the levels of release of some hormones;
- Burst-pause firing pattern in several major brain areas;
- Certain areas of the brain actively produce NREMS
- Decrease in the turnover of acylcholine; norepinephrine, and serotonin;
- An increase of many types of pathogens in the body cause NREMS to increase;
- Selective deprivation causes more attempts to enter it NREMS and NREMS rebound occurs when uninterrupted sleep is resumed;
- Awakening from NREMS results in sleep inertia.

Overall, there have been relatively few studies of selective NREMS deprivation, so most of the hypotheses about its functions are derived from its characteristics. They are divided into hypotheses about restoration, conservation, and preparation for REMS.

Restoration

As indicated in the discussion about sleep in general, a very old and prevailing notion is that sleep provides some kind of rest and restoration. This process is most often thought to occur during NREMS.

NREMS benefits the body. NREMS functions to restore or recover some aspects of bodily functions worn down during wakefulness. This homeostatic notion is old and very prevalent (see above). Many lines of evidence are marshaled in support of this hypothesis, but not always without qualifiers or alternate explanations.

- The longer you are awake, the more intense your subsequent SWS. Conversely, SWS intensity decreases exponentially with the length of sleep (see Chapter 1). An explanation is that the longer you are awake, the greater the wearing down of the body and/or using up of vital resources which can only be built back up during SWS. However, this explanation is weak, because the relationship between the length of being awake and subsequent SWS is not found in all animals.

- During NREMS, there is a decrease of catabolic hormones and an increase of anabolic hormones in the body (Chapter 5). The anabolic hormones tend to build up and restore the body while the catabolic hormones tend to wear the body out.
- Growth hormone is present only during the first SWS period of the night in adult humans. It is even more prevalent during SWS in children. However, it has been pointed out that growth hormone may not always do what its name implies (Horne, 1988), and the relationship between SWS and growth hormone has not been found in most other mammals.
- Sleep deprivation, or deprivation of SWS, results in a rebound during subsequent undisturbed sleep (Chapter 3), showing that the body has a need for SWS and will make an effort to obtain it even if the opportunity is delayed, which implies SWS has an homeostatic function.
- Likewise, if deprived of SWS early in the night, there will be more of it later in the night.
- There is a high amount of SWS in children, with slow declines during adulthood and much less or no SWS at all in retirees (Chapter 1). This decline parallels that of metabolic rate in humans. In other species with no decline in SWS with advancing age, there is no decline in metabolic rate.
- However, the increase of SWS following exercise sometimes reported in the past research is no longer viewed as supportive evidence, because these effects are mediated by the resulting increase in body temperature (Carskadon, 1993).
- There are increases in the capability of the immune system that occur during NREMS (Chapter 5). Further, many illnesses cause enhanced sleepiness, and the resulting extra sleep has been shown to be beneficial to the recovery from illness (Chapter 5).

SWS primarily benefits the brain.   Other hypotheses focus on the brain rather than the body as the beneficiary of SWS. Slowing down of brain activity allows repairs. Horne (1988) points out that in larger, more advanced animals, the body does not need a special period of rest, because it gets enough from quiet wakefulness. Smaller animals spend most of their waking active and may need sleep to get rest. However, this does not apply to the cerebrum, which is constantly active during wakefulness; it may need sleep to rest and rejuvenate. Horne also points out that extra brain stimulation during waking increases SWS but has no effect on REMS. Even in animal experiments that show increased REMS following learning something new during the day (see Chapter 13), there is also an increase in NREMS and total sleep time.

Cerebral metabolic rate is high during infancy and childhood when SWS is also high (Horne, 1988; Wauguier, Dugovic, & Radulovacki, 1989) and there is more brain organization and information processing occurring. Horne (1992) seems to argue that SWS in humans is most important for the functioning of the prefrontal part of the cortex, since sleep deprivation results in reversible deficits in functions typically associated with this area of the brain. Also, people with psychological disorders known to involve the frontal cortex have less SWS. In short, SWS is a kind of off-line maintenance for the brain.

There is some evidence that NREMS is important for memory. McNaughton's research (c.f. Wilson & McNaughton, 1994) showed that hippocampus cells that are active during a new experience when awake are also active during subsequent NREMS. However, this activity could merely be a carryover of activity from waking. To this point, there is only a little evidence that such reactivation has any subsequent consequences.

Born's group (e.g. Plihal & Born, 1999) has reported that sleep early in the night, that is dominated by NREMS, is important for declarative memory—such as paired associate learning or mental spatial rotation—but not for procedural memory. Other research results suggest that just the SWS component of NREMS is important for declarative memory. Human SWS may also be involved with human non-declarative tasks, but it is not clear if it is exclusive to SWS. Details of brain mechanisms that underlie memory consolidation in SWS are reviewed by Sejnowski & Destexhe (2000).

Other studies have shown that NREMS, like REMS, may increase after positive reinforcement conditioning (Peigneux et al., 2001). For example, rats that failed a two-way avoidance learning task showed improvement on day 2 in proportion to the duration of their NREMS episodes. In humans, it has been observed that intense maze learning and learning a virtual environment both increased sleep spindles and time in stage 2 during subsequent sleep.

Conservation

Earlier the hypothesis that all sleep has a conservation function was discussed. Some researchers maintain that only NREMS or only SWS serves that function, not all of sleep. Specifically they posit that NREMS functions to conserve energy by reducing metabolic rate, energy expenditure, and temperature.

In support of metabolic conservation, they cite as supporting evidence the fact that several studies in humans and other mammals show a high correlation between metabolic rate and amount of NREMS suggesting that as metabolism increases, so does the need to conserve. However, critics say that these data are confounded by equally high correlations of these factors with body size and feeding habits. In altricial species, i.e., those born relatively immature, the development of metabolic rate and SWS parallel each other. Also, some animals increase SWS during times of fasting caused by the reduced availability of food.

A temperature regulation function of NREMS is supported by the fact that:

- NREMS is a time of regulated, controlled, active cooling of the body (Chapter 5) by a decrease in heat production coupled by changes in mechanisms that allow increased loss of body heat. This process is in contrast to REM, which is a time of uncontrolled body temperature regulation (see Chapter 5).

- One theory sees the development of NREMS occurring during evolution about the time that warm-blooded animals evolved (see Box 1 in Chapter 1). This development is not viewed as a coincidence, but rather a necessity to prevent negative effects resulting from being too warm for too long.

- It has been argued that SWS is the first stage on a continuum toward hibernation (Box 1 in Chapter 1). While hibernation conserves maximal amounts of energy by maintaining minimal metabolic levels, SWS does so, too, only to a lesser extent.

- The recent work of Rechtschaffen and colleagues at the University of Chicago shows the major effects of prolonged sleep deprivation in rats (see Box 31), which is eventually lethal, to be a disruption of energy metabolism and temperature regulation. However, these conclusions are for all of sleep, not just for NREM.

- Heating the body just a degree or two increases the amount of subsequent SWS (see Chapter 5). It is as if the body is using the cooling that accompanies SWS to balance off the increased heating of the body when awake, in an effort to maintain a constant daily average body temperature.

- Heating the basal forebrain area, which includes portions of the nearby anterior hypothalamus, increases SWS. This mechanism may regulate average daily body temperature just mentioned above.

- During free-running conditions (see Chapter 2), SWS occurs during the peak of the circadian body temperature rhythm.

- Extended sleep of 12 hours or more often includes the return of some SWS, when circadian body temperature is again on the rise.

- To be sure, some of the decrease in body temperature during NREMS is due to its typical co-occurrence with the low of the circadian body temperature rhythm and to the typical recumbent, reduced activity position typically assumed during sleep. However, a significant part of the decrease is due to NREMS sleep itself and occurs whenever NREMS sleep happens.

Other

See also the discussion of how NREMS is thought to prepare for REMS presented in the Chapter 13.

Slow waves indicate that the brain is not processing informational input that is complex (Meddis, 1975). Also, it is most difficult to awaken humans or animals from SWS and elicit behavioral responses. SWS is a time of enforced behavioral inactivity.

Stage 2

Little attention has been paid to attributing function to stage 2 sleep (called "light quiet sleep" in cats and some primates (see Box 1 in Chapter 1), probably because it is harder to manipulate (see Chapter 3). However, Meddis (1975) has speculated, more than concluded from data, about the functions of this stage of sleep.

Light quiet sleep, or stage 2, is seen only in cats and primates, thus it is most likely of more recent evolutionary development. In cats, it is similar to SWS except for less amplitude of the slow waves. This fact accounts for the lower behavioral thresholds of light quiet sleep. In primates, K-complexes are a kind of isolated slow wave with a characteristic shape. Spindles and K-complexes have been observed to occur in response to stimuli and might serve to jam out stimuli not important enough to need to attend to or to cause arousal (see Chapter 2).

If these things are true, then it follows that stage 2 sleep is a more advanced way of maintaining the behavioral quiescence of SWS while simultaneously sustaining a higher level of selective vigilance. Indeed, those primates who are more vulnerable while asleep have more light quiet sleep, which would keep them more vigilant.

Chapter 13 continues where this chapter leaves off. It will focus on the functions of REMS and dreaming.

Box 33

Core and Optional Sleep

Jim Horne, psychologist and long time sleep researcher of Loughbrough University in England, has a novel and interesting notion of sleep (Horne 1983b; 1983c; 1988). He posits that sleep is of two functional types that he calls core sleep and optional sleep.

Core sleep is necessary to obtain first. It consists mainly of restorative, homeostatic, and other internal benefits, especially those involving brain mechanisms. Core sleep contains a high proportion of SWS but also some other NREMS stages and a bit of REMS. The need for this kind of sleep builds with wakefulness especially waking brain effort. It is a "deeper sleep" necessary for normal functioning.

Optional sleep is secondary to core sleep and more flexible. It can be extended or reduced in accordance with environmental demands. It is more for safety, energy conservation, and efficiency kinds of functions. It can also function as relief from boredom but may accommodate brain restitution if necessary. Optional sleep contains a high proportion of REMS. It is on a circadian schedule but may also be governed by "behavioral drive." It may vary with the seasons to act as a time occupier when the environment is less habitable.

These two kinds of sleep have different proportions in different animals—especially animals that occupy different branches of the phylogenetic tree. Core sleep is more important for animals higher up in the phylogenetic tree, with their more advanced brains. Although these higher animals can and do engage in relaxed wakefulness, relaxed wakefulness can only relax the muscles. It cannot "relax" the brain; only sleep can. Optional sleep is more important in smaller, less advanced insectivores and rodents, that is, animals that tend to have high levels of activity when awake, in order to conserve energy. For them and others, a safety function may also be an important aspect of optional sleep. Other factors that determine the relative proportions of core and optional sleep include immaturity, safe sleeping habitat, and body size. For example, vulnerable animals have less NREMS (Meddis, 1983).

According to this theory, both core and optional mechanisms are operating at sleep onset in all animals. However, core sleep starts with greater strength early in the sleep period but then declines, leaving primarily optional sleep later in the sleep period. The rate of decline of core sleep varies between animals. Figure 40 summarizes the factors affecting core and optional sleep in different kinds of animals.

Human core sleep appears to be about three NREM/REM sleep cycles (about 6 hours) but with a lot of individual variation (Benoit, 1985). It is the minimum necessary sleep in adults, but children need more. The optional component can be varied by 1–2 hours per nychthemeron via napping or lengthening the main sleep period (Horne, 1983c). According to this theory, human optional sleep probably originally developed to provide a time of safety, yet was flexible enough to enable humans to accommodate their daily sleep/wake schedule to the seasonal changing durations of daily light at the more extreme latitudes.

Others agree with Horne that there are these two kinds of sleep but do not agree that optional sleep is as optional as its name implies (Benoit, 1985; Stampi, Moffitt, & Hoffman, 1990). To some, optional sleep may more properly be described as "necessary but flexible" (Benoit, 1985, p. 438). That is, it can be foregone for a while, but eventually it needs to be recovered. Other optional sleep may be a way of occupying time that is unproductive and does need not to be recovered if missed, but may help us feel our absolute best. Or, perhaps, we can do without optional sleep in the short run, but not in the long run (Stampi, Moffitt, & Hoffman, 1990).

In contrast to absolute differences between core and optional sleep, Bonnet and Arand (1995) posit a more gradual logarithmic change of the benefits of sleep with large benefits occurring in early sleep but increasingly small benefits as the sleep period goes on.

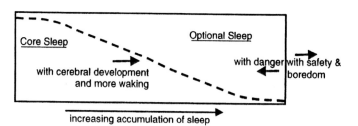

Figure 40. The relationship of core to optional sleep and some factors that effect the amount to optional sleep. (Based on Horne, 1983c.)

There are several lines of criticism that have been leveled against the core/optional theory.

(1) Dement and others cite MSLT and other data showing the level of and problems with chronic sleep deprivation in the Western world. Six hours is just not enough sleep for most people. Chronic sleep deprivation leads to many negative effects (see Chapters 3 and 9).

(2) Experiments show that people who, for a couple of nights, get more, not fewer, hours of sleep than they typically get show a brief sleep inertia upon awakening but increased alertness, better psychomotor performance, and improved mood during the rest of the day (Carskadon, 1993).

Functions of REMS and Dreaming[53]

This chapter continues where Chapter 12 left off. It will focus on the functions of REMS and dreaming.

THE FUNCTIONS OF INDIVIDUAL SLEEP STAGES (CONTINUED)

REMS

REMS characteristics that may imply functions:

- Rapid eye movements
- Additional phasic as well as tonic events
- Usually follows NREMS
- Deprivation of REMS causes "REM pressure" and REMS rebound
- Motor output is inhibited
- Some parts of the brain are the most active during REMS more than any other state but a few less active
- REM-on and REM-off areas of the brain
- Brainwaves indicate cortical arousal
- Theta waves are prevalent in the hippocampus
- High use of acetylcholine but low use of norepinephrine and serotonin in the brain
- Brain temperature is increased
- Heart rate, blood pressure, and respiration are irregular
- Penile erections and vaginal engorgement
- Lack of body temperature regulation

Parts of this chapter was adapted from Moorcroft, 1993 with permission of the publisher.

- Rich and copious dreaming
- Lack of reflective thought
- Percent of REMS varies greatly between species, yet there are generally higher amounts of REMS in altricial species early development and in adulthood. Animals with a safe sleeping site typically have more REMS, and smaller animals typically have more REMS.
- Unlike NREMS, REMS appears to be dispensable; vulnerable animals have less, there is only limited rebound of lost REMS, and people on certain drugs, get along quite well without it.

There has been more research and speculative focus on REMS than on the other sleep states, probably because of its paradoxical nature (see Chapter 1). An early idea was that REMS was needed to prevent hallucinations and mental illness. However, this notion was soon refuted. In fact, REMS deprivation can even help some people with severe depression. Unlike NREMS, which is proportional to prior wakefulness, REMS seems related to the circadian temperature rhythm; the propensity for REMS increases when body temperature is at its nadir but shows the least likelihood when body temperature is at its acrophase and for a few hours thereafter (Borbély, 1986).

Box 34

REMS is a Syndrome, not a State

We treat REMS as if it is a single, unified entity. It is certainly easier to do it that way, and, for the most part, it makes little difference that we do this. However, in reality, REMS may be more complex and be not so much a unified state as a convenient assemblage of components (McCarley & Massaquoi, 1992a) that need to be recruited in a specific order (Hobson et al., 1986). Not only is this concept shown by the fact that various and separable brain systems are involved but also because various components of REMS occur before the onset of full-blown REMS. For example, the neck muscle potential may decrease several seconds or more before the onset of other polysomnographic signs of REMS, and there is a decrease of sweating 2–3 minutes prior to polysomnographic onset of REMS, indicating turning off this thermoregulatory mechanism. Several of the components of REMS can be dissociated using experimental techniques in the lab (Morrison & Reiner, 1986; Siegel, 1989). For example, REM without muscle paralysis can be produced by brain damage in the brainstem near the locus coeruleus, and muscle paralysis without REM can be produced by extra acetylcholine in these same brain areas. Additionally, a drug called reserpine can cause PGO waves to occur during waking. In reality, REMS is the coordinated concurrence of several phenomena rather than a unified state.

Yet, this explanation cannot entirely account for REMS. Rebound of this stage occurs following deprivation, suggesting that it is too important to be missed. Something is both necessary and uniquely, or at least most easily, obtained by this stage of sleep, yet there is no severe psychological deterioration if it is missed.

Cohen (1980) has emphasized that some of the functions of REMS seem to be preparatory, while others are adaptive. That is, some functions anticipate future needs and insure that the organism is ready, while others respond to what the organism has experienced and attempt better or more efficiently to utilize that experience. The preparatory functions he includes are the stimulation of the brain for proper growth, the repair and maintenance of the brain, and the exercising of brain circuits for genetically based behaviors. These functions help insure that the brain is ready to respond appropriately in the future when called upon. The adaptive functions include memory work on new learning, modulation of emotions, and the psychological benefits of dreams.

REMS as Preparatory

Growth and Restoration.   REMS seems to facilitate brain development (c.f. Turek & Zee, 1999; Shaffery et al., 2002). It is widely recognized from studies of sensory systems, especially vision, that stimulation of the growing brain is necessary for normal synaptic connections to be made between cells. In fact, the immature brain has too many neurons and synapses. Only those that are shown to be functionally useful through use are maintained. But, external stimulation may not be enough. Or, it may be too random and irregular. Or, it may not be handled well enough by the immature nervous system to insure appropriate connections with other brain areas (Chase, 1986). An internal source of stimulation that is more controlled and more predictable is necessary to stimulate the growing nerve tissue appropriately and speed its structural growth and physiological maturation. It is proposed that REMS provides this stimulation. High REMS early in life causes auto-stimulation necessary to facilitate useful synaptic connections. REMS later in life is needed to maintain synaptic connections. In this way, REMS is additive and complimentary to sensory input during waking.

Experimental evidence supports this hypothesis. Research shows that when REMS is artificially curtailed during infancy in animals, as adults they manifest anatomical brain abnormalities, behavioral abnormalities, and abnormalities in REMS. Additional research shows that by using drugs to deprive rat pups of REMS during critical weeks of brain growth, both permanent changes in brain structure and adult behavior result—especially differences in emotional, sensory, and sleep functions (Corner et al., 1987; Mirmiram, 1986). REMS deprivation in kittens worsens adult visual deficits produced by abnormal early sensory input (Oskenberg, 1987). Also, if PGO spikes are surgically suppressed in kittens, functioning of the visual areas of the nervous system develops abnormally (Davenne & Adrien, 1987).

However, it is possible that the high amount of REMS in immature animals occurs simply because the brainstem, where REMS sleep is controlled, matures before the forebrain, where NREMS is controlled (Nicolau et al., 2000). That is, the immature animal is simply not capable of producing NREMS until the forebrain matures.

Typically, REMS decreases in the adult from what it had been during development but it does not disappear (see Chapter 1). While it no longer facilitates brain growth and development, it may be necessary in brain maintenance. It is a predictable source of internal stimulation that maintains and self-corrects the functional pathways of interaction between brain cells. Supportive observations (Oswald, 1980) include the decrease in REMS during senility, less REMS in mentally retarded individuals, an increase in REMS following brain poisoning (presumably while the brain is trying to repair the damage), and a decline in REMS in elderly persons with organic brain dysfunction (Kryger, Roth, & Dement, 1989). Other researchers have shown that the decrease in the amount of REMS sleep is correlated with the decline in the level of cognitive ability in the elderly but not in young people (Prinz, 1980).

Levels of some neurotransmitters, especially catecholamines, may be replenished during REMS (Turek & Zee, 1999). Likewise, activity in the locus coerulus is much curtailed during REMS, giving it a chance to upregulate its catecholamine receptors. There may be a similar effect in other parts of the brain involving other norephinephrine, dopamine, and serotonin receptors. REMS deprivation causes a large reduction of the amplitude of inhibition in the brainstem caused by noradrenalin. However, while deprivation of REMS for 1 to 3 days lowers the levels of norepinephrine in the brain, chronic sleep deprivation does not have much effect on these receptors (Turek & Zee, 1999).

Maintenance.   REMS has been hypothesized to contribute to the maintenance of inherited behaviors, brain circuits for innate behaviors, and the brain's internal reward system.

I. Maintenance of Inherited Behaviors. REMS may contribute to the maintenance of inherited behaviors (Jouvet, 1998). Lower animals without REMS, or very little of it, do not need to have their inherited behaviors (behaviors involved with feeding, fighting, fleeing, and fornicating) refreshed, because they are using them frequently when awake. Higher animals, however, that rely on learning only irregularly use their inherited behaviors. Without regular use, the neural networks underlying inherited behaviors may weaken and eventually not be ready when needed. REMS allows these networks to be regularly stimulated and therefore maintained and ready for use.

Evidence for this idea comes from cats with lesions in a specific part of the brainstem, resulting in no inhibition of the muscles of movement during REMS. These animals do not show a random cross section of possible behaviors but seem to be acting out certain kinds of genetically programmed behaviors that occur during emotional states. It is as if they are tuning up their fight/flight response (Horne, 2000).

II. Orienting Response. Adrian Morrison (Horne, 1988; Morrison & Reiner, 1985; Morrison, Ball, Sanford, Mann, & Ross, 1990) has compared the features of REMS to the components of the orienting response found in awake animals. The orienting response is the name for behavioral and physiological responses made by an animal when alerted by unexpected or novel stimuli. During the orienting response, the animal freezes for a few moments in a state of heightened alertness. The muscle inhibition of REMS may be similar to freezing of muscle activity during orientation, and the low voltage fast brain activity with PGO spikes and hippocampal theta rhythm of REMS may correspond to the heightened brain alertness of the orienting response. Additionally, the low activity in the sympathetic nervous systems and the suppression of homeostatic responses, such as the restriction of body temperature regulation, that occur during REMS seem also to be components of the orienting response. Consistent with this comparison between REMS and the orienting response is the observation that awakening out of REMS, compared to awakening from NREMS, results in higher levels of arousal for 30 or more minutes (Lavie, 1989). The major difference between REMS and the orienting response is the sustained duration of the former compared to the transient nature of the latter. Perhaps REMS is a substitute for wake by maintaining brain activation while also maintaining sleep.

III. Erections of the Penis and Wet Dreams. On a related note, REMS erections and wet dreams may be an outward manifestation of brain circuit checks for innate behaviors. The only other functional speculation for these phenomena appeared in a paper about the memory effects of REMS, by Crick and Mitchison (1986) that mentioned erections in a section entitled "Side Effects of REMS." They first point out that erections are not a result of the erotic content of dreams and then continue with: "There seems no obvious reason why erections should not also be inhibited in sleep. One may wonder whether this phenomenon might have selective advantage in evolution. It would not, after all, be too surprising if this particular state of male readiness for sexual intercourse contributed to the number of offspring fathered. However, this assumes that the female of the species will be in easy proximity to the male during or shortly after sleep. One wonders, therefore, if REMS penile erection has been observed in animals such as tigers, which are solitary except for brief periods of sexual intercourse, as opposed to lions, which constantly sleep in close proximity to each other" (p. 245).

Another novel idea for penile erections during REMS came from an undergraduate essay. Perhaps, it said, they are the antenna for psychic dreams.

IV. Reward System. REMS has also been hypothesized to activate periodically the brain's internal reward system to keep it active (Ellman & Weinstein,

1991). The high amount of REMS in immature mammals is thought to keep this system in a state of readiness in the face of insufficient external stimulation.

Sentinel Function.   REMS has also been hypothesized to prepare the brain for awakening, the so-called Sentinel Function (Snyder, 1966). There is greater sensory awareness of the external environment during REMS than during NREMS, and the brain can decide if external stimuli are familiar or unfamiliar, safe or threatening. Brain electrical responses to sensory stimuli during REMS are more like those of waking than they are during NREMS. Animals arouse more quickly and more completely from REMS than from NREMS and are more ready to cope with danger (Horne, 2000). REMS increases toward the end of the night as waking approaches, which could prepare the brain for awakening but could also be an effort of the brain to counteract the propensity to wake (Horne, 2000). Countering this notion is the fact that rats sleeping near cats have less REMS, not more. Also there is a negative correlation (-0.69) between the amount of REMS independent of total sleep time and exposure to danger (Horne, 2000). Additionally, the sentinel hypothesis does not address why there is the muscle paralysis of REMS.

REMS as Adaptive

Brain Temperature.   REMS functions to keep the brain warm during sleep, while much of the rest of the body cools (Wehr, 1992). Correlational data suggest a relationship of REMS with altriciality and endothermy. REMS is found in all endothermic mammals, but it is not clear that it is present in reptiles and lower animals that are ectothermic. Brain temperature does increase during REMS, and there is some increase in REMS in cool conditions. However, there are data that are inconsistent with this idea, such as cats having less REMS at lower room temperatures without subsequent REMS rebound (Horne, 2000). Also, this notion does not explain the muscle paralysis seen during REMS (Horne, 2000).

Drives.   REMS has been postulated to modulate the expression of drives. This modulation allows the waking animal more flexibility and adaptability in its waking drive gratification. Evidence comes from studies that show REMS deprived rats show more elevated drive behaviors. But these experiments involved stimulated or extreme responses and therefore may be limited to extremes. Casual observation of human behavior suggests REMS deprivation disinhibits aggressive, sexual, or eating behaviors.

Memory.   REMS may play an important role in memory (Maquet, 2001; Peigneus et al., 2001; Siegel, 2001; Stickgold et al., 2001). Sleep may be necessary for consolidation of memories, because it is permissive to brain plasticity. Consolidation is the well-accepted concept in psychology of a process that converts temporary working memory into more permanent long-term memory. In the process, it also helps the animal adapt its behavioral responses to recent environmental experiences. Kavanau (2001) holds this occurrence can only happen during REMS, when the brain is free from competitive use of the brain areas needed for consolidation.

The high rate of protein synthesis during REMS is consistent with maintenance of neural circuitry for memories. Also, the flow of information between the neocortex and hippocampus reverses during REMS, such that information is now going from the neocortex to the hippocampus (Stickgold, personal communication, June, 2001).

There are three lines of research that have been utilized to see if REMS plays an important role in consolidation of memories: (1) learning something new increases subsequent REMS, (2) memory consolidation is diminished by REMS deprivation, and (3) replays of recently learned information occur during REMS. We will explore each of these in turn.

I. REMS increases after learning. If REMS is important for consolidating newly learned material into long-term memory, then it is reasonable to expect an increase in some aspect of REMS following a significant amount of new learning. An example of this type of research was done by Smith & Lapp (1991). For this experiment, several honors psychology majors had their sleep monitored a few days after final exams, as well as during the summer before and the summer after. They were not sleep deprived at the time. Their sleep was compared to a similar group of students who did not have final exams and were working at the time. The sleep following exams showed more rems and a higher density of rems. Sleep at other times was similar to that of students not taking exams, was similar, with a lower level of rems and rem density.

Many other experiments in both humans and laboratory animals have verified increases in some aspect of REMS after learning something new. These changes may be in the overall amount of REMS, duration of REMS, number of REMS periods, rem density, or number of rems. Such changes occur more often for implicit learning of performance tasks, such as learning to adapt to glasses that invert the visual field and learning to use a trampoline, but also for other types of tasks such as learning Morse code, foreign language learning, learning a computer program language, studying a textbook passage, and conditioning in 6-month-old children. However, there are some reports of negative results.

In general, there have been positive results in animal studies for sufficiently learned complex tasks, but not for simple tasks. Furthermore, an increase in REMS at a critical stage of the learning predicts better memory. The amount of REMS returns to normal once the task has been mastered. For example, in an experiment in which learning was distributed over a number of sessions the learning peak was reached just after the greatest increase in REMS. If a subsequent modification to the task was introduced, there was another increase in REMS about the time it was learned (Peigneus et al., 2001).

A difficulty with these kinds of studies is the assumption that the only thing the subject is learning is the imposed new task. It is as if the mind of the subject is otherwise blank and idle, which much evidence suggests it is not. Another problem is that more is going on when the subject is learning a new task than simply the learning. Usually there is some kind of stress involved, whether it is from a negative reinforcer, such as mild but unpleasant electric shock in the animal studies, or uncertainty about receiving a positive reinforcer—such as an animal being rewarded by food with correct responses, or a person trying not to look like a fool when learning something new. Studies have show that stress alone can sometimes increase REMS. However, controls undergoing much the same procedure have shown no significant REMS increase when the task was not learned or when there was nothing new to learn. Another criticism is that species that need to learn a lot of things in order to survive do not necessarily have the most REMS.

It may be discovered in the future that the measures that have been looked at so far, such as changes in the absolute or relative duration of REMS, the number of REMS periods, and the number or density of REMS may be too crude really to determine the role of REMS in consolidation of memories. Other, more refined measurements, may reveal more in the future.

II. Memory consolidation diminished by REMS deprivation. If REMS is necessary for consolidation of recently learned tasks, then blocking REMS after new learning should interfere with the memory for that task.

An example of this kind of research was done by biopsychologist Carlyle Smith of Trent University of Peterborough, Ontario, Canada, who developed the concept of REM windows (cf. Smith, 1996). A REM window is a period of time during the several days following complex cognitive learning when the occurrence of REMS is crucial for the maximal retention of learning.

For example, rats were to learn to swim to a platform they could stand on that was submerged and not visible just below the surface of a large tank of cloudy water (this equipment is known as the Morris water maze). The animals deprived of 4 hours of REMS after a 4-hour delay following the end of the training session showed memory deficits for the task the next day. The memory deficit did not occur if the 4 hours of REMS sleep deprivation occurred either immediately following the end of training or begun after an 8-hour delay. The results were interpreted as consolidation of memory which this task took place only during the second 4 hours of REMS, i.e. the "REM Window," following the learning experience (Smith & Rose, 1996).

Other experiments have shown REM windows for other tasks in both animals and humans, but the timing of the window varies with the task and other influences. Also, Smith has shown that during critical REM windows, manipulations of brain chemistry interfere with retention. Similar manipulations of brain chemistry at other times during sleep have no such effect.

As in the REMS increase studies, in animals, simple tasks with relatively few things to learn were not much affected by REMS deprivation including passive avoidance, one-way active avoidance, and simple mazes. However, more complex tasks were affected such as shuttle box, discrimination learning, probabilistic learning, complex mazes, instrumental conditioning, and spatial reference memory. In these tasks, greater behavioral adaptation and change is needed, thus there is more to consolidate. Similar research in humans has shown that sleep late in the sleep period (when more REMS occurs) improved procedural memory but not declarative memory (Born & Fehm, 1998).

Many human studies do not clearly show that REMS apart from NREMS is responsible for memory. In some cases, it looks like NREMS followed by REMS is necessary for consolidation (see below). Additionally, there are discrepant results. Yet, a lot of evidence does show that REMS deprivation, but not NREMS deprivation, interferes with the recall of sentences, prose passages, short stories, and lists of words in categories.

Other evidence shows that emotional material is recalled better after REMS, but NREMS is without effect. For example, Cartwright (1974) gave subjects crossword puzzles, word-associations, and story completions to do. They ranged from neutral to emotional. Half of the subjects then stayed awake, and the other half had REMS between the time they started working on the problems and when they finished them. The more emotional the problem, the more REMS influenced performance. REMS, but not wake, changed the way the subjects saw the emotional problems.

Criticisms of this category of research include the fact that in many of these experiments the REMS window is defined by looking at the data after the experiment is done and that the location of the window changes with changes in the task or even the strain of the rat used. That is, there is little predictive value in the concept of the REMS window. It also has been pointed out that REMS deprivation involves considerable stress and other effects that could interfere with post-deprivation testing. Support for this criticism comes from an experiment that deprived rats of REMS by gently rocking them. No learning deficit resulted, but when more stressful deprivation procedures were used, a learning deficit was noted. Yet, other studies have shown performance decrements 20 hours after REMS deprivation that were not seen during intervening times when the effects of stress should be stronger.

Additional criticism is that the deprivation procedure can disrupt circadian rhythms. Thus, any effect observed on memory of the task cannot simply be attributed to the disruption of consolidation by REMS deprivation. Also, it has been pointed out that there are no clinical signs of memory problems in people who have taken drugs for years with the side effect of severely reducing if not eliminating REMS.

REMS deprivation seems to disrupt newly learned implicit memory tasks (procedural tasks) or those described as "ego threatening" but not intentional tasks such as verbal learning or paired associated learning. It has been pointed out that if this is so, then REMS has little to do with what is unique about human intellect. However, other studies show a role for REMS in language learning.

III. Memory replay during REMS. Part of the process of memory consolidation could involve the replay in the brain of recently learned information. An example of this research involved recording the activity of hippocampal cells during sleep in rats by McNauton's group following experiencing something new during the prior waking period. In one experiment (Poe et al., 2000), brain activity of rats was recorded while they ran a rectangular track for food. Each part of the track was represented in the hippocampus by activity in specific cells, so, as each rat ran about the track, the pattern of activity in the hippocampus kept changing in a repetitive pattern. Some days the animal kept running the same familiar track, but, on other days, novel portions were opened and traversed. Patterns of activity in the hippocampus that were seen when the animal was running the track were also seen during subsequent REMS. Also, there was a difference in the replay from the familiar portions compared to the novel portions in that only the replay of the novel was timed in such a way to strengthen their synaptic connections.

Other research has found evidence for replays during sleep of something newly learned in the cat cortex (Amzica, Neckelmann, & Steriade, 1997) and, using PET scans, in the human cortex (Laureys et al., 2001). However, it has been pointed out that replay during sleep of neuronal patterns that occurred during prior learning when awake does not necessarily mean that consolidation is taking place. It simply may be a continuation of the activity that began during waking. There is, as of yet, only preliminary evidence that this replay has an effect on subsequent behavior.

Kavanau (c.f. 1997) has a related theory. He posits that both sleep and memory are dependent upon the evolution of mechanisms that augment and sustain the effectiveness of synapses. This process cannot be done during waking because of interference from sensory input and disruptive body movements. It can happen during REMS because the inhibition of muscles prevents movement from disruption and sensory input is attenuated.

Others see the influence of REMS on memory as being more specific. During REMS, new experiences from waking are selected, sorted, and consolidated, then linked with old experiences (Hobson, 1988; Koukkou & Lehmann, 1983). REMS may reorganize memories by simultaneously activating old and new ones in the absence of distractions. Or it may integrate new information into the personality structure of the person (Webb, 1983).

This process might be viewed as a kind of off-line reprogramming that is both a consolidation of past learning and a preparation for future learning.

To some sleep experts, the evidence is not solid enough to conclude firmly that sleep plays a general role in the consolidation of memory. While there is no role for sleep for certain kinds of memories such as simple declarative memory, the evidence suggests there is consolidation during sleep for implicit learning, foreign language learning, and intensive student studying, as well as for emotional memories and memories for complex logic games. Others have meticulously detailed the problems with certain key studies and whole groups of certain kinds of studies (c.f. Siegel, 2001). Yet, while such weaknesses exist, when the results of many studies using several very different methods point to the same conclusion, and the weaknesses of one method are not found in the other methods, then it is reasonable to conclude positively that sleep plays a role in memory consolidaion.

Emotions.   REMS has also been postulated to play an important role in the regulation of mood and emotions. It has been thought to result in "enhanced effective adjustment" and "greater interpersonal skill and inventiveness" (Cohen, 1980, p. 315). REMS is said to tame or modulate drives by reducing drive-motivated behaviors. Included by some in this context (see for example Webb, 1983) is Freud's discharge model (see Chapter 8) of dreams, which states that dreams act as a safety valve for repressed drive. Others see this emotional function as due to REMS itself and not its accompanying dreams. For example, Vogel (1979) asserts that REMS lessens wakening drive-motivated behaviors. He infers this assertion from the effects of REMS deprivation on depressed individuals. Vogel maintains that REMS deprivation increases many drive-motivated behaviors as a result of increasing excitability in many brain structures, including those important for drive. The result is that REMS tames or modulates drives by reducing drive-motivated behaviors. This brain excitation, hence anti-depressive effect, however, is easily and quickly reversed by even a little subsequent REMS. What might be the purpose of this effect? REMS sleep may normally serve to modulate or tame the drives, leaving a person more flexible and adaptive when awake (Horne, 1988). The person who is depressed already has a low drive level and REMS only further reduces it. Without REMS, drives in the depressed person are more activated and approach a more normal level.

Other observations show an increase in REMS time after days of stress, worry, and intense learning (Greenberg, 1981; Hartmann, 1973). Generally, this increase will occur following a large variety of emotionally demanding events, both positive and negative, during the day. It can be seen in exaggerated form in variable length sleepers (see Chapter 3).

Other data show that the amygdala has high activity during REMS, possibly related to memories charged with emotions, but this high activity may also be blocking emotions since adrenaline and cortisol are unchanged during dreams and there are few of the changes in heart rate and blood pressure that accompany waking emotion (Horne, 2000).

Other adaptive aspects of REMS.   The rems of REMS have prompted speculation about function. One function has to do with binocular vision. Complex organization and neural processing is necessary in order for the brain to receive and properly process coordinated input from two eyes. During early maturation, the rems of REMS may facilitate the proper growth of the brain mechanisms for binocular vision. Later in life, they may sever to maintain function in these areas. Support for these related ideas is seen in the high REMS in species with a lot of crossing of the optic nerves but much less in species with little crossing. There is also some evidence that binocular coordination is better at the end of REMS. However, it has been pointed out that there are many exceptions to this generalization, and there is REMS in species with few or no eye movements.

David Maurice, affiliated with the Columbia University Department of Ophthalmology, advanced the hypothesis that the rems of REMS are to stir the fluids in the eye to keep them from not stagnating. This process is necessary, because these fluids are the only source of oxygen to the cornea during sleep, since the cornea does not have a blood vessel supply of its own and is shut off from air when the eyelids are closed. Experimental evidence shows that when the eyelids are closed and the eyes not moving, the fluid in the eye does become stagnant. Furthermore, evidence shows that eye movements are sufficient to prevent the stagnation and the fluids in the eye are oxygenated by blood vessels. Experiments in animals demonstrated that the cornea shows signs of disease when the eyeballs are prevented from moving for a few days.

NREMS–REMS Sequence

The fact that REMS most often follows NREMS suggests that something happens during REMS that is in response to something that happens in NREMS (Benington & Heller, 1994). Support comes from the facts that REMS percent is related to amount of NREMS, not the amount of waking, and the interval between REMS periods is dependent on the amount of elapsed NREMS regardless of the amount of intervening waking.

Exactly what REMS responds to from NREMS is not entirely clear. One possibility is to maintain a level of arousal in the cortex by compensating for the low level of arousal during NREMS (Vertes & Eastman, 2000), serving to reduce the vulnerability of the sleeper to underarousal, while it might also function to get the brain ready to be awake, since REMS is prominent close to the end of sleep. Another notion is that the cellular activity of REMS warms the brain after a period of cooling during NREMS (Wehr, 1992).

Additionally, REMS may provide a regularized system check that can, in part, help determine the adequacy of repair done in NREMS and locate where more maintenance is needed during the subsequent NREMS episode (McGrath & Cohen, 1978). Early in the night, the need is for macro restoration and adjustment that requires only brief testing, thus NREMS is long and REMS is short. Later, however, the restoration and adjustment becomes more and more refined and delicate—a kind of micro restoration—which requires longer and more detailed evaluation that is possible only in REMS. For this reason, late in the night, NREMS is short, and REMS is long. REMS may also be randomly testing the rest of the nervous system beyond the brain, resulting in the bodily concomitants of REMS such as irregular activation of the respiratory system, cardiovascular system, and other functions controlled by the automatic nervous system. In this case, it is important, for safety's sake, to prevent the muscles of movement from being activated while their nervous system controlling units are being tested.

On the other hand, REMS may provide a periodic respite from NREMS as a substitute for waking (Horne, 2000; Rial, 1997). It may be a wake substitute, or "pseudowake," rather than a state of sleep per se. In adults, it occurs at a time when an animal is not productive, not stimulated, and not endangered. In the very young, who are unable to take care of themselves when awake, high amounts of REMS helps keep them safer. NREMS drives us deep into unconsciousness but REMS merely distracts us from it. Arousal is easier from REMS in the presence of stimuli indicating danger or other emotional significance. Greater amounts of REMS near the end of sleep, or when sleep is extended, may substitute for wakefulness when NREMS, for unstated reasons, cannot be sustained, yet it is desirable to remain asleep rather than to wake up. However, research shows that allowing unlimited NREMS during the day in humans, which reduces NREMS at night, has no effect on REMS the following night. If REMS were a "filler," then there should be more of it in this situation.

The sequence of NREMS–REMS may be necessary for consolidation of some kinds of learning. An example is in the research on discrimination learning by Robert Stickgold of Hobson's group at Harvard. In one experiment (Stickgold, James, & Hobson, 2000), subjects were trained on a visual discrimination task that required them to identify the orientation of three short diagonal lines imbedded in a field of short horizontal lines flashed on a computer screen for a fraction of a second. There was no improvement until the subjects got sleep. In a subsequent experiment, one-half of the subjects were not allowed to sleep during the night following the training but got two full nights of sleep after that. The remaining subjects were allowed to sleep on all three nights. On the fourth day, all subjects were tested on the task. Those not deprived of sleep performed the task more rapidly than they had on the training day, but those deprived for the one night after training displayed no improvement. Subsequent selective deprivation experiments showed that memory enhancement took place in a two-stage process during the night following the training: both early NREMS followed by late REMS during the same night of sleep are required. It has been pointed out, however, that a different group of researchers, using the same task, found the same improvement over time whether or not the subjects slept, but they did find that selective deprivation of REMS reduced memory for doing the task.

This NREMS–REMS sequential stage finding is similar to Guiditta's earlier notion that information first processed in NREMS is then finished in REMS (Guiditta et al., 1995). Guiditta posits that NREMS strengthens "adaptive memories" and weakens "non-adaptive memories," and the subsequent REMS stores the results. Alternatively, he says, during SWS the memories to be strengthened are selected. Then, during REMS, the actual strengthening occurs. Yet, this theory does not account for why SWS diminishes as sleep progresses through the night and REMS increases.

Horne, in a review of the literature, concludes that, in the end, there is no solid evidence that REMS provides any unique, positive benefits (Horne, 2000). Rather the benefits of sleep come from NREMS. Obviously, more research on the functions of sleep is needed.

Box 35

Is REMS Phylogenetically Older than NREMS?[54]

Reptiles, amphibia, and fish sleep (see Box 1 in Chapter 1). However, unlike birds and mammals, their sleep is of only one kind which leads to an important question: Is this one kind of sleep comparable to REMS, NREMS, or neither? Whatever the answer to this question might be, another logically follows: what are the evolutionary steps between this unified primitive sleep in lower vertebrates and the multiple types of alternating sleep of higher vertebrates?

A widely held view is that NREMS is older. Most of the support comes from studies of brain waves during sleep in reptiles that, to some researchers, closely resemble only NREMS. It is only higher animals that also have REMS, thus NREMS must be older and REMS a later development during evolution.

Others hold that REMS is older. First, they see the brain wave data from sleeping reptiles as indicating a kind of REMS, not NREMS. They also point to the fact that the first sleep in infant mammals is REMS and that NREMS only gradually supplants much of it with maturity. Additionally, Rial and colleagues (1997) point to the fact that the control for REMS is in the brainstem, SWS in the midbrain[55], and waking is in the cortex. This progression is the order of development of the brain during evolution. Thus, they maintain that REMS is older than SWS. Further, they continue, REMS is equivalent to waking in cephalocordates, such as the lancet, and SWS is equivalent to waking in poikilotherms. As such, true waking came along only later in evolution.

A third view, developed by Karmanova, holds that neither REMS nor NREMS is oldest but that both emerged together out of older, sleep-like states (Karmanova, 1982). Ida Gavrilovna Karmanova has a doctorate in biological sciences and is retired director of the Laboratory of Wake-Sleep Evolution at the I. M. Sechenov Institute of

Evolutionary Physiology and Biochemistry in St. Petersburg, Russia. Based on her decades of study of sleep in various phylogenetic levels of animals, she believes that both NREMS and REMS evolved somewhat simultaneously out of more primitive rest states that she calls "sleep-like states." From these primitive states, she has traced the evolutionary development of sleep from "primary sleep" in fish and amphibians through "intermediate sleep" in reptiles to "true sleep" in birds and mammals by studying some remnants of these stages in currently living animals. Seigel (cf., Siegel, 1997), based on his studies of the primitive echidna (see Box 1 in Chapter 1), comes to a similar conclusion that both NREMS and REMS evolved from a primitive mixture of the two.

Obviously, there is currently no consensus to which type of sleep is the oldest. Perhaps, with more sleep research we shall someday know and agree on the answer.

THE FUNCTIONS OF DREAMING

Why do we spend so much time dreaming? Why does our mind put forth the effort to create dream after dream night after night? Surely there must be good purpose for such an endeavor. Through the ages, there have been many ideas about what dreams are (see Chapter 6). Some of these ideas are related to functions. Rather than review all of these ideas, we shall focus our attention here on theories that give primary importance to dream function and that are also in the forefront of current consideration.

At the beginning of the 20th century, Freud changed the focus of the realm of the function of dreams to a focus on an individual, psychological, internal orientation. Prior to Freud, the prevailing notion was that the source of dreams came from outside the individual. Because of Freud, during the first half of 20th century, much of the Western world came to believe that dreams functioned as an individual's emotional drive, or instinct, relief valves. Pent-up pressure from basic drives and wants that could not be manifested while awake because of personal and societal constraints could be released during dreams in disguised forms. It was believed that if this pressure did not release, then severe psychological problems would result. During this time, there were others, collectively known as post-Freudians, who accepted Freud's basic foundation but modified his details.

The discovery of REMS in the middle of the 20th century led to the rapid demise of the details of the Freudian and post-Freudian views, for it was found when people were deprived of sleep, or specifically REMS, hence major dreaming, they did not go crazy. REMS deprivation does not even cause a change in NREMS mentation (Kahn, Fisher, & Edwards, 1978). Subsequently, there were a number of new putative functions for dreams, but all in the realm of the internal and the personal. As of yet, there is neither convincing evidence nor consensus about the correctness of any one of the theories of dream functioning. It may be, as with sleep itself, that several functions of dreaming coexist. The leading candidates today are that dreams benefit the emotions of the dreamer, generate creative solutions to problems, and/or play a role in consolidating memories.

Essentially, what many of these theories say is that you dream about things that are important to you, in the sense of being emotionally arousing or effectively significant (Fiss, 1979). The process is adaptive, since you focus on your problems and seek solutions (Cartwright, 1990). These solutions may subsequently be assimilated into existing memory structures (Cartwright, 1990) and may be of help for waking behaviors. Dreams, then, are involved in the processes of self-regulation and self-reflectiveness (Moffitt, 1987). They function like a gyroscope to keep the self on a steady course in the face of the vicissitudes of daily life. Other theories, or corollaries to the main theories, conclude that dreams are for play, rehearse responses to potential threats, and/or distract our attention while asleep.

Still, there are many who believe that dreams have no functions; they are merely epiphenema generated as the brain is attending to some other function (c.f. Domhoff, 1985; Flanagan, 1995, 2000; Foulkes, 1999). In this regard, dreams are similar to the noise the heart makes when it pumps blood. The noise does not have a function; it does not help pump blood. It is a by-product, or, more properly, an epiphenomon, of the pumping activity of the heart. Similarly, dreams are seen as a by-product of the activity of the brain as it goes about its other (real) functions during sleep. Many theories of dreams that come out of cognitive neuroscience are of this type, such as The Activation-Synthesis theory and Foulkes's cognitive theory of dreaming. Yet Hall—Van de Castle analyses of series of dreams show there is consistency in dreams, hence meaning.

Others counter that dreams are much more organized than disorganized, have too much temporal progression, and focus too much on the dreamer in the world for them to be meaningless random epiphenomena (Revonsuo, 2000). They point to studies of the experiences that result when the brain is randomly stimulated, such as epileptic seizures of the temporal lobe. These experiences are quite different from those of dreaming. They contain varying perceptions that do not form a coherent world, no story-line and poor perceptual detail. Dreams, of course, contain all of these aspects.

It should be noted that speculations about the functions of dreams rarely differentiate between the dreams of REMS and the mentations of NREMS. The theories either are directed at only REMS dreaming or at any dreaming and mentation that occur during any stage of sleep. There are no dominant theories specific to NREMS mentation.

Several aspects of REMS dreams have been influential in formulations about their functions:

- Emotional content—many dreams have noticeable emotional contents, mainly negative
- Bizarreness—many aspects of dreams are frequently bizarre including characters, settings, and activities, as well as the sequential flow

- Personalness—much of what a person dreams about is recognizable to the dreamer including characters, settings, and objects. For the most part, they are things that are a part of the individual's current life but also include things that are a part of the individual's biographical memory. They are mostly first person experiences
- Lack of voluntary control—the dreamer is typically in control of its content while other cognitive processes are maintained
- Realistic—while we are dreaming, the things in the dream seem very realistic and we unquestioningly accept what is in them; they have a narrative structure
- There is a complete involvement in the experience while we are dreaming. This experience differs from waking when we are often distracted by other stimuli or thoughts
- Dreams occur between two periods of waking—the contents of our dreams are influenced by our recent waking experiences and can have an effect on our subsequent waking
- We have many more dreams than we remember

Before we explore the putative functions of dreaming in more detail, we need to keep a couple of things in mind. It is difficult to test the veracity of many of the theories of the functions of dreaming. First, as mentioned in Chapter 6, our only access to the content of people's dreams is via their description of what they remember of their dreams. The dream report may not be entirely accurate. Also, there may be whole categories of dreams that seldom, if ever, reach waking consciousness. As a result, we cannot be sure that our theories of functions of dreams are accurate and complete.

Second, it is necessary but difficult to show that dreams make a difference. One way to do so is to provide an adequate control group when doing research on the theories. Such control groups might be people who do not dream or dream differently than the experimental group. There are people who say they never dream, but in most cases what really is happening is that they do not spontaneously remember their dreams. There are those with damage to specific areas of the brain who, as far as can be determined, do not dream (Solms, 1997), but any differences between them and people who dream might be primarily caused by the brain damage itself rather than the lack of dreaming. Without an adequate control group, it is difficult to separate any effect of dreaming from sleep itself. Thus, the theories of dreams tend to be even more speculative, relying more heavily on logic and intuition than theories involving other aspects of sleep. That is, the fact to assumption ratio is often quite low, and the research attempting to test one or another of these theories has provided only weak support or contradictory results (Cartwright, 1989). Nevertheless, many of the contemporary theories are interesting, instructive, and seem to have at least elements that are plausible. We will examine some of these elements.

The best research, to date, on the functions of dreaming compares different qualities of dreams, and the best example is the research of psychologist Rosalind Cartwright of Rush Medical College in Chicago. She showed that those who dream more about an ex-spouse in early days of divorce were coping much better a year later. Details of this research are presented below.

Emotional Adaptation

The fact that dream content is heavily emotional leads to the notion that dreams play some kind of a role in emotional adaptation. In other words, dreaming helps individuals cope with the turmoil of their current waking life. This popular view has its origin in Jung's notion that dreaming helps maintain psychic balance, as well as Adler's view of a personal problem-solving function in dreaming. More recent studies, using functional imaging of the brain during sleep, lend some support. These studies show activation during REMS of the brain areas involved with emotions, suggesting that emotions may be important in shaping the content of dreams (Hobson, Pace-Schott, & Stickgold, 2000).

One way that dreaming might provide emotional adaptation is by preserving our identity (Cartwright, 1977). They retell who we are. They act like an emotional gyroscope (Kramer, 1987) making corrections to get us back toward an ideal. They bring a balance into our lives. They can also act like a safety valve allowing us to "let off" built up emotional pressure.

In this regard, dreams are best viewed as occurring between two periods of wake (Fiss, 1979; Kramer, 1987; 1990). The preceding period of wake affects the mood of the subsequent dream, or, put another way, the dream reflects the preceding period of wake. But the dream then affects the subsequent period of wake as a kind of mood regulator.

There is an advantage in dealing with emotions in dreams, for there is an absence of inhibition from logic and no fear of ridicule while dreaming. We can relate our waking stresses to past memories of a similar nature without being disturbed by the interruptions that are frequent when we are awake. We are then freer to try out different solutions, because we are free from the consequences and social constraints of waking life (Koulack, 1991). We are also freer to mix ideas while dreaming than when we are awake. So, unlike when awake, our mind can work more directly on the emotional problem on its own terms. It is often more successful to do so when dreaming than trying to deal with them when in the waking mode of thought. The end result is that when our dreams are working well, we can assimilate the emotional problem into our psyche in a way that promotes overall well being. Mark's dreams two nights before his piano recital are an example of this assimilation.

> On May 9, I dreamt that I could see myself practicing my part. I could see my hands on the keyboard the way one would, seated at a piano, but, every once in a while, I would switch and be someone at the door looking in at myself through a window in the door.

On May 10, I dreamt a vague and indistinct dream. I don't remember seeing much except clouds and a bust of Mozart (who wrote the piece), but I heard the entire piece (actual playing time: 35 minutes) from beginning to end with all instruments present. I woke up feeling much more confident and relaxed.

Laboratory studies showed that there is a measurable change in certain aspects of mood after dreaming; what psychologist Milton Kramer calls the mood regulatory hypothesis (Kramer, 1993). He finds that mood is generally better and less variable following dreaming. Furthermore, behavior is changed as a result. These studies have also shown that it is the dream content, especially the characters in the dream, that is related to the mood change. And, while some aspects of mood are affected by sleep physiology, such as "clear thinking," others are affected by the dreaming, such as "unhappiness."

In order to test Kramer's (1993) mood regulatory hypothesis, Cartwright and associates (Cartwright, Young et al., 1998) report their findings of research on 61 volunteers undergoing divorce who completed the study. Subjects were awakened in the sleep lab several minutes into each REMS period for dream collection. Those undergoing divorce who were not depressed had a low percent of negative dreams throughout the night. Those who were depressed at the time of the divorce, but were not a year later, had a lot of negative dreams early in the night, but fewer as the night went on. Those who were depressed both at the time of the divorce and a year later had a few negative dreams early in the night, but more as the night went on. In this last group, the dreaming process may have failed because the negative mood was too intense or because of some other reason.

Cartwright and colleagues (Cartwright, Luten et al., 1998) also did similar research with a non-depressed group of "normal" people. Sixty students, 30 males and 30 females, at a medical college were selected from a group of volunteers because of having no current or past major depression. They regularized their sleep on a 23.00 to 7.00 schedule for two weeks before coming to the sleep lab. Before and after each night of sleep, they filled out a mood scale. On the second night in the lab, they were awakened after several minutes of each REMS period and asked to report what they had been experiencing. Those who showed a moderate amount of depressed mood at bedtime showed better mood after dreaming. Also, the first dreams of the night were influenced by the presence of negative mood before sleep. They contained more negative affect and less positive affect early in the night, with the negative diminishing and the positive increasing as the night went on, suggesting a "working through" of the problems by the dreams. This pattern was not seen if the dreamer did not start the night with negative mood. Cartwright's conclusion from these data is that a function of dreams appears to be to modulate mood when negative mood is moderate.

In a related theory, Boston psychiatrist Ernest Hartmann maintains that dreams are guided by our emotions and emotional concerns and then help us deal with them (Hartmann, 1998). This function is most easily seen in people who have experienced psychological trauma, since it is much clearer what emotion is involved with the dreams. However, Hartmann believes the same process occurs with all emotions, even ones we may not be consciously aware of. What dreams do is make emotions into visual metaphors. These metaphors help explain things better. Minor parts of the dream are used to connect the metaphors by weaving together similar traumas, stresses, and life events to make them into new material. In this way, new neural networks are created.

For Hartmann, dreams thus help us by providing relief of the current trauma or emotion and, at the same time, prepare us for future trauma, stress, and problems of life all within the safety of the dream. Also, when sleeping, the brain is able to broadly reach out more to make the new connections than is possible when awake. In this way, dreaming can be therapeutic. Dreams are a kind of "built in psychotherapy" that occurs in a safe place. And, it all happens whether we remember the dream or not.

Modern thinkers have seen the relationship of dreams to the dreamer's waking life in one of two ways—complementary or continuous (Cartwright, 1977, 1978). Complementary dreams contain things that compensate for or are supplementary to what has recently occurred in waking life in an attempt to bring overall balance or harmony. For example, when Paul had been severely criticized for making an error at work, which he believed may have jeopardized his chances for promotion, he subsequently dreamed that he was competing in pre-Olympic track trials and was doing quite well and was "still in the running." Jill during the day had been bragging about being selected as one of 10 finalists in a contest by a popular teen magazine for a modeling feature in a future issue. That night, her dreams contained an image of a group of strangers pruning rose bushes ("cutting them down to size").

Continuous dreams, on the other hand, are those in which the themes, concerns, and events of waking life are continued in our dreams. Jerry had recently been working nights and weekends at his job, hoping to make a good impression and be rapidly promoted. After an argument with his wife about his "never being home," he had a dream that he was in a hot air balloon race in which he was "rising fast but on a collision course with a house that looked like mine."

Which is correct? Do our dreams take an active role in attempting to compensate for our waking lives in an effort to bring balance to our psyche? Or, is the focus of our dreams continuous with the cares and events of our waking lives? Probably, both are correct. Our mind may choose one or the other depending on current need, or perhaps the created dream may contain an element of each. The choice seems to depend upon where the greatest need exists in a person's life at the moment.

Overall, however, the empirical evidence for the emotionally adaptive function of dreaming is only correlational and relatively weak according to Revonsuo (2000). While the evidence is clear that much of the reported content of dreams is related to current emotional problems of the dreamer, there is little convincing evidence that dreaming of such problems has a salutatory effect on our waking psyche, since, he maintains, few causal relationships between dream content and waking adjustment have been established. Revonsuo also states that if this is indeed the function of dreaming, it is strange how often it fails given the high proportion of negative dreams that amplify the negative experiences, rather than those that overtly comfort and heal.

Creativity

Dreams are creative by their very nature. Every night each of us puts together several very original and unique dreams, a very creative process. Other aspects of the creativity of dreams carry over into our waking lives in several ways.

Your dreams may also suggest solutions to your everyday personal problems (Koulack, 1987) or suggest solutions to puzzles. They do so, because they allow less constrained associations between memories and cognitive processes than are allowed when awake (Stickgold et al., 1999b), by providing access to our recent and remote memories tying them to alternate cognitive strategies, followed by assimilation or accommodation into our existing memories and/or personality (Cartwright, 1990). Stickgold and associates (1999b) awakened people from REMS or NREMS and immediately gave them a semantic priming task while the brain was thought to be functionally organized as it was during the preceding stage of sleep. In this task, subjects were shown a series of words mixed with non-words one at a time and had to identify as quickly as possible whether or not they were seeing a word. Before each word (for example "wrong") or non-word ("wronk") was shown, the subjects were primed with a word unrelated to the word ("paper"), weakly related ("thief"), or strongly related ("right") was shown. The results showed that following NREMS awakenings, strong primes were very effective, but weak ones were not. However, the opposite is true following REMS awakenings, showing that associations are more remote then, allowing more creativity. Creativity in our dreams, it seems, come about because weak associations are facilitated during REMS.

The creativity in dreams can help us with our personal, emotional problems. In dreams, we can creatively relate our current stresses to similar ones in our past experience, and then we are freer to try out different solutions (Koulack, 1991). We are free from the interruptions that occur during wakefulness, free from social constraints, and freer to mix ideas than when awake. During dreams, we are also free from social requirements and self-criticism and can deal with our waking experiences creatively (Strauch & Meier, 1996). Here we engage in novel experiences and playfully deal with the world, all happening easily and unconsciously in our dreams.

But, there seem to be natural constraints on the solution to puzzles in dreams. First, you must be working on the problem or, in some other way, have the need for such a dream during your waking life. Second, you need to be able to recognize that the dream is offering a solution. Third, such dreams appear to be rather unpredictable, meaning that you cannot pick and choose when they will occur, and that you have to be ready to record and use them when they do come. The following excerpt from Tom's dream shows these things.

> Before this dream, I'd been having trouble deciding how to work out a color scheme on a particular woodcut for art class. In my dream, consequently, I somehow worked out an idea and woke up knowing what I was planning to do next. I also had short conversations

with the class professor in my dream, although I don't remember exactly what was discussed. This class, where I work with my hands and tools a lot, is often included in my dreams.

Watt's lead shot dream presented in Chapter 6 is another excellent example of all of the factors involved with creative dreams. It was an important problem that he had been working on during his waking life, yet he had to have the dream several times before he recognized what it was saying to him. We can only wonder what new discoveries have been lost because dreamers did not pay attention to what their dream might have been trying to tell them.

Yet, this research is not conclusive (c.f. Revonsuo, 2000). Achieving waking creative solution, which may be correlated with a dreamed solution, does not indicate a causal relationship. It is just as likely that the solution was arrived at when awake, and the dream simply reflects this.

Cognitive

Just like REMS, dreaming is thought to facilitate memory reorganization and maintenance. It has been hypothesized that during dreaming, memories are reorganized by associating and integrating the past with the present (Hobson, 1989). Dreaming also helps us master new experiences by assimilating them into the structure of preexisting memories helping keep our memories more efficiently organized. A related idea is that dreams are important for reprocessing waking experiences into our memories that are important for our survival (Winson, 1990) (see Chapter 7). For animals, the survival value of dreams involves memories for things like where to obtain food or where to escape from predators. In this way, dreams are biologically relevant. For humans, the survival value of dreams is more involved with the complex interrelationships of humans and the complexities of human personality.

Foulkes (1983) also focuses on a memory function of dreaming. He was struck by the parallel between cognitive development in children and the development of their dreams (see Chapter 6). As a result, he developed a theory that states that dreams help integrate our knowledge—especially that knowledge available to conscious recall. This integration occurs both within types of memory and between types of memory, such as semantic and episodic, recent and distant, verbal and visual-spatial. To Foulkes, the integration occurs even though we do not remember much of our dreams. As a result, we are left with: (1) an increase in the range of our experiences that even includes unrealistic things, (2) greater reality testing, since when we awaken, we know that much of what we dreamed was not real, and thus we can more easily recognize that our minds are capable of creating things that are not real, and (3) better self-knowledge because of combining motor memories with recognition memories giving us more flexibility.

Then again, perhaps the association of dreams with memory processes is more apparent than real. Jerome Siegel (2001) doubts that dreams reflect the consolidation of recent waking events, because so little of dream content is related to a recently intensive learning task or other recent experiences. And even those dreams that do seem to incorporate experiences from recent waking seldom are an exact rehearsal of the experiences or learned tasks but more about the situation related to the experience or learning. It is possible that dreams are epiphenomona of brain processes as they activate and then recombine memories and emotions (Stickgold et al., 2001), and the dreams themselves do nothing to aid in the process.

On a different note, one theory that has received a lot of notice, more because one of its originators is a Nobel Laureate, although in chemistry. It states that dreaming during REMS subtracts something from the memory stores of the brain rather than adds something (Crick & Mitchison, 1986) (see Chapter 7). According to this theory, a cleaning up of the memory banks occurs by the brain ridding itself of unwanted, useless, and even confusing associations, leaving what remains clearer, cleaner, and more meaningful. The experienced dream is composed of those memories that are being weakened. Remembering and interpreting dreams is not good because it is counterproductive to this process. The major problem with this theory is that there is a low ratio of facts to assumptions to support it. In fact, there is no good evidence for it (Benington, 2000), but there is ample evidence against the theory. Memories and functions in the brain fade with disuse, not by being activated.

Cartwright (1989) has incorporated some of these ideas about dream functions into the current understanding of how the brain works. The result is her Parallel Distributed Processing Model of dreaming. To Cartwright, our mind is composed of patterns of cognitions resulting from experiences while trying to meet our biological and psychological needs, including self-esteem. Affect accompanies these experiences concerning how successful we are in getting our needs met. All of these factors are stored in different places in the brain, that is they are distributed, at about the same time, in parallel, with interconnections between them of varying strengths. The result is different from what might occur when awake because of a different brain organization when asleep. Other related memories and past associations may also be stimulated in the process. The end result is the dream that we are aware of.

Play

Several investigators of dreams, such as Kelly Bulkeley (1999), have likened their function to that of play. Play is fanciful, yet important. It is enjoyable, but also useful. It can be creative and exploratory. It is done for its own sake in a semi-real realm of its own making. Play involves strong emotions. Play tends toward exaggeration, variation, and nonsensical yet is governed by some rules that often differ from that of non-play behavior. It is free, unpressured experimentation with possibilities and potentials. Play enables trying out various possibilities of experience. It allows safe experience with different skills and behaviors. It gives us the opportunity to experience things and social relationships differently from in our serious life. In play, there may be exaggerated, bizarre imagery. We are free to explore and interact differently than we are in real life. In all of these ways, play can result in our enhanced flexibility and prepare us for the future.

So in dreams, we can sometimes play. This idea encompasses both the emotion and creativity aspects of dreaming. It can be important.

Other

There are a few other theories about dreaming that deserve to be noted in passing. One is that dreams act to distract the brain's attention to keep us from waking up (Horne, 2000). This process intensifies as the end of the sleep period gets nearer, because we are more likely to awaken early then. Another is that dreaming provides for, or results from, necessary stimulation of the brain from within, compensating for the loss of stimulation from the environment or complementing waking stimulation.

Revonsou (2000) views the functions of dreams from an evolutionary standpoint. In order to understand the primary function of dreaming, we have to take into account that the environment in which our ancestors lived was full of threats. Anything that gave a survival advantage allowing for the increased possibility to reproduce would eventually tend to be favored by eons of evolution.

Revonsou maintains that, when we dream, we rehearse perceptions of threats and ways to avoid them. These process may be "threat scripts" from our ancestral past or in response to recently experienced threats during waking. This response is a safe way to enhance the probability of surviving such threats, thus being able to produce offspring. In this way, dreaming became established during evolution. Rather than alleviating emotional problems and thereby contributing to mental health or comfort, they aid reproductive success in much the same way that pain and suffering do. They do so, even if not remembered.

Revonsou (2000) supports this theory with a thorough and comprehensive review of the dreaming literature backed up by relevant information from psychology, evolutionary biology, and cognitive neuroscience. He focuses on the normative content of dreams, children's dreams, recurrent dreams and nightmares, PTSD dreams, and REM Behavior Disorder. He includes the dreams of people in hunter-gatherer societies of today that are preferentially filled with the kinds of threats that our ancestors would have experienced in their waking lives but have far fewer of the kinds of things only experienced by contemporary humans. He finds that our dreams more often contain negative content such as misfortunes, aggression, and threatening strangers and animals than pleasant experiences. They do not contain much of experiences our evolutionary ancestors would not have had, such as working at a computer, reading, or calculating. He also points out that the areas of the brain that subserve emotional and perceptual experience are activated during REMS.

This theory has been said to be too narrow (Moorcroft, 2000). While it seems adequate to explain the primal function of dreaming, it does not allow enough latitude of other functions that may be applicable today. Also, it begins with the assumption of the veracity of the relatively new field of behavioral biology to be able to explain the source of all behavior. Flanagan (1995, 2000) also takes an evolutionary approach to the function of dreaming but concludes that dreaming is an epiphenomenona without function. At this point in time, it is premature to accept fully the exclusiveness of the explanations of behavioral biology and the theories of dreaming by Revonsou and Flanagan.

Conclusion to the Functions of Dreaming

Careful analysis of most of these functions proposed for dreaming shows the central importance of emotions in dreams. The creative and play dreams can be said to involve emotions. The creative dreams involve things that are important or necessary to the dreamer—things in which the dreamer has invested much of his or her recent waking life. Even the play that occurs in dreams can be said to have an emotional basis and benefit, just as awake play does. Memory consolidation often involves memories that have an emotional component to them. Even the behavioral biology based theory of Revonsou focuses on emotions. This point is important in understanding dreams; that regardless of whatever else they may be, they have an emotional focus or core.

If the dreams are successful in fulfilling many of the proposed purposes, the dreamer awakens better able to cope and be more productive. If, however, the dream was unsuccessful or provided only partial success, subsequent dreams may deal with the subject matter again, or the actual dream may be repeated again. But, not all dreams successfully accomplish what they were intended to do; (Cartwright, 1991) some fail, some are trivial, and some are noxious. "Just as not all sleep is physiologically restorative, so not all dreams are necessarily psychologically restorative" (Fiss, 1979, p. 64).

Epilogue

As a way of summing up this book, I would like to present some of my views, especially those on the functions of sleep. Sections I and II of this book showed us that sleep is not just a passive shut down of the brain and body with nothing important going on other than to recharge our batteries. Rather, sleep is actively produced with many important things going on. Section III revealed that knowledge and understanding about dreams and dreaming has been harder to grasp compared to the knowledge and understanding about sleep. But, like sleep, dreams are actively produced and seemingly important.

In these sections, we have seen that much has been learned about sleep and dreaming, especially since the discovery of REMS in 1953. Certainly, enough has been learned to fill a textbook such as this one. But the quest is not over. There is still a lot to be learned, and, in order to learn it, there is a need for more sleep and dream research, which means there is also a need for more sleep and dream researchers. Perhaps you will be a part of this quest. A background in the biological, chemical, or psychological sciences is an excellent preparation prior to graduate school, focusing on the study of sleep or dreams. There is a National Multi-Site Training Program for Basic Sleep Research involving six universities in the United States (UCLA, University of Chicago, Harvard, University of Pennsylvania, Stanford, the University of Texas) that provides interdisciplinary training for predoctoral and postdoctoral students with full tuition and financial aid. Contact the Sleep Research Training Program, Brain Research Institute, University of California, Los Angeles, California 90024-1746. Also, many other graduate schools have someone on the faculty who is doing sleep or dream research and can help you get special training in these areas. See who is publishing research in an area you might be interested in and contact them to see if they have a post-graduate program you might be able to join. Meanwhile, see if there is someone at your college or university, or at a local sleep disorders center, who is doing sleep research and whom you could volunteer to help.

Section IV reviews some of the more common problems people have with their sleep or dreams. By the end of the 20th century, much had been discovered about these problems and how to treat them effectively. At the beginning of the 21st century, there are sleep disorder centers in almost every moderate sized city in the United States, and growing numbers in other parts of the world, where people with sleep or dream problems can have them diagnosed and treated. This opportunity has led to great improvements in the quality of life, and sometimes the longevity of life, for many people. Additional information about sleep disorders can be obtained from The National Sleep Foundation, 1522 K Street, NW, Suite 500, Washington, DC 20005; 202/347-3471; nsf@sleepfoundation.org; e-mail: www.sleepfoundation.org. This resource is excellent for professionals and non-professionals alike, who would like to obtain more information about sleep and sleep disorders.

Perhaps you might consider a career in this area. Any support you can give to these efforts will help bring adequate treatment to many people and very possibly to someone you know and love. Perhaps you may want to enter the expanding field of Sleep Disorders Medicine yourself as a Polysomnographic Technician or a M.D. board-certified in Sleep Medicine. Or, after earning a Ph.D. in clinical or counseling psychology, obtain appropriate training to become an accredited practitioner in the emerging field of Behavioral Sleep Medicine. For more information on any of these careers, contact the Associated Professional Sleep Societies, One Westbrook Corporate Center, Suite 920, Westchester, IL, 60514; 708-492-0930;www.apss.org.

Section V explored the functions of sleep and dreaming from a variety of perspectives. In addition to learning more about dreaming and dreams, the search has been on for the primary function of sleep that caused its evolution. It is thought, based on evolutionary theory, that this one function gave its possessors an advantage that enabled them to live more successfully and reproduce, thus passing this trait on to their offspring. Later, additional functions were added to sleep, because it was already present and convenient (Sleep Research Society, 1997), and they, in turn, may have added to reproductive success.

However, research to date has not convincingly found this primal function of sleep among all the candidates. It is possible that the over the eons, the original function of sleep was lost, and only the added functions remain. It is also possible that more than one function of sleep coevolved (Arden, 1996; Nicolau et al., 2000). This view maintains that no single function by itself was advantageous enough to be the cause of the evolution of sleep, but several functions evolving collectively may have provided the advantage and thus sleeping and dreaming evolved. Given our current state of knowledge, this idea seems the most reasonable to me.

Efficiency

The well-known symptoms of sleepiness may not point the way to the functions of sleep. Instead they may be the way that the body gets us to seek sleep for another less obvious purpose (Rechtschaffen, 1998). This concept is similar to the symptoms of hunger (rumbling stomach, light headedness, sensory appeal of food, etc.) that may draw our attention to the need to eat but do not reflect the real reason we need to eat. In this regard, it is possible that the urge to sleep produces the inefficiency rather than, as most commonly assumed, the other way around (Meddis, 1979).

My own view of the functions of sleep, which is similar to that of Feinberg and Floyd (1982), but also includes dreaming, incorporates most of the ideas presented in Chapters 12 and 13. Yet, I am struck by evidence that sleep does not seem to be absolutely necessary for anything. People and animals can do without it for long periods of time. Only work from Rechtschaffen's lab (see Box 33 in Chapter 12) has shown that sleep deprivation can have lethal consequences in rats, but this conclusion was drawn only after a few weeks of continuous sleeplessness. People and animals can survive a few days, or even a week, of sleep deprivation, then recover after only a couple bouts of normal sleep. This suggests that because many things that occur during sleep can occur when we are awake, or we can do without them. Aspects of sleep brain waves, muscle inhibition, PGO waves, and so on have been found to occur outside of sleep in, for example, narcoleptics, people who sleep-walk, and people who are severely sleep deprived. Likewise, the following have been demonstrated regarding REMS and its components (Sakai, 1985):

- REMS without PGO waves in animals with lesions in a specific part of the brainstem;
- REMS without muscle paralysis in humans with REM behavior disorder;
- REMS without its characteristic brain waves following administration of the drug atropine.

Each of the aspects thus appears to be an independent process for which sleep is not necessary and, therefore, not the cause (Fiss, 1979).

Yet, without an adequate amount of quality sleep, there is a deviation from the optimal, normal level of functioning. In short, we do not do as well without sleep. Perhaps, then, sleep has no function other than to orchestrate various components and provide a convenient time when they can occur most easily and most *efficiently* (Adam & Oswald, 1983; McGaugh et al., 1979). This statement is not to belittle this function; efficiency is important and in the long run may even be essential, as the Rechtschaffen research shows. But, in the short run, it can be sacrificed for other, more pressing needs.

Sleep has a rhythmic character (Chapter 2). In this respect, it is no different from many other rhythms seen in life on our planet and may have evolved out of them. Specifically it may have evolved out of a simple rest/activity cycle seen in other animals (Box 1 in Chapter 1), primarily as a behavioral strategy to keep its practitioner out of harm's way and to conserve a little energy at the same time. As warm-blooded animals evolved, sleep may have become more important in the regulation of body temperature. Still later, with the evolution of bigger and more complex brains, sleep also assumed importance in the development and maintenance of this very delicate, yet complex structure. Likewise, sleep, thus evolved, could be a convenient time to perform some cognitive and emotional housekeeping Thus, dreams were added.

Remnants of this evolutionary history are evident today in present species that have different places on the evolutionary tree (Horne, 1988). Remnants are also evident within individual higher species since, during evolution, existing functions of sleep were not simply replaced but new functions were also added. Later, these add-ons may have gained primary importance, with the others becoming secondary, or even discarded.

Sleep may be likened to an American university. There are many aspects and functions of universities—education, research, extension services, and athletics, to name a few. Each helps define the university and make it what it is; yet, each aspect can exist apart from the university. The assemblage of these various, potentially autonomous, entities not only defines the university but also lends a certain efficiency to each of its parts. Yet, the university can be recognized even if some of its parts are absent. So, too, with sleep. Sleep may, in the end, just be the "recruitment and coupling" of potentially independent elements, including dreams (McGinty, 1985).

Just as at the university, teaching may be considered a primary function and athletics a secondary function, some of the functions of sleep may be more primary and others secondary (Meddis, 1979). Also, the function of the university may differ at different times in history—at one time the primary function of many universities was to produce teachers and preachers—just as the function of sleep has differed throughout evolution (Horne, 1983c).

Also, the function of the university may differ for different students depending on their attributes and needs. The more musically gifted may value the music courses and organizations more than they value the academic and athletic functions. In contrast, another student with intellectual abilities may value the classroom and library much more. All of these students may also participate in other things while at the university, because they are available and convenient, but they are of more or less secondary importance. So, too, with sleep. The extent to which sleep is for safety, energy conservation, restoration, or whatever may depend on such interrelated things such as the size of the body, degree of cerebral development, and constituents of the diet (Horne, 1988). The same is certainly true of other characteristics of animals. Some animals have claws, others hooves, and still others fingers. Some have fins, and others have no appendages at all. We can also see differences among animals' behaviors. Some rely heavily on fixed inherited instincts, while others rely on learned behaviors. Some animals live in very structured social groups, while others are mostly solitary.

Likewise, different types of animals may have different functions for sleep according to their own unique needs.

Finally, the function of the university may change for an individual student during the course of study. It is not unusual for U.S. students to change majors, or perhaps they were attracted to the university primarily because of its social and extracurricular activities but discovered the joy of serious study by the time they graduated. In a similar way, the function of sleep may change during the course of its nightly duration (Horne, 1988). The greater amounts of SWS early in the human sleep period followed by more REMS toward the end of the sleep period certainly support such a notion.

In the end, then, the function of sleep may be to provide optimal circumstances for many diverse functions. Its function may be summed up in one word— EFFICIENCY.

This statement does not imply that sleep is unimportant. As Webb (1971) said very well,

> My position views sleep as a process which evolved to aid us to adapt our behavior to an environment of eons ago. The sleep of Babylon is the sleep of today. For those times and places it functioned effectively as a biological system. But, modern times have brought the Edison Age of electric lights and is abolishing the natural rhythm of night and day, the jet aircraft tosses sleep across multiple time zones, and drugs have given promises of bending sleep to our momentary demands. Pervasively, we raise our strident cries and push our self-centered demands that sleep be subservient to our whimsy, bend to our needs, pressures and terrors. We ominously move toward viewing our failures of sleep to be "illnesses" to be "cured."
>
> My view point is to the contrary. In a reasonably natural and stable environment sleep will serve its function as a silent and well-trained servant. It is rather our "misbehaviors" in relation to sleep, goaded by a changed environment and a thoroughly anthropomorphic arrogance about "nature", which "fails" sleep as it is pushed beyond its natural limits. From my perspective, anchored in my adaptive theory of sleep, we must rather than learn the proximal causes of sleep, learn the laws of sleep. In turn we must teach ourselves to act in accord with these laws. I agree with Francis Bacon of 500 years ago: "Nature cannot be commanded except by being obeyed.

Notes

1. Specific references to statements in this chapter that can be found in multiple, widely available sources are not included in the text. A selection of these sources is listed below and can also be consulted for verification or more detail.
   Kryger, Roth, & Dement, 2000
   Lee-Chiong, Satela, & Carskadon, 2002
   Moorcroft, 1993
   Sleep Research Society, 1997
2. In this book rem is not capitalized when it indicates the rapid eye movements themselves but capitalized when indicating the sleep stage.
3. A nychthemeron (nick-sthem-er-on) is a full period of a night and a day or 24 hours. In everyday use "day" can mean 24 hours or the portion of every 24 hours that is light. In science we need to be more precise so we eliminate ambiguity when we use nychthemeron to refer to a 24 hour cycle and reserve the term "day" to refer to the light portion of this cycle.
4. Specific references to statements in this chapter that can be found in multiple, widely available sources are not included in the text. A selection of these sources is listed below and can also be consulted for verification or more detail.
   Kryger, Roth, & Dement, 2000
   Lee-Chiong, Satela, & Carskadon, 2002
   Moorcroft, 1993
   Sleep Research Society, 1997
   Turek and Zee, 1999
5. Homeostasis is the process of trying to compensate for deviations from a standard or norm. The thermostat in your home engages in homeostasis when it turns on the furnace or air conditioner if the room becomes cooler or warmer than the desired temperature you have set on it.
6. You probably have experienced a brief loss of electrical power that temporarily shuts everything off (including your computer). This occurrence is similar to microsleeps that are intrusions of a few seconds of sleep causing the absence of alertness in the midst of waking. During a microsleep, a person appears to be staring off into space or the head may droop a bit.

7. Specific references to statements in this chapter that can be found in multiple, widely available sources are not included in the text. A selection of these sources is listed below and can also be consulted for verification or more detail.

   Kryger, Roth, & Dement, 2000

   Lee-Chiong, Satela, & Carskadon, 2002

   Moorcroft, 1993

   Sleep Research Society, 1997

8. Specific references to statements in this chapter that can be found in multiple, widely available sources are not included in the text. A selection of these sources are listed below and can also be consulted for verification or more detail.

   Kryger, Roth, & Dement, 2000

   Lee-Chiong, Satela, & Carskadon, 2002

   Moorcroft, 1993

   Sleep Research Society, 1997

   Turek and Zee, 1999

9. From Siegel, 1989.

10. At this point you may be questioning how an area of the brain that is important for waking is also key to sleeping. The answer is like members of very different political parties who may be neighbors but have very different influences on political processes by whom they contact and what they say when they contact them. Similarly, in the brain, cells that perform one function may exist in the same area with cells that perform the opposite function because their communication with other neurons differs both in where their axons travel and what neurotransmitters they release there.

11. PGO waves were discovered in animals but are thought to occur also in humans. These waves are phasic clusters of up to 6 sharp electrical peaks closely related to the occurrence and direction of rems. They originate in the pons, then travel to the lateral geniculate nuculeus in one side or the other of the thalamus, and from there to the cerebral cortex, especially the occipital cortex, on the same side. Since their discovery, they have been found to involve more portions of the brainstem, cerebellum, and cortex than their name implies. They are probably triggered by the hypothalamus and forebrain during REMS when the cortex has few sensory inputs.

12. You might wonder why these areas are mutually inhibitory and how this process would work. When the VLPO is activated and initiating sleep, its activation would inhibit the wake promoting systems and thus remove their inhibition from the VLPO, which facilitates sleep and tends to maintain it once it has begun. Likewise, arousing inputs to the wake-promoting areas would reduce their inhibition coming from the VLPO, thereby facilitating and maintaining wakefulness. In this way, the VLPO could emphatically flip-flop between sleep and waking but tend to maintain whatever state is currently being produced.

13. From Siegel, 1989.

14. Specific references to statements in this chapter that can be found in multiple, widely available sources are not included in the text. A selection of these sources are listed below and can also be consulted for verification or more detail.

    Carskadon M A (Ed.), 1993

    Kryger, Roth, & Dement, 2000

    Lee-Chiong, Satela, & Carskadon, 2002

    Moorcroft, 1993

    Sleep Research Society, 1997

    Turek and Zee, 1999

15. From Copinschi, Leproult, & Van Cauter, 2001; Steiger et al., 1998.

16. C.f. Roehrs & Roth, 2001.

17. Specific references to statements in this chapter that can be found in multiple, widely available sources are not included in the text. A selection of these sources is listed below and can also be consulted for verification or more detail.

    Moorcroft, 1993

    Carskadon, 1993

    The entire sixth issue of volume 23 of the journal Behavioral and Brain Sciences.

18. Specific references to statements in this chapter that can be found in multiple, widely available sources are not included in the text. A selection of these sources is listed below and can also be consulted for verification or more detail.

    Domhoff, 1996

    Moorcroft, 1993

    Sleep Research Society, 1997

    Strauch and Meier, 1996

19. This summary of Freud's theories on dreaming is from his wonderful and groundbreaking book *The Interpretation of Dreams* published in 1900. It is interesting and relatively easy to read.

20. The censor, for the same reason, also causes poor retention of dreams.

21. Over his 49-year professional career, Freud used secondary revision in different ways including: (1) putting finishing touches on the dream to make it more story-like and (2) revising the manifest content of the dream when retelling it to make it smoother and more logical. To illustrate this second type of secondary revision, recall your own experiences of waking up and reviewing your own dreams. Perhaps you dreamed of a casual acquaintance being in your class. But you believe the person was your friend, and your mind changes the memory of the dream to be consistent with your belief. Now when you recall the dream, it was your friend who was in class.

22. Psychoanalysts, including Freud, have denied the popular conception of an overemphasis on sex in psychoanalytic theory and practice. To some extent they are correct in that there is more to the theory and practice than just sexual motives, yet sex is a heavy emphasis.

23. The synopsis of Jung's theories is derived from his books *Dreams* (1974) and *Man and His Symbols* (1964). Also used were Mahoney's (1966) review of Jung's work, *The Meaning in Dreams and Dreaming: The Jungian Viewpoint*, and portions of Bulkeley, 1997 and Delaney, 1998.

24. Sources for the section on Adler include Bulkeley, 1997; Carskadon, 1993; and Weiss, 1986.

25. Sources for the section on French and Fromm include from Bulkeley, 1997; Weiss, 1986.

26. The information for this section on Boss was taken from Bulkeley, 1997; Delaney, 1998; and Domhoff, 1985.

27. In 1966, Hall wrote a short and easy to read book about his dream theory called *The Meaning of Dreams*.

28. From Delaney, 1996 and 1998.

29. From A. Siegel, 2001; Savary, Berne, & Williams, 1984.

30. From Foulkes, 1999.

31. Derived from Bulkeley, 1994, 1997 and Hunt 1989.

32. From Hartmann's 1998 book, *Dreams and Nightmares: The New Theory on the Origin and Meaning of Dreams*.

33. From Association of Sleep Disorders Centers, 1997.

34. Much of the information for this chapter can be found in sources like Kryger, Roth, & Dement, 2000 and Lee-Chiong, Satela, & Carskadon, 2002.

35. From Dinges, 2002; Harrison & Horne, 2000.

36. From Horne & Reyner, 1998.

37. For more information see Krauss, Chen, DeArmond, & Moorcroft (2003).

38. From Carrier, 2001; Sleep As We Grow, 2001.

39. From Lipman, 1996.

40. From, Cartwright & Lamburg, 1992; Krakow & Neidhardt, 1992.

41. Kryger, Roth, & Dement, 2000; Shapiro & Smith, 1997.
42. From Arkin, 1981.
43. Thanks to Mark W. Mahowold, M.D., A.C.P., Director of the Minnesota Regional Sleep Disorders Center in Minneapolis for his very careful reading of an early draft of these chapters and many helpful suggestions.
44. Most of the information in this chapter can be found repeated in a number of sources including Kryger, Roth, & Dement, 2000; Lee-Chiong, Satela, & Carskadon, 2002, & on the Net at http:// www.sleepfoundation.org/ so specific references are not given for much of this material.
45. All of the names used in this chapter are fictitious. The case histories are based on real patient histories with embellishments and additions for clarity and completeness. Many of the case histories presented were derived by combining the case histories of several patients.
46. Thanks to Mark W. Mahowold, M.D., A.C.P., Director of the Minnesota Regional Sleep Disorders Center in Minneapolis for his very careful reading of an early draft of these chapters and many helpful suggestions.
47. Most of the information in this chapter can be found in a repeated in a number of sources including Kryger, Roth, & Dement, 2000; Lee-Chiong, Satela, & Carskadon, 2002, and on line at http://www.sleepfoundation.org/ so specific references are not given for much of this material.
48. From Involuntary Eating, 2001.
49. From Borbley, 1986 and Horne, 1988.
50. Much of the information in this chapter can be found repeated in a number of sources including Kryger, Roth, & Dement, 2000; Nicolau et al., 2000; and Rechtschaffen, 1998.
51. From Lee-Chiong, Satela, & Carskadon, 2002 and WFSRS, 1999.
52. From Chase & Roth, 1990. See also McGinty & Szymusiak, 1990.
53. Most of the information in this chapter can be found repeated in a number of sources including Kryger, Roth, & Dement, 2000; Maquet, 2001; Nicolau et al., 2000; Rechtschaffen, 1998; and Siegel, 2001; Stickgold, Hobson, Fosse R., & Fosse M., 2001.
54. Adapted and updated from Moorcroft, 1993 with permission of the publisher.
55. Most others would place it in the diencephalous and lower telencephalous.

References

AASM. (2001). Sleep as we grow older. Brochure produced by the American Academy of Sleep Medicine, Rochester, MN, 2001.

Achermann, P., & Borbély, A. A. (1990). Simulation of human sleep: Ultradian dynamics of electroencephalographic slow-wave sleep. *J Biol Rhythms, 5*, 141–157.

Achermann, P., & Borbély, A. A. (1990). Modeling the ultradian dynamics of EEG slow-wave activity and REM sleep. *Sleep Research, 19*, 127.

Adler, T. (1993). Speed of sleep's arrival signals sleep deprivation. *American Psychological Association Monitor, 24*, 20.

Akerstedt, T. (1995). Work hours and sleepiness. *Neurophysiologie Clinique, 25*, 367–375.

American Academy of Pediatrics. (1997). Task Force on Infant Position and SIDS. Does bed sharing affect the risk of SIDS? *Pediatrics, 100*, 272.

American Psychiatric Association. (2000). *Diagnostic and Statistical Manual of Mental Disorders DSM-IV-TR (Text Revision)*. Washington, DC: American Psychiatric Association.

American Sleep Disorders Association. (1997). *International Classification of Sleep Disorders, Revised: Diagnostic and Coding Manual*. Rochester, MN: American Sleep Disorders Association.

Amzica, F., Neckelmann, D., & Steriade, M. (1997). Instrumental conditioning of fast (20- to 50-Hz) oscillations in corticothalamic networks. *Proceedings of the National Academy of Sciences of the United States of America, 94*, 1985–1989.

Anch, A. M., Browman, C. P., Mitler, M. M., & Walsh, J. K. (1988). *Sleep: A Scientific Perspective.* Englewood Cliffs, New Jersey: Prentice Hall.

Antrobus, J. S. (1983). REM and NREM sleep reports: comparison of word frequencies by cognitive classes. *Psychophysiology, 20*, 562–568.

Antrobus, J., Hartwig, P., Rosa, D., Reinsel, R., & Fein, G. (1987). Brightness and clarity of REM and NREM imagery: Photo response scale. *Sleep Research, 16*, 240.

Arden, J. B. (1996). *Consciousness, Dreams, and Self: A Transdisciplinary Approach.* Madison, Connecticut: Psychosocial Press.

Arkin, A. M. (1981). *Sleeptalking: Psychology and Psycholphysiology.* Hillsdale, NJ: L. Erlbaum Associates.

Aserinsky, E., & Kleitman, W. (1953). Regularly occurring periods of eye motility and concommitant phenomena during sleep. *Science, 118*, 273–274.

Backhaus, J., Hohagen, F., Voderholzer, U., & Riemann, D. (2001). Long-term effectiveness of a short-term cognitive-behavioral group treatment for primary insomnia. *European Archives of Psychiatry and Clinical Neurosciences, 251*, 35–41.

Badia, P. (1990). Memories in sleep: Old and new. In R. R. Bootzin, J. F. Kihlstrom, & D. L. Schachter (Eds.), *Sleep and Cognition* (pp. 67–76). Washington: American Psychological Association.

Baratte-Beebe, K. R., & Lee, K. A. (1999). Sources of midsleep awakenings in childbearing women. *Clinical Nursing Research, 8*, 386–397.

Barrett, D. (1993). The "committee of sleep": A study of dream incubation for problem solving. *Dreaming, 3*, 115–122.

Benington, J. H. (2000). Sleep homeostasis and the function of sleep. *Sleep, 23*, 959–966.

Benington, J. H. (2001). Determinants of recuperation during sleep. Presentation at the Annual Meeting of the Associated Professional Sleep Societies, Chicago.

Benington, J. H., & Heller, H. C. (1994). Does the function of REM sleep concern Non-REM sleep or waking? *Progress in Neurobiology, 44*, 433–449.

Benington, J. H., & Heller, H. C. (1995). Restoration of brain energy metabolism as a function of sleep. *Prog. Neurobiol. 45*, 347.

Benoit, O. (1985). Homeostatic and adaptive roles of human sleep. *Experientia, 40*, 437–440.

Berger, R. J. (1963). Experimental modification of dream content by meaningful verbal stimuli. *Br J Psychiat, 109*, 722–740.

Berger, R. J., & Phillips, N. H. Energy conservation and sleep. (1995). *Behav Brain Res, 69*, 65–73.

Blagrove, M., & Akehurst, L. (2000). Personality and Dream recall frequency: Further Negative Findings. *Dreaming, 10*, 139–146.

Boivin, D. B., Czeisler, C. A., Dijk, D. J., Duffy, J. F., Folkard, S., Minors, D. S., Totterdell, P., & Waterhouse, J. M. (1997). Complex interaction of the sleep-wake cycle and circadian phase modulates mood in healthy subjects. *Archives of General Psychiatry, 54*, 145–152.

Bonnet, M. H. (1986). Performance and sleepiness as a function of frequency and placement of sleep disruption. *Psychophysiology, 23*, 263–271.

Bonnet, M. H., & Arand, D. L. (1995). Are we chronically sleep deprived. *Sleep, 18*, 908–911.

Borbély, A. A. (1986). *The Secrets of Sleep*. New York: Basic Books.

Born, J., & Fehm, H. L. (1998). Hypothalamus-pituitary-adrenal activity during human sleep: a coordinating role for the limbic hippocampal system. *Exp Clin Endocrinol Diabetes, 106*, 153–163.

Born, J., Hansen, K., Marshall, L., Molle, M., & Fehm, H. L. (1999). Timing the end of nocturnal sleep. *Nature, 397*, 29–30.

Bremer, F. (1935). Cerveau "isolé" et physiologie du sommeil. *C R Soc Biol* (Paris), *118*, 1235–1241.

Bremer, F. (1936). Cerveau. Nouvelles recherches sur le mecanisme du sommeil. *C R Soc Biol., 122*, 460–464.

Bulkeley, K. (1994). *The Wilderness of Dreams*. Albany, NY: State University of New York Press.

Bulkeley, K. (1996). *Among All These Dreamers*. Albany, NY: State University of New York Press.

Bulkeley, K. (1997). *An Introduction to the Psychology of Dreaming*. Westport, Connecticut: Praeger.

Bulkeley, K. (1999). *Visions of the Night*. Albany, New York: State University of New York Press.

Busink, R., & Kuiken, D. (1996). Identifying Types of Impactful Dreams: A Replication. *Dreaming, 6*, 97–119.

Carrier, J. (2001). Sleep in the later years of life. *Sleep Review, 2*, 48–50.

Carskadon, M. A. (1993). (Ed.) *Encyclopedia of Sleep and Dreaming*. New York: Macmillian.

Cartwright, R. D. (1974). Problem solving: waking and dreaming. *Journal of Abnormal Psychology, 83*, 451–455.

Cartwright, R. D. (1977). *Night Life: Explorations in Dreaming*. Englewood Cliffs, New Jersey: Prentice-Hall.

Cartwright, R. D. (1978). *A Primer on Sleep and Dreaming*. Reading, Mass: Addison-Wesley.

Cartwright, R. D. (1979). The nature and function of repetitive dreams: a survey and speculation. *Psychiatry, 42*, 131–137.

Cartwright, R. D. (1989). Dreams and their meaning. In M. H. Kryger, T. Roth, & W. C. Dement (Eds.), *Principles and Practice of Sleep Medicine* (pp. 184–190). Philadelphia: Saunders.

Cartwright, R. (1990). A network model of dreams. In R. R. Bootzin, J. F. Kihlstrom, & D. L. Schacter (Eds.), *Sleep and Cognition* (pp. 179–189). Washington: American Psychological Association.

Cartwright, R. D. (1991). *Who needs dreams?* Presented at The Upper Midwest Sleep Society Meeting, St Paul, Minnesota.

Cartwright, R. D., & Lamberg, L. (1992). *Crisis Dreaming: Using Your Dreams to Solve Your Problems.* New York, NY: HarperCollins.

Cartwright, R., Luten, A., Young, M., Mercer, P., & Bears, M. (1998). Role of REM sleep and dream affect in overnight mood regulation: a study of normal volunteers. *Psychiatry Research, 81*, 1–8.

Cartwright, R., Young, M. A., Mercer, P., & Bears, M. (1998). Role of REM sleep and dream variables in the prediction of remission from depression. *Psychiatry Research, 80*, 249–255.

Cauffield, J. S., & Forbes, H. J. (1999). Dietary supplements used in the treatment of depression, anxiety, and sleep disorders. *Lippincotts Primary Care Practice, 3*, 290–304.

Chase, M. H. (Ed.) (1986). Overview of sleep research, circa 1985. *Sleep, 9*, 452–457.

Chase, M. H., & Roth, T. (1990). (Eds.) *Slow Wave Sleep: Its Measurement and Functional Significance.* Los Angeles: Brain Information Service/Brain Research Institute.

Cohen, D. B. (1980). The cognitive activity of sleep. *Progress in Brain Research, 53*, 307–324.

Coren, S. (1996). *Sleep Thieves.* New York: The Free Press.

Corner, M. A., Mirmiran, M., Bour, H. L. M. G., Boer, N. E., van de Poll, H. G., van Oyen, M. A., & Uylings, H. B. M. (1980). Does rapid-eye-movement sleep play a role in brain development. In P. S. McConnel, G. J. Boer, H. J. Romijn, N. E. van de Poll, & M. A. Corner (Eds.), *Adaptive Capabilities of the Nervous System* (pp. 347–356). Amsterdam: Elsevier.

Crick, F., & Mitchison, G. (1983). The function of dream sleep. *Nature, 30*, 111–114.

Czeisler, C. A., Duffy, J. F., Shanahan, T. L., Brown, E. N., Mitchell, J. F., Rimmer, D. W., Ronda, J. M., Silva, E. J., Allan, J. S., Emens, J. S., Dijk, D. J., & Kronauer, R.E. (1999). Stability, precision, and near-24-hour period of the human circadian pacemaker Science. *Science, 284*, 2177–2181.

Davenne, D., & Adrien, J. (1987). Lesion of the ponto-geniculo-occipital pathways in kittens. I. Effects on sleep and on unitary discharge of the lateral geniculate nucleus. *Brain Research, 409*, 1–9.

Dawson, D., & Reid, K. (1997). Fatigue, alcohol and performance inpairment. *Nature, 388*, 235.

Delaney, G. (1996). *Living Your Dreams.* San Francisco: HarperSanFrancisco.

Delaney, G. (1998). *All About Dreams.* New York: HarperCollins.

Dement, W. C., & Kleitman, N. (1957). Cyclic variations in EEG during sleep and their relation to eye movements, body motility, and dreaming. *Electroencephalogr Clin Neurophyusiol, 9*, 673–690.

Dement, W. C. (2001, Winter). Reducing America's Sleep Debt. *Sleep Review.*

Dement, W. C., & Vaughn, C. (1999). *The Promise of Sleep.* New York: Delacorte Press.

Dement, W. C., & Wolpert, E. (1958). The relation of eye movements, body motility, and external stimuli to dream content. *J Exp Psychol, 55*, 543–554.

Dijk, D. J., & Czeisler, C.A. (1994). Paradoxical timing of the circadian rhythm of sleep propensity serves to consolidate sleep and wakefulness in humans. *Neurosci Lett, 166*, 63–68.

Dinges, D. F. (1989). The nature of sleepiness: causes, contexts, and consequences. In A. J. Stunkard, & A. Baum (Eds.), *Eating, Sleeping, and Sex* (pp. 147–180). Hillsdale, New Jersey: Erlbaum.

Dinges, D. (2002). *What it means to be awake.* President's address given at the annual meeting of the Associated Professional Sleep Societies, Seattle, Washington, June 10, 2002.

Dinges, P. F., & Powell, J. W. (1989). Sleepiness impaires optimum response capability—it's time to move beyond the lapse hypothesis. *Sleep Research, 18*, 366.

Domhoff, G. W. (1985). *The Mystique of Dreams.* Los Angeles: University of California Press.

Domhoff, G. W. (1996). *Finding Meaning in Dreams: A Quantative Approach.* New York: Plenum.

Domhoff, G. W. (1999). *Using Hall/Van de Castle Dream Content Analysis to Test New Theories: an example using a theory proposed by Ernest Hartmann.* Paper presented to the annual meeting of the Association for the

Study of Dreams, Santa Cruz, CA. http://psych.ucsc.edu/ dreams/Articles/ domhoff_1999 e.html accessed 11/27/01.

Domhoff, G. W. (2001). A new neurocognitive theory of Dreams. *Dreaming, 11*, 13–33.

Domhoff, G. W. (2003). *The Scientific Study of Dreams: Neural Networks, Cognitive Development, and Content Analysis.* Washington, DC: American Psychological Association Press.

Domhoff, G. W., & Schneider, A. (1999). Much ado about very little: the small effect sizes when home and laboratory collected dreams are compared. *Dreaming, 9*, 139–151.

Donath, F., Quispe, S., Diefenbach, K., Maurer, A., Fietze, I., & Roots, I. (2000). Critical evaluation of the effect of valerian extract on sleep structure and sleep quality. *Pharmacopsychiatry, 33*, 47–53.

Drago, D. A., & Dannenberg, A. L. (1999). Infant mechanical suffocation deaths in the United States, 1980–1997. *Pediatrics, 103*, e59.

Drummond, S. P. A., Gillin, J. C., & Brown, G. G. (2001). Increased cerebral response during a divided attention task following sleep deprivation. *J. Sleep Research, 10*, 85–92.

Drummond, S. P., Brown, G. G., Gillin, J. C., Stricker, J. L., Wong, E. C., & Buxton, R. B. (2000). Altered brain response to verbal learning following sleep deprivation. *Nature, 403*, 655–657.

Drummond, S. P., Brown, G. G., Stricker, J. L., Buxton, R. B., Wong, E. C., & Gillin, J. C. (1999). Sleep deprivation-induced reduction in cortical functional response to serial subtraction. *Neuroreport, 10*, 3745–3748.

Eich, E. (1990). Learning during sleep. In R. R. Bootzin, J. F. Kihlstrom, & D. L. Schachter (Eds.), *Sleep and Cognition* (pp. 88–108). Washington, DC: American Psychological Association.

Ellman, S. J., & Weinstein, L. N. (1991). REM sleep and dream formation: a theoretical integration. In S. J. Ellman, & J. S. Antrobus (Eds.), *The Mind in Sleep: Psychology and Psychophysiology, Second Edition* (pp. 446–488). New York: 1991.

Empson, J. (1993). *Sleep and Dreaming, 2nd edition.* Hertfordshire, England: Harvester Wheatsheaf.

Fiss, H. (1979). Current dream research: A psychobiological perspective. In B. F. Wolman (Ed.), *Handbook of Dreams* (pp. 20–75). New York: Van Nostrand Reinhold.

Fiss, H. (1991). Experimental studies for the study of the function of dreaming. In S. J. Ellman, & J. S. Antrobus, (Eds.). In *The Mind in Sleep: Psychology and Psychophysiology, 2nd ed.* (pp. 308–326). New York: Wiley.

Flanagan, O. (1995). Deconstructing Dreams: The spandrels of sleep. *The Journal of Philosophy, 92*, 5–27.

Flanagan, O. J. (2000). *Dreaming Souls: Sleep, Dreams, and the Evolution of the Conscious Mind.* New York: Oxford University Press.

Foulkes, D. (1978). *A Grammar of Dreams.* New York: Basic Books.

Foulkes, D. (1982). *Children's Dreams: Longitudinal Studies.* New York: John Wiley & Sons.

Foulkes, D. (1983). Cognitive processes during sleep: Evolutionary aspects. In A. Mayes (Ed.), *Sleep Mechanisms and Functions in Humans and Animals—an Evolutionary Prespective* (pp. 313–337). Berkshire, England: Van Nostrand Reinhold.

Foulkes, D. (1999). *Children's Dreams and the Development of Consciousness.* Cambridge, MA: Harvard University Press.

Freud, S. (1900). *Interpretation of Dreams.* New York: Modern Library.

Freud, S. (1958). *The Standard Edition of the Complete Psychological Works of Sigmund Freud, Vol. 12.* London: Hogarth.

Gamwell, L. 2000. (Ed.), *Dreams 1900–2000.* Binghamton, NY: Cornell University Press.

Gray, E. K., & Watson, D. (2002). General and specific traits of personality and their relation to sleep and academic performance. *Journal of Personality, 70*, 177–206.

Greenberg, R. (1981). Dreams and REM sleep: An intergrative approach. In W. Fishbein (Ed.), *Sleep, Dreams, and Memory* (pp. 125–133). New York: Spectrum.

Guiditta, A., Ambrosini, M. V., Montagnese, P., Mandile, P., Cotugno, M., Grassi Zucconi, G., & Vescia, S. (1995). The sequential hypothesis of the function of sleep. *Behav Brain Res, 69*, 157–166.

Guilleminault, C. (1982). (Ed.), *Sleeping and Waking Disorders: Indications and Techniques.* Menlo Park, California: Addison-Wesley.

Guilleminault, C., & Lugaresi, E. (1983). *Sleep-Wake Disorders: Natural History, Epidemiology, and Long-term Evaluation*. New York: Raven Press.

Hall, C. (1966). *The Meaning of Dreams*. New York: McGraw-Hill.

Harrington, J. M. (1994). Shift work and health—a critical review of the literature on working hours. *Ann Acad Med Singapore, 23*, 699–705.

Harrison, Y., & Horne, J. A. (1995). Should we be taking more sleep? *Sleep, 18*, 901–7.

Harrison, Y., & Horne, J. A. (1999). One night of sleep loss impairs innovative thinking and flexible decision making. *Organizational Behavior and Human Decision Making Processes, 78*, 128–145.

Harrison, Y., & Horne, J. A. (2000). The impact of sleep deprivation on Decision Making: A Review. *J Experimental Psychology: Applied, 6*, 236–249.

Hartmann, E. (1998). *Dreams and Nightmares: The New Theory on the Origin and Meaning of Dreams*. New York: Plenum Trade.

Hartmann, E. L. (1973). *The functions of sleep*. New Haven: Yale University Press.

Hauri, P. (1979). What can insomniacs teach us about the functions of sleep? In R. Drucker-Colin, M. Shkurovich, & M. B. Sterman (Eds.), *The Functions of Sleep* (pp. 251–271). New York: Academic Press.

Hauri, P. (1982). *The Sleep Disorders*. Kalamazoo, Michigan: Upjohn.

Hauri, P., & Linde, A. (1990). *No More Sleepless Nights*. New York: Wiley.

Hicks, R. A., Johnson, C., & Pellegrini, R. J. (1992). Changes in the self-reported consistency of normal habitual sleep duration of college students (1978 and 1992). *Perceptual and Motor Skills, 75*, 1168–1170.

Hicks, R. A., Lucero, K., & Mistry, R. (1991). Dreaming and habitual sleep duration. *Perceptual and Motor Skills, 72*, 1281–1282.

Hilakivi, L. (1987, June–July). *Sleep and Sleep Function in Mammalian Development*. Presented at the Fifth International Congress of Sleep Research, Copenhagen, Denmark.

Hobson, A., & McCarley, R. (1977). The brain as a dream state generator: an activation-synthesis hypothesis of the dream process. *American Journal of Psychiatry, 134*, 1335–1348.

Hobson, J. A. (1983). Sleep: order and disorder. *Behavioral Biology in Medicine, 1*, 1–36.

Hobson, J. A. (1988). *The Dreaming Brain*. New York: Basic Books.

Hobson, J. A. (1989). Dream theory: A new view of the brain mind. *The Harvard Medical School Mental Health Letter, 5*, 3–5.

Hobson, J. A., Pace-Schott, E., & Stickgold, R. (2000). Dreaming and the brain: Toward a cognitive neuroscience of conscious states. *Behavioral and Brain Sciences, 23*, 6, 793–842, discussion 904–1121.

Hong, C. C., Potkin, S. G., Antrobus, J. S., Dow, B. M., Callaghan, G. M., & Gillin, J. C. (1997). REM sleep eye movement counts correlate with visual imagery in dreaming: a pilot study. *Psychophysiology, 34*, 377–381.

Horne, J. A. (1983a). Human sleep and tissue restitution: Some qualifications and doubts. *Clinical Science, 65*, 569–578.

Horne, J. A. (1983b). Interacting functions of mammalian sleep. In W. P. Koella (Ed.), *Sleep 1982* (pp. 130–134). Basel: Karger.

Horne, J. A. (1983c). Mammalian sleep function with particular reference to man. In A. Mayes (Ed.), *Sleep Mechanisms and Functions in Humans and Animals—An Evolutionary Perspective* (pp. 262–312). Birkshire, England: Van Nostrand Reinhold.

Horne, J. A. (1988). *Why We Sleep*. New York: Oxford University Press.

Horne, J. A. (1989). Aspirin and nonfebrile waking oral temperature in healthy men and women: links with SWS changes? *Sleep, 12*, 516–512.

Horne, J. A. (1992). "Core" and "optional" sleepiness. In R. J. Broughton, & R. D. Ogilvie (Eds.), *Sleep, Arousal, and Performance* (pp. 27–44). Boston: Birkanser.

Horne, J. A. (2000). REM sleep—by default? *Neurosci Biobehav Rev, 24*, 777–797. http://www.websciences.org/cftemplate/NAPS/indiv.cfm?ID = 20002835

Horne, J., & Reyner, L. (1999). Vehicle accidents related to sleep: a review. *Occup Environ Med, 56*, 289–294.

Hunt, H. (1989). *The Multiplicity of Dreams: Memory, Imagination, and Consciousness.* New Haven: Yale University Press.

Hurovitz, C., Dunn, S., Domhoff, G. W., & Fiss, H. (1999). The dreams of blind men and women: A replication and extension of previous findings. *Dreaming, 9,* 183–193.

Iraki, L, Bogdan, A., Hakkou, F., Amrani, N., Abkari, A., & Touitou, Y. (1997). Ramadon diet restrictions modify the circadian time structure in humans. A study on plasma grastrin, insulin, glucose, and calcium and on gastric pH. *J Clin Endrorinol Metabol, 82,* 1261–1273.

Irwin, M., McClintick, J., Coslow, C., Fortner, M., White, J., & Gillin, J. C. (1996). Partial night sleep deprivation reduces natural killer and cellular immune responses in humans. *FASEB J, 10,* 643–653.

Johnson, D., Thorne, D., Rowland, L., Balkin, T., Sing, H., Thomas, M., Wesensten, N., Belenky, G. (1998). The effects of partial sleep deprivation on psychomotor vigilance. *Sleep, 21(3 Suppl),* 236

Jouvet, M. (1998). Paradoxical sleep as a programming system. *Journal of Sleep Research, 7 Suppl 1,* 1–5.

Jouvet, M. (1999). Sleep and Serotonin: An unfinished story. *Neuropsychopharmacology, 21,* 24S–27S.

Jung, C. G. (1933). *Modern Man in Search of a Soul.* New York: Harcourt, Brace and World.

Jung, C. G. (1964). *Man and His Symbols.* New York: Dell.

Jung, C. G. (1974). *Dreams.* Princeton, NJ: Princeton University Press.

Kahn, E., Fisher, C., & Edwards, A. (1978). Night terrors and anxiety dreams. In A. Arkin, J. S. Antrobus, & S. J. Ellman (Eds.), *The Mind in Sleep: Psychology and Psychophysiology* (pp. 533–542). Hillsdale, NJ: Erlbaum.

Karmanova, I. G. (1982). *Evolution of Sleep: Stages of the Wakefulness–Sleep Cycle in Vertebrates.* Basel: Karger.

Karmanova, I. G., & Oganesyan, G. A. (1999). *Sleep: Evolution and Disorders.* Lanham, MD: University Press of America.

Kavanau, J. L. (1997). Memory, sleep and the evolution of mechanisms of synaptic efficacy maintenance. *Neuroscience, 79,* 7–44.

Kavanau, J. L. (2001). Commentary: Brain-processing limitations and selective pressures for sleep, fish schooling and avian flocking. *Animal Behavior, 62,* 1219–1224.

Kleitman, N. (1972). *Sleep and Wakefulness.* Chicago: U of Chicago Press.

Koukkou, M., & Lehman, D. (1983). REM sleep dreams and the activation-synthesis hypothesis. *British Journal of Psychiatry, 142,* 221–231.

Koulack, D. (1987, June–July). *Dreams and Adaptation to Contemporary Stress.* Presented at the Fifth International Congress of Sleep Research, Copenhagen, Denmark.

Koulack, D. (1991). *To Catch a Dream: Explorations of Dreaming.* Albany, New York: State University of New York Press.

Kramer, M. (1987, June–July). *The Mood Regulatory Function of Dreaming: The dream as selective affective modulator.* Presented at the Fifth International Congress of Sleep Research, Copenhagen, Denmark.

Kramer, M. (1990). Nightmares (dream disturbances) in posttraumatic stress disorder: Implications for a theory of dreaming. In R. F. Bootzin, J. F. Kihlstrom, & D. L. Schacter (Eds.), *Sleep and Cognition* (pp. 190–202). Washington: American Psychological Association.

Kramer, M. (1993). The selective mood regulatory function of dreaming: An update and revision. In A. R. Moffit, M. Kramer, & R. F. Hoffmann (Eds.), *The Functions of Dreaming* (pp. 135–195). Albany, NY: State University of New York Press,.

Kramer, M., & Roth, T. (1979). The stability and variability of dreaming. *Sleep, 1,* 336–51.

Kramer, M., Roth, T., Arand, D., & Bonnet, M. (1981). Waking and dreaming mentation: A test of their interrelationships. *Neuroscience Letters, 22,* 83–86.

Krauss, D. A., Chen, P. Y., DeArmond, S., & Moorcroft, B. (2003). Sleepiness in the workplace: Causes, consequences, and countermeasures. In C. L. Cooper and I. T. Robertson (Eds.), *International Review of Industrial and Organizational Psychology.* New York: John Wiley & Sons, Ltd.

Kreuger, J. M. & Obal, F. J. (2002). Functions of sleep. In T. L. Lee-Chiong, M. J. Satela, & M. A. Carskadon (Eds.), *Sleep Medicine* (pp. 23–30). Philadelphia: Hanley & Belfus, Inc.

Kripke, D. F., Simons, R. N., Garfinkel, L., & Hammond, E. C. (1979). Short and long sleep and sleeping pills: Is increased mortality associated? *Archives of General Psychiatry, 36,* 103–116.

Krueger, J. M., & Karnovsky, M. L. (1995). Sleep as a neuroimmune phenomenon: a brief historical perspective. *Adv Neuroimmunol, 5*, 5–12.

Krueger, J. M., & Obal, F. Jr. (1993). A neuronal group theory of sleep function. *J Sleep Res, 2*, 63–69.

Krueger, J. M., ObáL, F. Jr., & Fang, J. (1999). Why we sleep: a theoretical view of sleep function. *Sleep Medicine Reviews, 3*, 119–129.

Krueger, J. M., Obal, F. Jr., Kapas, L., & Fang, J. (1995). Brain organization and sleep function. *Behav Brain Res, 69*, 177–185.

Kryger, M. H., Roth, T., & Dement, W. C. (1989). (Eds.) *Principles and Practice of Sleep Medicine.* Philadelphia: Saunders.

Kryger, M. H., Roth, T., & Dement, W. C. (2000). (Eds.) *Principles and Practice of Sleep Medicine, third edition.* New York: W.B. Saunders Company.

Laureys, S., Peigneux, P., Phillips, C., Fuchs, S., Degueldre, C., Aerts, J., Del Fiore, G., Petiau, C., Luxen, A., Van Der Linden, M., Cleeremans, A., Smith, C., & Maquet, P. (2001). Experience-dependent changes in cerebral functional connectivity during human rapid eye movement sleep. *Neuroscience, 105*, 521–525.

Lavie, P. (1989). To nap, Perchance to Sleep—Ultradian Aspects of Napping. In D. F. Dinges & R. J. Broughton (Eds.), *Sleep and Alertness: Chronobiological, Behavioral, and Medical Aspects of Napping* (pp. 99–120). New York: Raven Press.

Lee, K. A., McEnany, G., & Zaffke, M. E. (2000). REM sleep and mood state in childbearing women: Sleepy or Weepy? *Sleep, 23*, 877–895.

Lee, K. A., Zaffke, M. E., & McEnany, G. (2000). Parity and sleep patterns during and after pregnancy. *Obstetrics & Gynecology, 95*, 14–18.

Lee-Chiong, T. L., Satela, M. J., & Carskadon, M. A. (2002). (Eds.) *Sleep Medicine.* Philadelphia: Hanley & Belfus, Inc.

Leproult, R., Copinschi, G., Buxton, O., & Van Cauter, E. (1997). Sleep loss results in an elevation of cortisol levels the next evening. *Sleep, 20*, 865–870.

Lipman, D. S. (1996). *Snoring from A to ZZZ: Proven Cures for the Night's Worst Nuisance.* Portland, Ore.: Spencer Press.

Llinas, R.R., & Pare, D. (1991). Of dreaming and wakefulness. *Neuroscience, 44*, 521–35.

Maas, J. B. (1998). *Power Sleep: The Revolutionary Program that Prepares Your Mind for Peak Performance.* James B. Mass New York: Villard Books.

MacLean, A. W., Reiz, W. A., Austin, P., Coulter, M., Brunet, D. B., & Knowles, J. B. (1990). Psychophysiological correlates of lapses: Power spectral analysis of the EEG. *Sleep Research, 19*, 120.

Mahoney, M. F. (1966). *The Meaning in Dreams and Dreaming: The Jungian Viewpoint.* Seacaucus, NJ: The Citadel Press.

Mahowold, M. W., & Ettinger, M. G. (1990). Things that go bump in the night: the parasomnias revisited. *Journal of Clinical Neurophysiology, 1*, 119–143.

Mahowold, M. W., & Rosen, G. M. (1990). Parasomnias in children. *Pediatrician, 17*, 21–31.

Maquet, P. (1999). Brain mechanisms of sleep: contribution of neuroimaging techniques. *Journal of Psychopharmacology, 13*, S25–S28.

Maquet, P. (2001). The role of sleep in learning and memory. *Science, 294*, 1048–1052.

Masaya, T., & Heihachiro, A. (2000). Maintenance of alertness and performance by a brief nap after lunch under prior sleep deficit *Sleep, 23*, 813–819.

Mason, C. (2000, August). Sleep deprivation: The 24/7 sailor's dilemma. *Sail, 50*–53.

Maybruck, P. (1986). Contents of dreams of pregnant women. *Association for the Study of Dreams Newsletter, 3*, 8–9.

McAfee, T. (2000). Bed sharing is not a consumer product. *Arch Pediatr Adolesc Med, 154*, 530–531.

McCarley, R. W., & Massaquoi, S. G. (1986). A limit cycle mathematical model of the REM sleep oscillator system. *American Journal of Physiology, 257*, R1011–R1029.

McGinty, D. J., & Szymusiak, R. (1990). Hypothalamic thermoregulatory control of slow wave sleep. In M. Mancia & G. Marini (Eds.), *The Diencephalon and Sleep* (pp. 97–110). New York: Raven Press.

McGinty, D., & Szymusiak, R. (2000). The sleep-wake switch: A neuronal alarm clock. *Nature Medicine, 6*, 510–511.

McGrath, M. J., & Cohen, D. B. (1978). REM sleep facilitation of adaptive waking behavior: A review of the literature. *Psychological Bulletin, 85*, 24–57.

McKenna, J. J., & Gartner, L. M. (2000). Sleep location and suffocation: how good is the evidence? [letter] *Pediatrics, 105*, 917–99.

Meddis, R. (1975). On the function of sleep. *Animal Behavior, 23*, 676–601.

Meddis, R. (1979). The evolution and function of sleep. In D. A. Oakley & H. C. Plotkin (Eds.), *Brain, Behavior, & Evolution* (pp. 99–125). London: Methuen.

Meddis, R. (1983). The evolution of sleep. In A. Mayes (Ed.), *Sleep Mechanisms and Functions in Humans and Animals—an Evolutionary Prespective* (pp. 57–106). Berkshire, England: Van Nostrand Reinhold.

Mirmiram, M. (1986). The importance of fetal/neonatal REM sleep. *European Journal of Obstetrics, Gynecology and Reproductive Biology, 21*, 283–291.

Moffitt, A. (1987, June–July). *Experimental Studies of Individual Differences in Dream Recall and the Question of Dream Function.* Presented at the Fifth International Congress on Sleep Research, Copenhagen, Denmark.

Moorcroft, W. H. (1993). *Sleep, Dreaming, and Sleep Disorders: An Introduction, Second Edition.* Lanham, Md: University Press of America.

Moorcroft, W. H., Kayser, K. H., & Griggs, A. J. (1997). Subjective and objective confirmation of the ability to self-awaken at a self-predetermined time without using external means. *Sleep, 20*, 40–45.

Moorcroft, W. H. (2000). Sorting out additions to the understanding of cognition during sleep. *Behavioral and Brain Sciences, 23, 6*, 972–974.

Moore, R.Y. (1999). A clock for the ages. *Science, 284*, 2102–2103.

Morrison, A. R., Ball, L. D., Sanford, G. L., Mann, G. L., & Ross, R. J. (1990). Orienting can be elicited by tones in paradoxical sleep without atonia. *Sleep Research, 19*, 23.

Morrison, A. R., & Reiner, P. B. (1985). A dissection of paradoxical sleep. In D. J. McGinty, R. Drucker-Colin, A. Morrison, & P. L. Parmeggiani (Eds.). *Brain Mechanisms of Sleep* (pp. 97–110). New York: Raven Press.

Moruzzi, G. (1966). The functional significance of sleep with particular regard to the brain mechanisms underlying consciousness. In J. C. Eccles (Ed.), *Brain Mechanisms and Conscious Experience.* New York: Springer-Verlag.

Moruzzi, G., & Magoun, H. W. (1949). Brain stem reticular formation and activation of the EEG. *Electroencephalogr Clin Neurophysiol, 1*, 455–473

Murray, H. A., & Wheeler, D. R. (1937). A note on the possible clairvoyance of dreams. *Journal of Psychology, 3*, 309–313.

Nakamura, S., Wind, M., & Danello, M. A. (1999). Review of hazards associated with children placed in adult beds. *Arch Pediatr Adolesc Med, 153*, 1019–1023.

National Sleep Foundation. (2000). *Adolescent Sleep Needs: Research Report and Resource Guide.* Washington, DC: National Sleep Foundation.

National Sleep Foundation. (2002). Sleep in America Poll. Washington, DC March, 2002. http://www.sleepfoundation.org/img/2002SleepInAmericaPoll.pdf. Accessed June 26, 2002.

National Sleep Foundation. (2001). Sleep in America Polls, 1995, 1998, 1999, 2000, 2001. Washington, DC Copyright 2001. http://www.sleepfoundation.org/publications/sleeppolls.html. Accessed June 26, 2002.

National Traffic Safety Administration, (no date) Washington, DC (no revision date; accessed 6/28/2002) http://www.nhtsa.dot.gov/people/perform/human/drows_driving/

Nicolau, M. C., Akaarir, M., Gamundi, A., Gonzalez, J., & Rial, R. V. (2000). Why we sleep: the evolutionary pathway to the mammalian sleep. *Progress in Neurobiology, 62*, 379–406.

Nielsen, T. A. (2000). A review of mentation in REM and NREM sleep: "covert" REM sleep as a possible reconciliation of two opposing models. *Behav Brain Sci, 23*, 851–866.

Nikles, C. D. 2nd, Brecht, D. L., Klinger, E., & Bursell, A. L. (1998). The effects of current-concern- and nonconcern-related waking suggestions on nocturnal dream content. *J Pers Soc Psychol, 75*, 242–255.

Obal, F. Jr. (1984). Thermoregulation and sleep. In A. A. Borbely & J. L. Valat (Eds.), *Sleep Mechanisms* (pp. 157–172). New York: Springer-Verlag.

Ogilvie, R. D., Wilkinson, R. T., & Allison, S. (1989). The detection of sleep onset: Behavioral, physiological, and subjective convergence. *Sleep, 12*, 458–474.

Orr, W. C., Shadid, G., Harnish, M. J., & Elsenbruch, S. (1997). Meal composition and its effect on postprandial sleepiness. *Physiol Behav, 62*, 709–712.

Oskenberg, A. (1987). *Sleep and Sleep Function in Mammalian Development: REM Sleep and CNS Development in the Visual System of the Kitten.* Presented at the Fifth International Congress on Sleep Research, Copenhagen, Denmark.

Oswald, I. (1980). Sleep as a restorative process: Human clues. *Progress in Brain Research, 53*, 279–288.

Parmeggiani, P. L. (2000). Influence of the temperature signal on sleep in mammals. *Biol Signals Recept, 9*, 279–282.

Patton, D. V., Landers, D. R., & Agarwal, I. T. (2001). Legal considerations of sleep deprivation among resident physicians. *Journal of Health Law, 34*, 377–417.

Peigneus, P., Laureys, S., Delbeuck, X., & Maquet, P. (2001). Sleeping brain, learning brain. The role of sleep for memory systems. *Neuroreport, 12*, A111–A124.

Penn, P. E., Bootzin, R. R., & Wood, J. M. (1991). Nightmare frequency in sexual abuse survivors. *Sleep Research, 20*, 313.

People in traditional societies sleep in eye-opening ways. (1999, September 25). *Science News*, pp. 205–207.

Pigarev, I. N., Nothdurft, H. C., & Kastner, S. (1997). Evidence for asynchronous development of sleep in cortical areas. *Neuroreport, 8*, 2557–2560.

Plihal, W., & Born, J. (1999). Memory consolidation in human sleep depends on inhibition of glucocorticoid release. *Neuroreport, 10*, 2741–2747.

Poe, G. R., Nitz, D. A., McNaughton, B. L., & Barnes, C. A. (2000). Experience-dependent phase-reversal of hippocampal neuron firing during REM sleep. *Brain Research, 855*, 176–180.

Powell, N. B., Schechtman, K. B., Riley, R. W., Li, K., Troell, R., & Guilleminault, C. (2001). The road to danger: The comparative risks of driving while sleepy. *Laryngoscope, 111*, 887–893.

Prinz, P. N. (1980). Sleep changes with aging. In C. Eisdorfer, & W. E. Fann (Eds.), *Psychopharmacology of Aging* (pp. 1–12). Jamaica, NY: S P Medical & Scientific Books.

Rechtschaffen, A. (1978). The Single-Mindedness and Isolation of Dreams. *Sleep, 1*, 97–109.

Rechtschaffen, A. (1983). Dream Psychophysiology and the Mind-Body Problem. In M. Chase & E. D. Weitzman (Eds.), *Advances in Sleep Research, vol. 8, Sleep Disorders: Basic and Clinical Research.* New York: S P Medical and Scientific Books.

Rechtschaffen, A. (1998). Current perspectives on the function of sleep. *Perspectives in Biology and Medicine, 41*, 359–390.

Rechtschaffen, A., & Bergmann, B. M. (2002). Sleep Deprivation in the Rat: An update of the 1998 paper. *Sleep, 25*, 18–24.

Rechtschaffen, A., Bergmann, B. M., Everson, C. A., Kushida, C. A., & Gilliland, M. A. (1989). Sleep deprivation in the rat: X. Integration and discussion of the findings. *Sleep, 12*, 68–87.

Rechtschaffen, A., & Buchignani, C. (1983). Visual dimensions and correlates of dream images. *Sleep Research, 12*, 189.

Redwine, L., Hauger, R. L., Gillin, J. C., & Irwin, M. (2000). Effects of Sleep and sleep deprivation on interleukin-6, growth hormone, cortisol, and melatonin levels in humans. *J Clin Endocrinol Metab 85*, 3597–3603.

Revonsuo, A. (2000). The reinterpretation of dreams: an evolutionary hypothesis of the function of dreaming. *Behav Brain Sci, 23*, 877–901, discussion 904–1121.

Reyner, A., & Horne, J. A. (1995). Gender- and age-related differences in sleep determined by home-recorded sleep logs and actimetry from 400 adults. *Sleep, 18*, 127–134.

Rial, R. V., Nicolau, M. C., Gamundi, A., Rossello, C., & Akaarir, M. (1997). The evolution of waking states. In O. Hayaishi & S. Inoué: *Sleep and Sleep Disorders: From Molecule to Behavior* (pp. 99–112). Tokyo: Academic Press.

Roehrs, T., & Roth T. (2001). Sleep, Sleepiness, and alcohol use. *Alcohol Research and Health, 25*, 101–109.

Rosekind, M. R., Gander, P. H., Gregory, K. B., Smith, R. M., Miller, D. L., Oyung, R., Webbon, L. L., & Johnson, J. M. (1996). Managing fatigue in operational settings. 2: An Integrated Approach. *Behavioral Medicine, 21*, 166–170.

Rosenberg, K. D. (2000). Sudden infant death syndrome and co-sleeping. *Arch Pediatr Adolesc Med, 154*, 529–530.

Sanchez, R., & Bootzin, R. R. (1985). A comparison of white noise and music: Effects of predictable and unpredictable sounds on sleep. *Sleep Research, 14*, 121.

Savary, L. M., Berne, P. H., & Williams, S. K. (1984). *Dreams and Spiritual Growth: A Christian Approach to Dreamwork*. Ramsey, NJ: Paulist Press.

Schenck, C. H., Bundlie, S.R., Patterson, A. L., & Mahowold, M. W. (1987). Rapid eye movement sleep behavior disorder: A treatable parasomnia affecting older adults. *Journal of the American Medical Association, 257*, 1786–1789.

School Start Time Study, University of Minnesota's Center for Applied Research and Educational Improvement (2000). Minneapolis. August 20, 2001. (http://education.umn.edu/carei/Programs/start_time/). Accessed June 26, 2002.

Schredl, M. (2001). *Factors of Dream Recall*. Presented at the annual meeting of the Association for the Study of Dreams, Santa Cruz, California, July.

Sejnowski, T. J., & Destexhe, A. (2000). Why do we sleep? *Brain Research, 886*, 208–223.

Seligman, M. E. P., & Yellen, A. (1987). What is a dream? *Behavior Research and Therapy, 25*, 1–24.

Shaffery, J. P., Sinton, C. M., Bissette, G., Roffwarg, H. P., & Marks, G. A. (2002). Rapid eye movement sleep deprivation modifies expression of long-term potentiation in visual cortex of immature rats. *Neuroscience, 110*, 431–443.

Shapiro, C., & Smith, A. McC (1997). *Forensic Aspects of Sleep*. New York: Wiley.

Shiyi, L., & Inoué, S. (1995). *Sleep: Ancient and Modern*. Shanghai: Shanghai Scientific & Technological Literature P. H.

Siegel, A. (1983). Expectant father's dreams. *Dream Craft, 2*, 5–7.

Siegel, A. (2001). *A Mini-course for Clinicians and Trauma Workers on Posttraumatic Nightmares*. (Copyrighted 2001). http://www.asdreams.org/magazine/articles/seigel_nightmares.htm accessed 9/24/01.

Siegel, J. (2001). The REM sleep-memory consolidation hypothesis. *Science, 294*, 1058–1063.

Sleep Research Society. (1997). (Copyright 1997 WebSciences International and Sleep Research Society) *Basics of Sleep Behavior*. http://www.sleephomepages.org/sleepsyllabus/.

Smith, C. (1996). Sleep states, memory processes and synaptic plasticity. *Behavioural Brain Research, 78*, 49–56.

Smith, C., & Lapp, L. (1991). Increases in number of REMS and REM density in humans following an intensive learning period. *Sleep, 14*, 325–330.

Smith, C., & Rose, G. M. (1996). Evidence for a paradoxical sleep window for place learning in the Morris water maze. *Physiology and Behavior, 59*, 93–97.

Smith, C. S., Reilly, C., & Midkiff, K. (1989). Evaluation of three circadian rhythm questionnaires with suggestion for an improved measure of morningness. *Journal of Applied Psychology, 74*, 728–38.

Snyder, F. (1966). Toward an evolutionary theory of dreaming. *American Journal of Psychiatry, 123*, 121–136.

Solms, M. (1997). *The Neuropsychology of Dreams: A Clinico-anatomical Study*. Laurence, NJ: Erlbaum.

Solms, M. (2000). Dreaming and REM sleep are controlled by different brain mechanisms. *Behavioral and Brain Sciences, 23*, 843–50; discussion 904–1121.

Spiegel, K., Leproult, R., & Van Cauter, E. (1999). Impact of sleep debt on metabolic and endocrine function. *Lancet, 354*, 1435–1439.

Stampi, C., Moffitt, A., & Hoffman, R. (1990). Leonardo Da Vinci's polyphasic ultrashort sleep: a strategy for sleep reduction? *Sleep Research, 19*, 408.

Steiger, A., Antonijevic, I. A., Bohlhalter, S., Frieboes, R. M., Friess, E., & H. Murck (1998). Effects of hormones on sleep. *Hormone Research, 49*, 125–130.

Stewart, K. R. (1951). Dream Theory in Malaya. *Complex, 6*, 21–33.

Stickgold, R. (unpublished manuscript). The Death of the Dreamer: activation-synthesis revisited.

Stickgold, R., Hobson, J. A., Fosse, R., & Fosse, M. (2001). Sleep, Learning, and Dreams: Off-line Memory Reprocessing. *Science, 294*, 1052–1057.

Stickgold, R., James, L., & Hobson, J. A. (2000). Visual discrimination learning requires sleep after training. *Nature Neuroscience, 3*, 1237–1238.

Stickgold, R., Scott, L., Rittenhouse, C., & Hobson, J. A. (1999). Sleep induced changes in associative memory. *Journal of Cognitive Neuroscience, 11*, 182–193.

Strauch, I., & Meier, B. (1996). *In search of dreams. Results of experimental dream research.* Albany, NY: State University of New York Press.

Strecker, R. E., Morairty, S., Thakkar, M. M., Porkka-Heiskanen, T., Basheer, R., Dauphin, L. J., Rainnie, D. G., Portas, C. M., Greene, R. W., & McCarley, R. W. (2000). Adenosinergic modulation of basal forebrain and preoptic/anterior hypothalamic neuronal activity in the control of behavioral state. *Behav Brain Res, 115*, 183–204.

Stukane, E. (1985). *The Dream Worlds of Pregnancy.* New York: Quill.

Stuss, D., & Broughton, R. (1978). Extreme short sleep: Personality profiles and a case study of sleep requirement. *Waking and Sleeping, 2*, 101–105.

Takahashi, M., & Arito, H. (2000). Maintenance of alertness and performance by a brief nap after lunch under prior sleep deficit. *Sleep, 23*, 813–819.

Thiedke, C. C. (2001). Sleep disorders and sleep problems in childhood. *American Family Physician, 63*, 277–284.

Thomas, M. L., Sing, H. C., Belenky, G., Shepanek, N., Thorne, D. R., McCann, U. D., Penetar, D. M., Fertig, J., & Redmond, D. P. (1990). EEG changes following 48 hours of sleep deprivation in humans. *Sleep Research, 19*, 358.

Thorne, D. R., Thomas, M. L., Russo, M. B., Sing, H. C., Balkin, T. J., Wesensten, N. J., Redmond, D. P., Johnson, D. E., Welsh, A., Rowland, L., Cephus, R., Hall, S. W., & Belenky, G. (1999). Performance on a Driving-Simulator Divided-Attention-Task during One Week of Restricted Nightly Sleep. *Sleep, 22(1 Suppl)*, 301.

Thorne, D., Thomas, M., Sing, H., Balkin, T., Wesensten, N., Hall, S., Cephus, R., Redmond, D., Russo, M., Welsh, A., Rowland, L., Johnson, D., Aladdin, R., & Belenky, G. (1998). Driving-simulator accident rates before, during and after one week of restricted nightly sleep. *Sleep, 21(3 Suppl)*, 235.

Toth, L., & Krueger, J. M. (1992). Clinical correlates of sleep patterns after bacterial challange. *Sleep Research, 21*, 315.

Trockel, M. T., Barnes, M. D., & Egget, D. L. (2000). Health-related variables and academic performance among first-year college students: implications for sleep and other behaviors. *J Am Coll Health, 49*, 125–131.

Turek, F. W., & Zee, P. C. (1999). *Regulation of Sleep and Circadian Rhythms.* New York: Marcel Dekker, Inc.

Ullman, M., & Zimmerman, N. (1979). *Working with Dreams.* New York: Dell.

Ullman, M., Krippner, S., & Vaughan, A. (1989). *Dream Telepathy: Experiments in Nocturnal ESP.* Jefferson, NC: McFarland.

Urade, Y., & Hayasihi, O. (1999). Prostaglandin D_2 and sleep regulation. *Biochimica et biophysica Acta, 1436*, 616–615.

Van Dongen, H. P. A., & Dinges, D. F. (2001). Modeling the effects of sleep debt: On the relevance of inter-individual differences. *SRS Bulletin, 7*, 69–72.

Van Reeth, O., Weibel, L., Spiegel, K., Leproult, R., Dugovic, C., & Maccari, S. (2000). Interactions between stress and sleep: from basic research to clinical situations. *Sleep Medicine Reviews, 4*, 201–219.

Vertes, R. P., & Eastman, K. E. (2000). The case against memory consolidation in REM sleep. *Behav Brain Sci, 23*, 867–876; discussion 904–1121.

Villablanca, J. (1965). The electrocorticogram in the chronic cerveau isolé cat. *Electroencephalogr Clin Neruophysiol, 19*, 576–586.

Vogel, G. W. (1979). A motivational function of REM sleep. In R. Drucker-Colin, M. Shkurovich, & M. B. Sterman (Eds.), *The Functions of Sleep* (pp. 233–250). New York: Academic Press.

Walker, J. M., & Berger, R. J. (1980). Sleep as an adaptation for energy conservation functionally related to hibernation and shallow torpor. *Progress in Brain Research, 53,* 255–278.

Wauquier, A., Dugovic, C., & Radulovacki, M. (1989). (Eds.) *Slow Wave Sleep: Physiological, Pathophysiological, and Functional Aspects.* New York: Raven Press.

Webb, W. B. (1975). *Sleep: The Gentle Tyrant.* Englewood Cliffs, NJ: Prentice-Hall.

Webb, W. B. (1979). Theories of sleep functions and some clinical implications. In R. Drucker-Colin, M. Shkurovich, & M. B. Sterman (Eds.), *The Functions of Sleep* (pp. 19–35). New York: Academic Press.

Webb, W. B. (1983). Theories in modern sleep research. In A. Mayes (Ed.), *Sleep Mechanisms and Functions in Humans and Animals—An Evolutionary Prespective* (pp. 1–17). Berkshire, England: Van Nostrand Reinhold.

Webb, W. B. (1992). *Sleep: The Gentle Tyrant, Second Edition.* Boston: Anker.

Wehr, T. A. (1992). A brain-warming function for REM sleep. *Neuroscience and Biobehavioral Reviews, 16,* 379–397.

Wehr, T. A. (1992). In short photoperoids, human sleep is biphasic. *Journal of Sleep Research, 1,* 103–707.

Weiss, L. (1986). *Dream Analysis in Psychotherapy.* New York: Pergamon Press.

Welsh, A., Thomas, M., Thorne, D., Sing, H., Rowland, L., Redmond, D., Peters, R., Wagner, E., & Belenky, G. (1998). Effects of 64 hours of sleep deprivation on accidents and sleep events during a driving simulator test. *Sleep, 21(3 Suppl),* 234.

Wesensten, N. J., Balkin, T. J., & Belenky, G. (1999). Does sleep fragmentation impact recuperation? A review and reanalysis. *Journal of Sleep Research, 8,* 237–245.

WFSRS (World Federation of Sleep Research Societies) Newsletter, (1996, vol. 5). What is the minimal component of the brain that is capable of sleep? http://www.wfsrs.org/newsletters/Newsletter5_1/Theoretical_Issues/Issues.htm (accessed May 26, 2002).

Williams, R. L., & Karacan, I. (1978). *Sleep Disorders: Diagnosis and Treatment.* New York: Wiley.

Wilson, M. A., & McNaughton, B. L. (1994). Reactivation of hippocampal ensemble memories during sleep. *Science, 265,* 676–679.

Winson, J. (1990). The meaning of dreams. *Scientific American, 263,* 86–96.

World Federation of Sleep Research Societies. (1999). Third International Congress, Dresden, Germany. Symposium: NREMS Brain Organization: Local vs Global, Thursday October 7, 1999.

Index

Printed in the United States
26969LVS00001B/187-204